The P53 Diet & Lifestyle

The P53 Diet & Lifestyle

Get Control Of Your Health

By David W. Brown

Introduction by
Dr. Jerry Summers

P53 Publishing

First Printing, 2023

DISCLAIMER

I am not a doctor. I have been researching a plant-based diet's role on the body for many years. The claims made in this book are backed by the scientific studies listed at the end of this book, and on the P53 Diet website. I do not provide medical advice per medical condition, I quote the research studies that made those claims. Eating a plant-based has been shown to aid in the reversal of certain cancers and ailments, as well as lowering the risk of certain cancers according to the scientists that made those claims. This book is intended to serve as an informational guide. Any testimonials made in this book are made from the authors of those claims who are real subscribers of the P53 Diet website.

Dedication

Lisa A. Peterson

Owner P53 Oregon Mobile Food Cart

P53 Oregon Catering

P53 Washington Catering

Thank you so much for being so supportive. You put up with me all the years I spent pulling my hair out doing this research and putting it all together. You are a wonderful person. I appreciate all your patience. Now we get to share good health with everyone!

INTRODUCTION

By Dr. Jerry Summers

I was introduced to Dave Brown, via a friend of mine shortly after being diagnosed with prostate cancer. When Dave told me that his P53 diet was a totally plant-based diet, I thought to myself this guy has got to be joking. He is asking me to give up meat, dairy, refined sugars, and alcohol, and recommended a 1,000 to 1,200-calorie-a-day diet. I thought what else needs to be eliminated from my life, sex? But alas, Dave, all kidding aside, as Dave explained his diet from a cellular level and how certain foods can enhance the body's ability to fight cancer, the logic became too hard to deny. Being a skeptical person, I questioned him about the concern that I'd be hungry all the time and whether the food tasted like grass clippings and mulch. Dave told me I'd enjoy the food and wouldn't be starving all the time, but I must reduce my weight by 50 lbs. I started the P53 diet on 3/20/2022 at 240.2 pounds. In Fifteen days, my weight dropped to 225.2 down 15 pounds. The food is terrific, and I feel so much better!

Dave is genuinely interested in helping people get healthy. He explained to me that he is not a doctor. He stated that he has been researching the role of a plant-based diet to help fight cancer and other health-related issues for many years. He has shared his research findings with me. He has changed my life and eating forever. I highly recommend this diet to anyone serious about getting healthy. If you're battling cancer you would be foolish to ignore the benefits of this plan. I started this plan with a healthy dose of skepticism and the attitude that I had nothing to lose, except weight. I was diagnosed with an aggressive form of prostate cancer in January 2022. After researching my options, it appeared there were only two available for me, surgery, or radiation, with all of my doctors telling me active surveillance wasn't a viable option, or that I would fail with active surveillance. My major worry was that the quality of life with both options carried the risk of urinary incontinence. The risk was relatively small for either option, but the thought of dealing with incontinence for a year or permanently didn't appeal to me.

This journey began in 2017 with my PSA levels rising over the next five years. My PSA results barely exceeded the normal range in 2020. My primary physician continued to monitor my results and referred me to a urologist when my PSA hit 5.5 in 2021. The urologist put me on a 30-day high-dose antibiotic hoping the rise was caused by a prostate infection. After 30 days, we tested my PSA level and it had risen to 6.68, indicating the probability of more aggressive prostate cancer. The cancer was confirmed with a needle biopsy, indicating two lesions on the right side of my prostate consuming approximately 35% of the prostate. Next came a meeting with an oncologist and surgeon and weighing options. This is when I was referred to Dave and the P53 diet. This referral came with a stern warning, before you do anything, talk to Dave, he has been helping people with cancer for decades. I ignored the recommendation, and then I received a telephone call from Dave, apparently, my friend knew more about me than I suspected. After several extensive conversations with Dave, I became convinced the P53 diet was worth a try and if it didn't work, I could opt for one of the two medical options suggested in the fall. In March 2022, I underwent an MRI with contrast which confirmed two lesions that basically mirrored the needle biopsy results. My surgeon ordered another PSA test for the end of April 2022.

NOW the **Amazing** part, my PSA had dropped to **3.81** registering within the normal range, and the only change had been my participation in the P53 Diet. I had not started any medical procedures. After

5 weeks, I had lost 20.6 pounds with my weight dropping from 240.2 to 219.6. Dave has contacted me several times a week since starting this diet to encourage me. If you're battling cancer, you would be foolish to ignore the benefits of this plan.

Basic Medical Facts:

Lipid Panel and Chol/HDL Ratio Comparison 8/ 2021 to 5/2022	**8/26/2021**	**5/1/2022**	**Reference Range**
Cholesterol	215 H	107	OPT:< 200ml/ dL
Triglycerides	310 H	115	30-150mg/dL
HDL	36.8 L	36.5 L	OPT:> 40 md/ dL
LDL	116 H	48	OPT: < 40 mg/ dL
VLDL	62 H	23	4-40 mg/dL
Chol/HDL	5.8 H	2.9	OPT: < 4.97
Non-HDL Chol	178 H	71	OPT:< 130 mg/ dL

In January 2023, I had a second MRI with contrast with my physician and was astonished when the MRI showed the small lesion was gone and the large or the two was reduced by approximately 20%.

My surgeon wanted to do another needle biopsy but couldn't convince me it was necessary given the MRI results. At this point in my journey, active surveillance is conducted successfully. I have stopped all medications, considering the above lab results. I continue active surveillance under my primary physician's supervision. The P53 way of life is real and incredibly effective. My view of health care has changed dramatically and will always involve my questioning the medical advice provided. If this offends your physician, then perhaps you need to find one who understands it's your body and you have the right to question and decide what is best for your life.

Stay healthy and eat right; that will always be P53 for me!

TABLE OF CONTENTS

1

Current State of Health in America

The state of human health in America is a multifaceted and complex issue that encompasses a wide range of factors, including nutrition, lifestyle choices, and environmental influences. In recent years, several health indicators have raised concerns, with obesity, cancer rates, diabetes, and other ailments emerging as prominent challenges. I will delve into the current state of these health issues in America, exploring the factors contributing to their rise. The question I posed to you is, with all the so-called new treatments, all the money thrown at this, and new pills on the market, why is the health crisis including cancer rates continuing to rise?

The Obesity Epidemic

Obesity has reached epidemic proportions in the United States, affecting individuals of all ages, ethnicities, and socioeconomic backgrounds. According to the Centers for Disease Control and Prevention (CDC), the prevalence of obesity among adults in the United States was 42.4% in 2017-2018. This represents a significant increase from previous decades and has far-reaching implications for overall health.

Several factors contribute to the obesity epidemic in America. The availability and consumption of high-calorie, high-fat processed foods contribute to excessive calorie intake. Additionally, sedentary lifestyles, characterized by increased screen time and a decrease in physical activity, play a pivotal role.

Obesity is associated with a myriad of health issues, including an increased risk of heart disease, stroke, type 2 diabetes, and certain types of cancer. The economic burden of obesity is substantial, with healthcare costs related to obesity estimated to be in the billions annually. Addressing the obesity epidemic requires a varied approach that includes promoting healthy eating habits, and increasing physical activity.

Cancer remains a significant public health concern in the United States, with a diverse range of cancers affecting millions of individuals each year. According to the American Cancer Society, an estimated 1.9 million new cancer cases were diagnosed in 2020.

While genetics can play a small role in cancer development, lifestyle factors, and environmental exposures are major contributors. Tobacco use, poor diet, lack of physical activity, and exposure to carcinogens in the environment are all associated with an increased risk of developing cancer.

Efforts to reduce cancer rates in America focus on prevention and early detection. Public health campaigns promote tobacco cessation, healthy eating, and regular physical activity. I will cover more on cancer in the Chapter *"Cancers & Other Ailments."*

Diabetes, particularly type 2 diabetes, has become a major health concern in the United States. The CDC estimates that over 34 million Americans have diabetes, and another 88 million have prediabetes.

Similar to obesity, sedentary lifestyles, and poor dietary habits contribute significantly to the rise in diabetes. Genetic predisposition, age, and ethnicity also play a role. The increasing prevalence of obesity, a known risk factor for type 2 diabetes, further exacerbates the diabetes epidemic.

Untreated or poorly managed diabetes can lead to serious complications, including cardiovascular disease, kidney failure, and vision loss. The economic burden of diabetes is substantial, with costs related to medical care, lost productivity, and disability. Prevention and management strategies include lifestyle modifications, early detection, and access to affordable healthcare services.

Beyond obesity, cancer, and diabetes, several other health issues contribute to the overall state of human health in America. Mental health disorders, substance abuse, and cardiovascular diseases are among the additional challenges facing the population.

Mental health disorders, including depression and anxiety, affect millions of Americans. The stigma surrounding mental health often impedes individuals from seeking timely and appropriate care. Toxins present in the body play a damaging role in our mental health. See the chapter "Toxins" for more in-depth information on toxins.

Cardiovascular diseases, including heart disease and stroke, remain the leading causes of morbidity and mortality in the United States. Risk factors such as high blood pressure, high cholesterol, and smoking contribute to the prevalence of cardiovascular diseases. Public health initiatives promoting a healthy diet, lifestyles, and community-based interventions are crucial in reducing the burden of cardiovascular diseases.

The state of human health in America is characterized by a complex interplay of factors, including diet, lifestyle choices, genetic predisposition, and environmental influences. Obesity, cancer, diabetes, mental health disorders, and cardiovascular diseases represent significant challenges that require comprehensive and collaborative solutions. The diet is the starting point to getting control of your health and understanding what is making the body unhealthy. This book will delve into the factors that could be making you ill as well as ways to improve your health.

High Cost of Being Unhealthy

Living an unhealthy lifestyle can have significant financial implications, stretching far beyond the immediate expenses of medical bills and prescription medications. One of the most prevalent consequences is obesity, a condition with varied costs that ripple through various aspects of an individual's life.

Firstly, let's look into the economic burden of obesity. According to the World Health Organization (WHO), obesity is associated with a higher risk of chronic diseases such as heart disease, diabetes, and certain cancers. Treating these conditions incurs substantial medical costs, ranging from routine check-ups to more complex interventions. Individuals grappling with obesity often find themselves frequenting doctors' offices, leading to a consistent drain on their financial resources.

Prescription medications are another financial strain on the unhealthy. Chronic conditions often necessitate long-term medication, contributing to an ongoing expense that can be particularly burdensome for those without adequate health insurance. The cost of pills, especially for conditions related to an unhealthy lifestyle, such as hypertension or diabetes, can accumulate over time, further exacerbating the economic toll. The P53 Diet goal is for you to no longer need to rely on pills for your health. Research studies have shown that eating a plant-based diet can reduce the need for pills.

The toll on productivity and missed workdays due to health issues cannot be overlooked. Unhealthy individuals are more prone to illnesses, leading to increased absenteeism from work. This not only impacts personal income but also contributes to a broader societal economic burden as businesses contend with decreased productivity.

The vicious cycle of poor health often extends to mental well-being. Individuals grappling with health issues may experience heightened stress and anxiety, leading to a potential decrease in work performance. This, in turn, can result in missed career opportunities and financial setbacks, creating a self-perpetuating cycle of health-related and economic challenges.

The societal costs of an unhealthy population extend to the healthcare system as a whole. Overburdened hospitals and clinics must allocate resources to manage preventable conditions, diverting attention and funding from more pressing healthcare needs. This strain on healthcare resources can lead to longer wait times, reduced quality of care, and an overall decline in the effectiveness of the healthcare system.

The economic impact of an unhealthy population isn't limited to direct healthcare costs. Industries catering to unhealthy habits, such as fast food and sugary beverages, may initially benefit economically but contribute to long-term health issues. As more individuals succumb to preventable illnesses, the burden on healthcare systems and, by extension, on taxpayers increases.

The high costs of being unhealthy extend far beyond the immediate financial burden of medical bills and prescription medications. From the societal level down to the individual, the consequences of an unhealthy lifestyle are pervasive, affecting productivity, mental well-being, and the overall economic fabric of communities. Prioritizing health and wellness isn't just a personal choice; it's an investment in a more resilient, economically vibrant society.

The Perils of Fad Diets: Problems and Pitfalls

In an era obsessed with quick fixes and instant gratification, fad diets have become ubiquitous, promising rapid weight loss and a path to the elusive ideal physique. These diets, characterized by their trendy nature and often extreme restrictions, captivate individuals seeking a shortcut to fitness. However, beneath the allure of rapid results lies a landscape riddled with problems and pitfalls. In this comprehensive exploration, I will delve into the multiple issues associated with fad diets, examining their impact on physical health, psychological well-being, and long-term sustainability.

One of the fundamental problems with fad diets is their tendency to advocate extreme and unbalanced nutritional approaches. Many fad diets promote the exclusion of entire food groups, leaving individuals susceptible to nutrient deficiencies. For instance, low-carbohydrate diets may lead to insufficient fiber intake, impairing digestive health and increasing the risk of constipation. Likewise, extremely low-fat diets may deprive the body of essential fatty acids crucial for brain function and overall well-being. The absence of nutritional balance in fad diets can compromise the body's ability to function optimally, jeopardizing long-term health.

Fad diets frequently induce rapid weight loss through mechanisms that can have adverse effects on metabolism. When individuals inevitably resume normal eating patterns, their metabolism may remain sluggish, leading to weight regain and, in some cases, surpassing the initial weight. This metabolic adaptation can create a challenging cycle where weight loss becomes increasingly difficult, perpetuating frustration and discouragement.

The psychological toll of fad diets extends beyond the physical realm. The relentless pursuit of restrictive eating patterns can foster an unhealthy relationship with food and body image. Constantly cycling between deprivation and indulgence can contribute to feelings of guilt, shame, and anxiety surrounding food. Moreover, the emphasis on external validation through rapid weight loss can erode self-esteem and self-worth. The societal pressure to conform to unrealistic body standards, exacerbated by the prevalence of social media, intensifies the psychological impact of fad diets, potentially leading to disordered eating patterns and the development of eating disorders.

Diets that exclude entire food groups may lead to an inadequate intake of essential vitamins and minerals. Deficiencies in nutrients such as iron, calcium, vitamin D, and B vitamins can have far-reaching consequences, affecting energy levels, bone health, and immune function. The long-term consequences of sustained nutrient deficiencies can manifest in chronic health conditions, emphasizing the importance of a balanced plant-based diet for overall well-being.

Fad diets often center around the concept of rapid weight loss as the ultimate marker of success. This singular focus on the scale neglects the broader aspects of health, such as body composition, muscle mass, and overall well-being. Rapid weight loss, particularly through extreme measures, may result in the loss of muscle mass and essential fluids rather than fat. This can lead to a false sense of accomplishment, as the number on the scale may not accurately reflect improvements in body composition or health. The myopic emphasis on weight as the primary measure of success perpetuates a narrow and potentially harmful perspective on health and fitness.

The popularity of fad diets is often fueled by aggressive marketing campaigns and celebrity endorsements, creating a sense of urgency and desirability. Celebrities, with their wide-reaching influence, can inadvertently contribute to the normalization of unhealthy eating patterns by endorsing restrictive diets that may not be sustainable or suitable for the general population. The allure of rapid results, coupled with the endorsement of well-known figures, can overshadow the scientific scrutiny that should precede any dietary recommendation. This influence-driven adoption of fad diets further underscores the need for critical evaluation and awareness of the potential pitfalls.

Fad diets typically prioritize short-term results over long-term health, promoting quick fixes that may come at the expense of overall well-being. The emphasis on rapid weight loss often overshadows the importance of establishing sustainable lifestyle habits that support long-term health. Individuals drawn to fad diets may overlook the potential risks and consequences, focusing solely on the immediate goal of shedding pounds. This myopic approach neglects the broader picture of health, including the importance of regular physical activity, mental well-being, and the adoption of habits that support a balanced and fulfilling life.

The problems associated with fad diets are various and extend beyond the realm of quick fixes. From the lack of nutritional balance and unsustainability to the potential for metabolic consequences and psychological impact, fad diets present a host of challenges that can compromise both physical and mental well-being. Recognizing the pitfalls of these diets is essential for fostering a more informed and balanced approach to health and fitness. Embracing evidence-based, individualized nutrition, coupled with sustainable lifestyle habits, offers a more holistic and enduring path to achieving and maintaining optimal health as offered with the P53 Diet. As we navigate the complex landscape of dietary choices, a nuanced understanding of nutrition, coupled with a commitment to long-term well-being, is paramount. The P53 Diet is not considered a fad diet, it is considered a lifestyle of health.

Germ Theory vs Terrain Theory

Germ theory and terrain theory are two contrasting perspectives in the field of medical science that seek to explain the origins and development of diseases. While both theories have contributed significantly to our understanding of health and illness, they offer divergent explanations for the causes of diseases and their progression. The differences between germ theory and terrain theory lie in their fundamental views on the role of microbes and the environment in the onset of illnesses.

Germ theory, which gained prominence in the late 19th century through the work of scientists like Louis Pasteur and Robert Koch, posits that specific microorganisms, such as bacteria, viruses, and fungi, are the primary agents responsible for causing infectious diseases. According to germ theory, diseases are transmitted through the invasion of the body by pathogenic microorganisms that reproduce and spread, leading to illness. This theory has been the cornerstone of modern medicine and has guided the development of antibiotics, vaccines, and other treatments aimed at targeting and eliminating specific pathogens.

On the other hand, terrain theory, although not as widely accepted in mainstream medicine, offers an alternative perspective on the origins of diseases. Terrain theory, also known as the cellular theory, suggests that the internal environment of the body, or the "terrain," plays a crucial role in determining an individual's susceptibility to diseases. Proponents of terrain theory, including figures like Antoine Béchamp and Claude Bernard, argue that the overall health of the body, including factors such as nutrition, pH balance, and the state of the immune system, influences the development of diseases. In this view, microbes are not the sole cause of illnesses but rather opportunistic entities that thrive in a weakened or imbalanced internal environment.

One key distinction between germ theory and terrain theory is their approach to treatment and prevention. Germ theory has led to the development of vaccines and antibiotics, which target specific pathogens to eradicate or control infections. The focus is on external interventions to eliminate the cause of the disease. In contrast, terrain theory emphasizes the importance of strengthening the body's internal environment through lifestyle changes, proper nutrition, and other holistic approaches to enhance overall health and resilience against diseases. Proponents of terrain theory argue that maintaining a healthy internal terrain is essential for preventing the onset of illnesses and promoting longevity.

It has been stated that Louis Pasteur on his deathbed said *"Bernard was right; the pathogen is nothing; the terrain is everything."* There also have been books published such as the 1995 book by historian Dr. Gerald Geison entitled *"The Private Science of Louis Pasteur"* where Dr. Geison stated, *" The conclusion is unavoidable, Pasteur deliberately deceived the public, including especially those scientists most familiar with his public work."* This book by Dr. Gerald Geison is worth a read to really see how we have been misled about certain medical issues. Another great book that also explains more on this issue is *"What Really Makes You Ill"* by Dawn Lester and David Parker.

Putting poison in the body in the form of vaccines and antibiotics makes no sense to me. The body has been given the blueprint in the form of our DNA that has the instructions for our overall health and survival. We just need to keep the toxins out of our bodies and put the right nutrients in our bodies in the form of essential amino acids that we get from fruits, vegetables, nuts, seeds, and whole grains, this is what the P53 Diet is all about.

Risks of High-Fat Diets

In recent years, high-fat diets have gained popularity for their potential benefits, including weight loss and improved satiety. However, as with any nutritional trend, it is crucial to examine the potential risks associated with such dietary choices. While fats are essential for bodily functions, an excess of dietary fat, especially from certain sources, can pose significant health risks. This book shows the risks of high-fat diets, shedding light on the potential pitfalls that individuals should consider when adopting a diet plan. The P53 Diet limits the daily fat intake to no more than 16 grams of fat per day.

High-fat diets typically involve consuming a significant proportion of daily calories from fats, often exceeding the recommended dietary guidelines. These diets may include various types of fats, such as saturated fats, monounsaturated fats, and polyunsaturated fats, each with different effects on health.

Contrary to the belief that high-fat diets aid weight loss, an excessive intake of calories, regardless of the nutrient composition, can lead to weight gain. Fats are energy-dense, providing more calories per gram than carbohydrates or proteins. Overconsumption of high-fat foods may contribute to an energy surplus, leading to an increased risk of obesity and related health issues.

One of the primary concerns associated with high-fat diets is their impact on cardiovascular health. Diets rich in saturated fats have been linked to elevated levels of LDL (low-density lipoprotein) cholesterol, often referred to as "bad" cholesterol. Elevated LDL cholesterol is a well-established risk factor for cardiovascular diseases, including heart attacks and strokes.

High-fat diets, particularly those high in saturated fats, have been associated with insulin resistance, a key factor in the development of type 2 diabetes. Insulin resistance occurs when cells become less responsive to insulin, leading to elevated blood sugar levels. This metabolic dysfunction can contribute to the onset and progression of diabetes.

Excessive fat consumption, especially saturated fats, can contribute to the development of non-alcoholic fatty liver disease (NAFLD). NAFLD is characterized by the accumulation of fat in the liver, which may progress to more severe conditions, such as liver inflammation (non-alcoholic steatohepatitis) and cirrhosis. High-fat diets have fueled prostate cancer progression through the over-expression of MYC.

Certain fats, particularly saturated fats, and trans fats, may trigger inflammatory responses in the body. Chronic inflammation is associated with various health conditions, including arthritis, autoimmune diseases, and an increased risk of certain cancers.

A diet excessively high in fats may lead to nutrient imbalances, as individuals might prioritize fatty foods over nutrient-dense options. This can result in deficiencies of essential vitamins and minerals, compromising overall health and well-being.

Emerging research suggests a potential link between high-fat diets and cognitive decline. Diets rich in saturated fats may contribute to the development of oxidative stress and inflammation in the brain, increasing the risk of neurodegenerative conditions such as Alzheimer's disease.

Moderation, balance, and an emphasis on the quality of fats consumed are key factors in maintaining a healthy dietary pattern. Following the P53 Diet's daily allowance for fat will help you achieve your desired health goals. The following chapters in this book will help to show you a plan to *"get control of your health."*

Keto Diet Organ Concerns

The ketogenic diet, characterized by high fat, low carbohydrate, and moderate protein intake, has gained popularity for its potential weight loss benefits. However, it's crucial to acknowledge that while the ketogenic diet may offer short-term advantages for some individuals, there are concerns about its potential impact on organ health over the long term.

One primary concern is the impact on the kidneys. The ketogenic diet induces a state of ketosis, where the body relies on ketones for energy instead of glucose. This shift may lead to an increased production of nitrogen, placing a higher burden on the kidneys to eliminate excess waste products. Prolonged stress on the kidneys could potentially contribute to kidney damage or dysfunction.

The high intake of saturated fats common in a ketogenic diet may pose a threat to cardiovascular health. Elevated levels of saturated fats can lead to an increase in LDL cholesterol, which is associated with a higher risk of heart disease. Though proponents argue that the diet can improve lipid profiles, the long-term consequences remain uncertain, and caution is warranted.

Organic acidosis is another concern. The process of ketosis can result in the accumulation of ketone bodies, leading to a condition known as ketoacidosis. While ketoacidosis is more common in individuals with diabetes, there is a potential risk for those following a ketogenic diet, especially if not monitored closely. Acidosis can disrupt the body's acid-base balance, impacting organ function and potentially leading to complications.

The restrictive nature of the ketogenic diet may contribute to nutritional deficiencies, affecting organ health indirectly. Limited intake of fruits, vegetables, and whole grains can result in insufficient vitamins, minerals, and fiber, which are essential for overall well-being. Such deficiencies may adversely affect the liver, which plays a vital role in nutrient metabolism and detoxification.

The brain, highly dependent on glucose for energy, might face challenges during extended periods of carbohydrate restriction. While ketones can serve as an alternative fuel source, the brain's optimal functioning may still require a balanced intake of carbohydrates. Prolonged adherence to a ketogenic diet could potentially impact cognitive function and mood.

It's important to note that individual responses to the ketogenic diet vary, and more research is needed to fully understand the long-term effects on organ health. Before embarking on any drastic dietary changes, individuals should consult with healthcare professionals to ensure that their chosen approach aligns with their health goals and is sustainable without causing harm to vital organs.

2

SAD (Standard American Diet)

Sad is definitely a way to describe how Americans eat. Diet could be the number one cause of cancer. We know that if we allow ourselves to eat the Standard American Diet, the risk of eating this way can lead to significant health problems for yourself and your children. One of the reasons this is SAD is that it is tough to find what a Standard American Diet is comprised of. There are so many people saying low carbs; and high fat is the way to go. The P53 Diet consists of 75 - 80% Carbs, 10 - 12.5% Proteins, and 10 - 12.5% Fat. The carbohydrates I consume are not simple carbohydrates they are complex carbohydrates, which means longer chains. These longer chains of carbohydrates take longer to metabolize. This is the way I now eat, and I am in the best health of my life. I don't eat or drink animal products. I get the intake of amino acids from fruit, vegetables, legumes, and whole grains. My blood work is a measuring stick for my health, and it is very close to perfect. I eat the opposite of the Standard American Diet; I am living proof eating the P53 Diet way works. Research also shows eating the way I eat can improve your overall health. Eating the standard American diet way can cause obesity, hypertension, high cholesterol, diabetes, stroke, gout, and cancer to name just a few. Every time you take the kids somewhere and say, I need to feed them, but I don't have time to feed them healthy foods, so I will just get some fast food. This is the problem with children's health issues.

The standard American diet refers to a diet that is:

1. High intake of processed foods
2. High in the intake of animal meat
3. High in the intake of dairy
4. High intake of cooking oils
5. High in the intake of sugar
6. High in the intake of salt
7. High in the intake of fried foods
8. Low in the intake of fruit
9. Low in the intake of vegetables
10. Low in the intake of legumes
11. Low in the intake of whole grains

We know through scientific evidence that eating a SAD diet is the biggest reason why people are overweight and obese. Not only are you overweight and obese eating the SAD diet, but you are also putting yourself at high risk of putting toxins in your body that can cause somatic mutations leading to cancer. Remember that 90 to 95 percent of all cancers are somatic. The toxins enter the body when we eat or drink animal products. Toxins can also enter the body by eating fruits and vegetables with pesticides. So please remove the pesticides as described in the previous chapter. According to the USDA 29% of vegetables eaten are potatoes (most are in the form of French fries). While a potato is good nutrition, putting it in a deep fryer with oils isn't. We as Americans consume on average 130 pounds of sugar per year (people that eat SAD). That is so disgusting to me. Parents if you are allowing your kids to consume this much sugar you are the reason for their failing health, low self-esteem, and other ailments. When you consume this much sugar, we are also tasking the pancreas to release more insulin which is very unhealthy as it can lead to diabetes. Another problem with SAD is the consumption of sodium chloride (NaCl), otherwise known as table salt. During my research, I was studying stomach cancer around the world and found countries that have a very high consumption of sodium chloride also have a very high rate of stomach cancer. Our bodies need salt in moderation. Every cell in our body needs salt and salt is just another term for "ions" or charged particles. Our bodies are electrical and need a certain amount of salt to make things like nerve cells fire; getting too much salt can cause high blood pressure, and stroke and increase the risk of heart disease. According to the Centers for Disease Control (CDC), adults consume 3400 mg of sodium (salt) daily. The CDC recommends for adults daily consumption of sodium should be less than 2,300mg. The P53 Diet plan is less than 1,500 per daily intake. According to the National Health and Nutrition Examination Survey in the United States 2009 -2010, about 43% of sodium eaten by people comes from just ten common food types:

- *Pizza*
- *Bread/Rolls*
- *Savory Snacks*
- *Sandwiches*
- *Cheese*
- *Chicken Patties/Nuggets, etc*
- *Pasta Mixed Dishes*
- *Soups*

- **Pizza** - While high in sodium, cheese brings toxins and high fats in the form of saturated fats, and processed meats carry high sodium, toxins, and animal proteins. Most pizza sauces bring a lot of sugar to the body. The dough in most pizzas has bleached flour and olive oils.
- **Burgers** - Most fast food burgers use added chemicals to help preserve the meat. Research shows us that the consumption of red meat can increase the risk of cardiovascular diseases. Other

studies show the consumption of red meat can increase the risk of kidney stones. Red meat also has high levels of uric acid.

- **Hot Dogs** - Studies show that people have a high risk of getting leukemia from eating hot dogs. Hot dogs contain nitrates and nitrites once digested can form nitrosamines, which have been linked to cancer.
- **Chicken** - In a 2013 study in the Journal of Environmental Health Perspectives found levels of arsenic in chicken from 10 American cities, this study included the organic chickens. Antibiotics are still found in chickens and are available in grocery stores. Chicken is very high in saturated fat.
- **Pork** - High levels of nitrosamines have been found in pork. Nitrosamines have been linked to cancer. Pork has high levels of Omega-6 fatty acids with links in some studies to liver disease. When meat is cooked at high a temperature, carcinogens like heterocyclic amines are formed which can lead to liver cancer.
- **Beef** – In studies I have seen, stated red meat could potentially cause colon cancer. Red meat has also been found to be linked to cardiovascular disease. Some scientists have found a relationship between red meat consumption and an increased risk of getting Alzheimer's.
- **Cheese** - Cheese has a high amount of sodium. It was also full of saturated fats. Cheese is also dangerous to the cardiovascular system. Cheese carries unwanted toxins into the body. Cheese has a high level of caseins. Cheese has a morphine-like compound. More on cheese and dairy in the chapter on *"Animal Products."*
- **Processed Meats** - Processed meats have been linked to an increased risk of getting chronic diseases. Process meats also contain nitrates and nitrites once digested can form nitrosamines, which have been linked to cancer. High levels of sodium are also found in processed meats. More on this in the chapter on *"Animal Products."*

- **Ice Cream** -Ice cream contains large amounts of sugar, which brings a risk of diabetes. Dairy products also carry unwanted toxins into the body. More on this in the chapter on *"Animal Products."*
- **Cooking Oils** - The average consumption of vegetable oils is 70 lbs per year per person. Some processes use a petroleum solvent to extract the oils. Cooking oils contain very high levels of polyunsaturated fats (PUFAs). They are easy to oxidize causing inflammation and can cause mutations in cells. Research has shown that oxidation can lead to cancer.
- **Fried Foods/French Fries** - Have been linked to obesity, heart disease, high blood pressure, high cholesterol, and cancer. Heating foods at high temperatures creates Acrylamide. When food is cooked at very high heat the amino acid asparagine reacts with sugars and produces Acrylamide. Acrylamide has been shown to cause cancer in animals. Potatoes have high sugars such as fructose which makes potatoes more likely to create acrylamide when exposed to high heat. The oils that most foods are fried in are rich in fats.
- **Processed Foods** - Most nutrients have been removed. They have additives, preservatives, and dangerous chemicals. Most have added sugars. Most of the fiber has been removed.
- **Soft Drinks** - Soft drinks are loaded with sugar which can cause an increased risk of stroke, obesity and it can also cause kidney damage and even cancer. The high sugar amounts can cause insulin resistance which can lead to diabetes. It can cause tooth decay and oxidative stress.
- **Candy** - Candy also has high amounts of sugar just like the case above with soft drinks. They both cause the pancreas to release insulin, which can cause diabetes. A lot of candy in stores today contain dyes like red 40, yellow 5, and yellow 6 that are known toxins, more on this in the chapter *"Toxins"* They contain no

nutrients and are high in calories. Too much sugar can cause tooth decay and oxidative stress.

To sum it up, if you allow yourself or your family to consume foods on this list on a daily basis then you should save your money you will need it to pay for all the medical bills you will see due to bad choices made with your health. Science can tell us a lot these days. We now have the ability to see how our bodies work from a cellular level. Please select whole plant-based foods for you and your family.

3

Basics of the P53 Diet & Lifestyle

Why Is It Called P53

The P53 gene is aptly referred to as the *"guardian of the genome"* due to its pivotal role in preserving the integrity and stability of an organism's genetic material. This gene acts as a critical regulator, orchestrating a complex network of cellular processes that are instrumental in preventing the development and proliferation of cancerous cells.

At its core, the P53 gene functions as a tumor suppressor. In response to various stressors, such as DNA damage, cellular hypoxia, or other abnormalities that could lead to genomic instability, P53 becomes activated. Once activated, P53 sets off a cascade of events designed to either repair the damaged DNA or initiate programmed cell death (apoptosis) if the damage is irreparable. This dual functionality is crucial in eliminating cells with compromised genetic material, thereby thwarting the potential formation of cancer.

The intricate mechanisms by which P53 operates contribute to its moniker as the *"guardian of the genome."* One of its primary functions is to halt the cell cycle, allowing time for DNA repair before cell division occurs. By acting as a checkpoint, P53 prevents the propagation of cells that might carry mutations or genetic abnormalities, thus maintaining the fidelity of the genome.

Moreover, P53 plays a central role in apoptosis, the programmed cell death essential for eliminating cells that pose a risk of becoming cancerous. When the DNA damage is beyond repair, P53 facilitates the activation of genes involved in apoptosis, ensuring that the damaged cell undergoes a controlled and orderly demise. This prevents the aberrant survival and replication of cells with faulty genetic material.

The significance of P53 in tumor suppression is underscored by its frequent mutation in various cancers. Dysfunctional P53, resulting from genetic mutations, compromises its ability to act as an effective guardian of the genome. In such cases, cells with damaged DNA may escape surveillance and continue to divide, contributing to the initiation and progression of cancer.

Beyond its direct involvement in DNA repair and apoptosis, P53 also influences a myriad of cellular processes, including metabolism, senescence, and angiogenesis. Its various regulatory functions highlight the comprehensive role it plays in maintaining genomic stability and overall cellular health.

The P53 gene's designation as the *"guardian of the genome"* encapsulates its indispensable role in safeguarding the integrity of an organism's genetic material. Through its intricate and versatile mechanisms, P53 acts as a sentinel, tirelessly monitoring and responding to potential threats to genomic stability, thereby playing a crucial role in the prevention of cancer and the maintenance of overall cellular health.

Wellness with P53 Diet

In a world inundated with health and wellness advice, discerning the path to genuine well-being can be a daunting task. Enter P53 Diet, a revolutionary approach that transcends conventional dieting norms by tapping into the inherent potential of the plant-based diet. P53diet.com is your comprehensive guide to understanding and embracing this groundbreaking nutritional philosophy. Moreover, the website offers an exclusive glimpse into the practical application of the P53 Diet by providing a valuable resource for those eager to witness the transformative impact of this approach firsthand.

Key Principles of P53 Diet

Antioxidant-Rich Foods:

• P53 Diet advocates for a diet rich in antioxidants, emphasizing the consumption of fruits, vegetables, and nuts. These antioxidants act as cellular bodyguards, neutralizing harmful free radicals and promoting a resilient cellular environment.

Anti-Inflammatory Nutrition:

• Chronic inflammation is a common denominator in many health issues. P53 Diet encourages the intake of anti-inflammatory foods, fruits, vegetables, and leafy greens, to counteract inflammation and support a balanced immune response.

Macronutrient Balance:

• Achieving a harmonious balance of macronutrients—proteins, carbohydrates, and minimal fats—is essential for optimal cellular function. P53 Diet provides practical guidelines for maintaining this balance, ensuring a sustainable and energy-efficient approach to nutrition.

Mindful Eating Practices:

• Beyond the specific foods recommended, the P53 Diet places emphasis on mindful eating. Being attuned to hunger and fullness cues, savoring each bite, and fostering a positive relationship with food are integral components of this approach.

A Hub of Knowledge and Support:

• P53diet.com serves as the hub for all things related to the P53 Diet, providing a wealth of information, practical resources, and a supportive community for individuals on their wellness journey. The website offers in-depth insights into the science behind the P53 gene, empowering users with the knowledge to make informed choices about their health.

Educational Materials:

• P53diet.com features a comprehensive array of educational materials that elucidate the intricate relationship between nutrition and cellular health. From articles and blog posts to videos and infographics, the website caters to diverse learning preferences, ensuring that users gain a deep understanding of the principles that underpin the P53 Diet.

Practical Guidance:

• Navigating a new dietary paradigm can be challenging, but the P53 Diet provides practical guidance to simplify the journey. Sample meal plans, delicious recipes, and expert tips are readily available to assist users in incorporating P53 Diet principles into their daily lives seamlessly.

Inspiring Success Stories:

• Real-world success stories from individuals who have embraced the P53 Diet grace the pages of P53diet.com. These narratives serve as powerful testimonials to the transformative potential of aligning with the principles of the P53 gene, offering encouragement and inspiration to those considering or embarking on their P53 Diet journey.

Community Engagement:

• Building a supportive community is integral to the P53 Diet philosophy. P53diet.com facilitates community engagement through forums, social media groups, and live events. Users can connect with like-minded individuals, share experiences, and draw motivation from the collective pursuit of optimal health.

A Window into Transformation:

• For those eager to experience the tangible benefits of the P53 Diet, p53diet.com is a treasure trove. This section of the website provides exclusive access to sample insights, allowing users to explore the practical application of the P53 Diet in a straightforward and accessible manner.

Sample Meal Plans:

• P53 Diet offers a variety of meal plans tailored to different preferences and dietary needs. From simple and quick options for busy individuals to more elaborate recipes for culinary enthusiasts, these meal plans provide a practical starting point for incorporating P53 Diet principles into daily life.

Delicious Recipes:

• The website features a collection of delicious recipes designed to showcase the diversity and flavor inherent in the P53 Diet. These recipes go beyond mere sustenance, offering a culinary experience that aligns with the nutritional principles of The P53 Diet.

Nutritional Guidance:

* The p53diet.com doesn't just provide recipes; it offers nutritional guidance to help users understand the rationale behind each ingredient. This insight enables individuals to make informed choices, fostering a sense of empowerment and autonomy in their dietary decisions.

Meal Preparation Tips:

• Efficient meal preparation is a cornerstone of sustainable dietary practices. P53 Diet shares practical tips and tricks for streamlining the cooking process, making it easier for individuals to incorporate the P53 Diet into their daily routines.

P53 Food Trucks:

• With the proven success of the P53 Diet, the demand to get P53 Diet recipes on the go has spawned the P53 Foods carts. Starting in the Pacific Northwest with 3 food carts today with more on the way. Please check p53diet.com for the current location of the P53 Food Carts.

The P53 Channel Podcast:

• The success of the P53 Diet has also had the clients of the diet ask me to produce a weekly podcast to cover more detailed up-to-date information. Starting in January 2024 *"The P53 Channel Podcast"* will be launched.

P53 Diet, as championed by P53diet.com, represents a paradigm shift in the realm of nutrition and wellness. By understanding and leveraging the power of plant-based foods, individuals can embark on a transformative journey toward optimal health. P53 Diet serves as a gateway for those curious about the practical application of the P53 Diet, offering a glimpse into the delicious and nourishing possibilities that await. Embrace the power within, explore the science-backed principles of the P53 Diet, and join a community that is redefining the path to holistic well-being. If you are interested in owning your P53 Food Cart or P53 Catering in your area please visit ***"The P53"*** website at thep53.com for all things P53 related.

20 Steps to the P53 Diet & Lifestyle

Step 1. Choose a calorie plan - To start your weight loss program you need to choose which calorie intake you feel comfortable with. You will lose weight faster on 1000 and 1200 calorie intake than you will on a 2000-calorie intake. In order to make this diet work, you must have the discipline to stick with the diet. No program will ever work unless you make the effort to make it work. In most people choosing this diet for weight-loss you should choose a 1200 calorie plan to start.

Step 2. 75 - 80% of calories should be from plant-based carbohydrates - Other diets say you should have low carbohydrates in your diets. The truth of the matter is, that our bodies need carbohydrates. We get the right kind of carbohydrates from whole plant foods, like fruit and veggies. Get the right carbohydrates, NOT the refined carbohydrates from processed foods. No less than 75% of calories should be from carbohydrates.

Step 3. 10 - 12.5% of calories should be from fats - Our bodies need fat in our diet, but the body needs the right kind of fat. We need to limit the saturated fats in our diet and have more unsaturated fats that are found in plant foods. No more than 12.5% of calories can be fats. Limit your fat intake to no more than 16 grams of fat per day.

Step 4. 10 - 12.5% of calories should be from proteins - Another myth out there is we need a lot of proteins. Well, research scientists have proven that too much protein can cause weight gain, and can harm the liver in the process. Researchers and scientists have stated that reducing protein intake is a healthier plan for the body. We can get the proteins we need from whole plant foods. No more than 12.5% of calories can come from proteins.

Step 5. You can not consume any animal products (meat, dairy, fish, eggs, or honey) - According to research by scientists from around the world, animal products bring unwanted health problems into our bodies. The best thing you can do for your body is to eliminate animal products, this means dairy, meat, eggs, fish, and even honey. All animal products bring toxins into our bodies. When you stop consuming animal products you will feel a difference in your overall health. I was one of those people. Please read more on this in the chapter entitled *"Animal Products."*

Step 6. You can not consume any food with food additives - Food additives can bring bad chemistry into our bodies and can cause gene mutations and other ailments. Food additives can cause oxidative stress in cells in the form of free radicals. We should all know by now our bodies don't like toxins. Keep all unwanted chemistry out of the body. Read your food labels and check on this website the list of known carcinogens.

Step 7. Keep added sugars close to zero - Too much sugar can cause an array of health problems for humans. I think we all know we need to reduce our sugar intake to be healthy people. Try to keep your added sugar intake close to zero. Your sugar intake should come from plant foods like fruits and veggies. Refined sugars are not good for our bodies. This means NO SODA POP AT ALL. This also means no diet soda either. Almost all soda pop contains bad chemistry. Processed sugars can cause oxidative stress in cells in the form of free radicals.

Step 8. Keep sodium intake under 1500mg per day - Sodium chloride is salt. Both sodium and chloride are electrolytes. We need salt in our diet for electrical signaling and fluid balance. Sodium also helps the body absorb amino acids, glucose, chloride, and H2O. Too much sodium can lead to high blood pressure and increase your risk of heart attacks and stroke. There is also research that I have seen that states too much sodium can lead to a higher risk of stomach cancer.

Step 9. Keep all toxins out of the body - Toxins can enter the body in many ways. If we keep the consumption of processed foods very low, then we are lowering our risk of having bad chemistry in our bodies that can harm us. Try to keep processed foods to under 5% of calories.

Step 10. Get daily exercise - Exercise is a major part of overall good health. Exercise helps the body in so many ways not just for weight loss. Studies have shown that the more you exercise, the more cancer cells go through apoptosis. Do a brisk walk of 2 miles each day! Too much exercise can create oxidative stress see Chapter 15 for more on exercise and oxidative stress.

Step 11. No fried foods - If you stop eating fried foods you will lower your risk of certain cancers according to research scientists. Fried foods increase your risk of diabetes and heart disease. When you heat a carbohydrate at high temperatures you create acrylamide. Acrylamide has been proven to induce mutations in mammalian cells. It has been labeled a dangerous genotoxic carcinogen. Potato chips have one of the highest levels of acrylamide. Fried foods increase your calorie intake and increase your fat intake.

Step 12. Take a plant-based vitamin B12 each day or Nutritional Yeast - If you follow this diet you will need to get your vitamin B12 from sources other than animal products. You can take a B12 supplement or you can get your vitamin B12 from nutritional yeast. Please check with your doctor on the amount you will need.

Step 13. Try to reduce cooking temperatures on all cooked foods - As stated in Step 11 heating carbohydrates at high temperatures can cause damage to our bodies. We can also cook out the vital nutrients by cooking on high heat. Try to steam vegetables and try lowering temperatures on all cooked foods, take a little more time it is worth it. Air fryers are still heating carbohydrates at a high temperature.

Step 14. Eat different colored plant-based food - We have all heard the phrase *"eat the rainbow"* and the reason is that different phytochemicals that our bodies need on a daily basis come in the color of our fruits and veggies. Try to eat the rainbow each day to ensure your body is receiving the phytochemicals it needs.

Step 15. Reduce the use of cooking oils to close to zero - Cooking oils bring too much fat into our bodies, which is very unhealthy for us and can play a role in obesity. Try reducing the use of cooking oils. Some cooking oils use hexane in the manufacturing process. Hexane is produced from crude oil.

Step 16. Get 8 hours of sleep each night - Sleep plays such an important role in our body's health. According to scientists, sleeping in a very dark room can release more melatonin. When more melatonin is released into the blood it inhibits the growth of most cancer cell lines. Get 8 hours of sleep a night and make the room dark.

Step 17. Alcohol use should be limited - We know alcohol is bad for the human body. Stopping the consumption of all alcohol is the best for weight loss and other health issues for most people, but this is an impossible task. Try to limit yourself to 1 drink per day if you feel the need, but again zero alcohol is the best way to achieve your weight loss and health goals.

Step 18. Eat mostly uncooked vegetables - We know that cooking certain fruits and vegetables can cook out the needed nutrients from the food. You should eat most of the fruits and vegetables raw, at least 60% should be uncooked. Try steaming some of your vegetables.

Step 19. Drink plenty of water - Try to consume 2 liters of water per day, that should be about 8, 8-ounce glasses of water per day. Try to drink the water cold. Make sure the pH of the water is 7.2 or higher. Make sure the water has no chlorine or fluoride.

Step 20. Reduce the stress in your life - Try to reduce the stress in your life. When you are stressed, your body releases a hormone called cortisol. Cortisol has been shown to weaken the immune system, increase blood pressure, create nerve problems, cause anxiety, headaches, and depression as well as cause weight gain. I know this is easier said than done.

Controlling your health is much like a business you need a good business plan to follow to be successful. Your health should have a plan to ensure you stay in good health. This is where the P53 Diet comes into play, follow the 20 steps in the plan on a daily basis and you will have good results, stick to the plan it works. If you want to only stick to 50% of the plan then you will only get 50% of the results. This is the way I have chosen to live my life and my health is the best it has ever been. I don't make hospital visits, I eat a plant-based P53 Diet and it works.

Building Muscle On a Plant-Based Diet

Building muscle on a plant-based diet has gained increasing attention in recent years as more individuals explore the benefits of plant-based lifestyles. Contrary to the misconception that muscle gain is exclusively linked to animal protein consumption, a well-planned plant-based diet can provide the essential nutrients needed for effective muscle development. I will delve into key aspects of building muscle on a plant-based diet, including protein sources, nutrient considerations, meal planning, and potential challenges.

Protein Sources in Plant-Based Diets

Protein is a cornerstone for muscle growth, and while animal products are traditionally rich sources, numerous plant-based options can fulfill this role. Legumes, such as lentils, chickpeas, and beans, are excellent protein sources and form the basis of many plant-based diets. Tofu and tempeh, derived from soybeans, are versatile and protein-dense options. Edamame, quinoa, and whole grains like brown rice and oats also contribute to the protein intake necessary for muscle building.

Nuts and seeds, such as almonds, chia seeds, and hemp seeds, are not only rich in healthy fats but also provide a protein boost. Including a variety of these plant-based protein sources in daily meals ensures a well-rounded amino acid profile, essential for effective muscle synthesis.

Nutrient Considerations for Muscle Growth

Apart from protein, other nutrients play crucial roles in muscle development. Calcium, found in fortified plant milk and leafy greens like kale and bok choy, supports muscle function and bone health. Iron, prevalent in lentils and spinach, is vital for oxygen transport to muscles, aiding endurance during workouts. Omega-3 fatty acids, sourced from flaxseeds, chia seeds, and walnuts, contribute to inflammation control, facilitating recovery after intense exercise.

Vitamin D, essential for calcium absorption and muscle function, can be obtained through sunlight exposure or fortified plant-based milk alternatives. A well-rounded intake of vitamins and minerals, obtained from a diverse array of plant foods, ensures that the body has the necessary tools for optimal muscle growth.

Meal Planning for Muscle Gain

Effective meal planning is key to building muscle on a plant-based diet. Distributing protein intake throughout the day helps provide a consistent supply of amino acids for muscle synthesis. Including protein-rich snacks like hummus with veggies, a handful of nuts, or a smoothie with plant-based protein powder can contribute to meeting daily protein goals.

Balancing macronutrients is crucial for overall health and muscle development. Incorporating complex carbohydrates, such as whole grains, fruits, and vegetables, provides sustained energy for workouts. Healthy fats from avocados and nuts support hormone production, including those involved in muscle growth.

Pre- and post-workout nutrition is particularly important. Consuming a protein-rich snack before exercise and a combination of protein and carbohydrates afterward supports muscle repair and replenishes glycogen stores. Plant-based protein shakes, almond butter on whole-grain toast, or a smoothie with fruits are excellent choices for these periods.

Challenges and Considerations

While building muscle on a plant-based diet is entirely feasible, some challenges need attention. One primary concern is ensuring an adequate intake of certain nutrients that are more commonly found in animal products. Vitamin B12, crucial for energy metabolism, can be obtained through fortified plant-based foods like Nutritional Yeast. Creatine, beneficial for strength and muscle gain, is found in smaller amounts in plant foods but can be supplemented if needed.

Another consideration is protein quality. Plant-based protein sources may lack one or more essential amino acids, but by combining different plant foods, individuals can achieve a complete amino acid profile. This is known as protein complementation and involves pairing foods like black beans and brown rice, or hummus and whole-grain bread.

Achieving Muscle Growth on a Plant-Based Diet

Building muscle on the plant-based P53 Diet is not only achievable but can also offer numerous health benefits. A thoughtful and well-planned approach to nutrition, incorporating a variety of plant-based protein sources and nutrient-dense foods, is essential. Strategic meal planning, attention to nutrient considerations, and addressing potential challenges ensure that individuals can thrive and build muscle effectively while embracing a plant-centric lifestyle, like what is offered on the P53 Diet website. As awareness grows and more research emerges, the viability and advantages of plant-based muscle building are likely to become even more evident in the realm of fitness and nutrition.

What is Meant by Gluten-Free?

Gluten-free has become a prevalent term in today's dietary lexicon, and it refers to a diet that excludes gluten, a protein found in wheat, barley, rye, and their derivatives. Gluten is responsible for the elasticity and structure of dough, giving bread its chewy texture and baked goods their characteristic shape. While gluten is harmless for most people, it can cause severe health issues for individuals with celiac disease, wheat allergy, or non-celiac gluten sensitivity. The science behind gluten-free diets revolves around understanding the impact of gluten on the digestive system and immune response.

Celiac disease is an autoimmune disorder characterized by an abnormal immune reaction to gluten. When individuals with celiac disease consume gluten, their immune system mistakenly attacks the lining of the small intestine. This immune response damages the intestinal villi, small finger-like projections that play a crucial role in nutrient absorption. As a result, individuals with celiac disease may experience malabsorption of nutrients, leading to various health issues, including anemia, osteoporosis, and fatigue. The only effective treatment for celiac disease is strict adherence to a gluten-free diet.

Wheat allergy is another condition that necessitates a gluten-free diet. Unlike celiac disease, which is an autoimmune disorder, wheat allergy is an allergic reaction to proteins found in wheat, including but not limited to gluten. Symptoms of wheat allergy can range from mild, such as hives or nausea, to severe, with anaphylaxis being a rare but life-threatening possibility. Individuals with wheat allergy must avoid all forms of wheat, which includes steering clear of gluten-containing products.

Non-celiac gluten sensitivity (NCGS) is a condition characterized by gastrointestinal and/or extra-intestinal symptoms related to the consumption of gluten in individuals without celiac disease or wheat allergy. The exact mechanisms underlying NCGS are not fully understood, and it remains a topic of ongoing research. Unlike celiac disease and wheat allergy, there are no specific diagnostic tests for NCGS, making it challenging to identify and manage. The primary treatment for NCGS is also a gluten-free diet.

The science behind gluten-free diets involves recognizing the intricate interactions between gluten, the immune system, and the digestive tract. The immune response triggered by gluten in susceptible individuals can have far-reaching consequences beyond the gastrointestinal system. Advances in research have led to a better understanding of the genetic and immunologic factors contributing to conditions like celiac disease, shedding light on why some individuals are more predisposed to gluten-related disorders than others.

Gluten-free diets, when properly managed, can improve the health and well-being of individuals with celiac disease, wheat allergy, or non-celiac gluten sensitivity. However, it's crucial for those adopting a gluten-free lifestyle for non-medical reasons to be aware that eliminating gluten without a medical necessity may lead to nutritional deficiencies. Many gluten-containing grains, such as wheat, barley, and rye, are significant sources of essential nutrients like fiber, B vitamins, and minerals.

The term gluten-free pertains to a diet devoid of gluten, primarily adopted by individuals with celiac disease, wheat allergy, or non-celiac gluten sensitivity. The science behind gluten-free diets involves understanding the autoimmune and allergic reactions triggered by gluten consumption and the resulting impact on the digestive system. While essential for managing certain medical conditions, a gluten-free diet requires careful consideration to ensure adequate nutrient intake for those without specific gluten-related disorders. There are a lot of gluten-free recipes on the P53 Diet website at p53diet.com you can even search for recipes that are gluten-free.

Testimonials

From ***Jammie Ashbrook*** subscriber:

"I started Dave's P53 Diet on 4/1/2022 at 263.7lbs. I was previously prescribed Eliquis for blood clots and Lisinopril for high blood pressure. I ate the P53 Diet for 6 weeks and lost 19.3lbs. I noticed the swelling in my legs stopped, my BP dropped from 150/95-100 to 100/65 and I was able to stop taking the Lisinopril as per my Cardiologist. I began noticing my neck, face, and chest shrinking. My shirts got looser. Friends and co-workers began noticing and commenting, at 5-6 weeks, asking me about what I was doing to lose weight. Saying I was looking good. And I felt great! Had more energy and was sleeping much better than before.

I do remember a few side effects that I noticed. In week 4, I tried a piece of pizza and after eating it I felt like my eyes were on fire. I also found that I slept really well initially, but in week 3 I started having "Restless Legs" at 10:30 pm every night. I had just been eating the P53 (plant-based) Diet, but not exercising daily. I initially thought that the walking I do at work would be enough, but then realized that I did need to get my cardio up for at least 35 min a day. I started walking 3-3.5mi/day after work and "Restless Leg" went away. Initially, it took me 45min to do this, and now I can do it in 35min. Another major change I noticed was the lack of brain fog, especially when I was at work. Much more mentally sharp. This has made project processes and completion much easier.

After having been on the P53 Diet and then going off of it a few times while vacationing this Summer, I can tell you I missed the benefits of being on it when I went off it. I just feel better when I'm eating exclusively Plant-Based and getting my daily cardio. For me this isn't a "diet", It's my new way of life. Living healthier! Feeling better! I might wander off the plant-based eating path occasionally for special occasions and vacays, but I don't want to go back to having less energy and having the ugly swelling in my legs. Also, acid reflux went away. This was a huge one for me. I would recommend Dave's P53 Diet to anyone wanting to make a positive lifestyle change."

J. Ashbrook

From ***Pat Chappell*** subscriber:

I grew up in a small town, Washougal Washington. I was an athlete during that time, and I learned at a young age that the combination of good nutrition and exercise was going to be vital for great health, and well-being in the long run of life. I learned through reading all of my mother's health books that she had accumulated over time. She pushed health and fitness, and I learned what vitamins and minerals did once they got into your system and the benefits they had.

I found out that plant-based nutrition is the best way to go. It has given me better energy, much better performance, and certainly overall better function from head to toe. I have been in and out of bodybuilding for years now, and I'm one hundred percent sold on using a plant-based nutrition plan to achieve a great body. The myth that you can't build a great body on plant-based nutrition is busted. I have done it and so have others.

By chance, I met Dave Brown. He introduced me to his P53 Diet Plan. He broke the plan down to me and gave me better insight than I already had. I totally believe in Dave's P53 Diet plan. I am a current member and will be for a long time. I have experienced and taken in all kinds of information on health in my life. I'm 64 years old now and this is literally the best information that I have seen. I load the recipes into my meal plan so I can have insight into all the nutritional values for that day. I am not using the P53 Diet and Lifestyle as a weight loss program, I am using it to build muscle the right way, NO SUPPLEMENTS and NO ANIMAL PRODUCTS.

I believe Dave has been ahead of the pack for years with his study and breakdown of nutrition. The amazing success Dave has had with all the cancer patients on the P53 Diet does not shock me at all. You talk about a guy that knows what he is talking about Dave is that guy. I would encourage all to get on the P53 Diet plan. Without a doubt, you will be on your way to a better life. The P53 Diet & Lifestyle just works!

Pat Chappell
Plant-Based
Exercise Trainer/Consultant

From ***Truett Standefer*** *subscriber:*

I spent most of my childhood in and out of hospitals and was diagnosed with Myasthenia Gravis (a Neuromuscular Disease) when I was 7. I was told that by the time I was 13, I would weigh over 200 lbs and would probably not live to see my 20's. I grew up doing absolutely everything the doctors said I would never do and beat the odds given me. As I have gotten older I have noticed that I fell in and out of remission more often. Nothing I was doing seemed to help the fatigue, the high blood pressure, the weight gain, and the overall feeling of exhaustion and depression. I met Mr. Dave Brown at a local coffee shop and struck up a conversation that has since changed my life. For a boy who grew up in Texas and lived on red meat and Dr. Pepper, the P53 Diet was a total shock to my system. After only a month of this new lifestyle, a visit to the Doctor confirmed, that my blood pressure had returned to normal, my energy level had gone through the roof and I was no longer as fatigued as I had been over the last 10 years. I am seeing health gains that I never thought were possible and I owe it all to Dave's incredibly easy P53 Diet system. You will not find a better system that teaches and guides you through the processes of putting the right foods into your body that allows your body to do exactly what it is designed to do and that is to heal itself!!

Truett Standefer

Restaurant Assistant General Manager

From ***Chris Swift*** *subscriber:*

It was the summer of 2019 when I got the long face from the doctor. He said I had a very aggressive form of prostate cancer. It was the same condition that killed my father. A couple weeks later I found myself on a camping trip up on Newberry Crater with Dave Brown. Dave was telling us about this book that he was working on and how his p53 diet could help fight prostate cancer from the research studies he found. I told him what the doctor had told me. He got up from where we were sitting, walked over to my cooler, and quickly threw away everything that was unhealthy. That was the moment I began a lifestyle of plant-based eating the P53 Diet way. I did that for 18 months while I was undergoing two surgeries, radiation, and lupron injections. It was surprising to me when the oncologist asked me what I was eating. He was curious because the treatments weren't making me sick. I told him I was eating a plant-based diet called the P53 Diet. He told me to keep it up. It was the best diet to fight cancer with. I am completely convinced that God and the P53 Diet way of eating saved my life while I waited for treatments during the pandemic.

I went from an eight on the Gleason scale all the way down to no disease detected. So, naturally, I thought hey, I can probably eat anything I want now. I couldn't have been more wrong. As I went back to eating a Western diet, my PSA numbers started to come up again. Indicating that something was growing. The doctors put me back on lupron injections every 4 months to kill my testosterone so that it would keep the cancer in check. The Good news is they can do this for the rest of my life. The bad news? Every 4 months I get injected with poison. I have to live a life of low testosterone, and no libido as a result. I also get to enjoy hot flashes like a woman going through the change. That's pretty much what happens when you take testosterone away from men.

The doctors watch the testosterone numbers. When they rise, the PSA numbers rise with them. And then you get another shot. More poison. My solution is to go back to the p53 lifestyle. I'll let God and good food take care of the disease. I believe with every fiber of my being, that this program will reverse the cancer. When the shot wears off, my testosterone will rise. And the good news? The PSA will not rise with it. I have an appointment when I'm 90 years old to go camping with Dave Brown. I plan to keep that appointment.

Chris Swift
Owner, Bull Mountain Coffee Roosters
Vancouver, WA

From ***Ryan Robinson*** *subscriber:*

Hi my name is Ryan, I am an avid surfer living in San Diego and this is my P53 story. I met Dave Brown on a visit to meet a childhood friend

I had not seen in forty years in Vancouver Washington. Later that day my friend asked me if I would like to meet a couple of her close friends. Of course I do and that's when I meet Dave. He talks a little about his diet and his food trucks which has me interested. Months go by and while surfing I am stung by a large adult stingray. This is the fourth time I have been stung in seventeen years and this one is bad. My foot swells up to the size of a football and my friend convinces me to go to urgent care and get antibiotics. They take my blood pressure and it is super high and they tell me to go see my primary care physician as soon as possible after giving me a prescription for antibiotics. It takes about two weeks for my appointment. The nurse takes my blood pressure and it is 205 over 125. My doctor finally comes in and tells me to go straight to the emergency room very rude tone. I get up walk out of her office and call my friend in Vancouver. She reminds me about Dave's diet and I give him a call about my hypertension. Dave and I have sort of clicked since day one as we are both watermen in different ways. This is a very disciplined diet, no more taco Tuesdays and ribeye Fridays. Dave told me once if you do this halfway way you will get half the results. I have told all my family and friends about the P53. When I first started this diet a family friend, who is on blood pressure medication told me you can only lose twenty-five to thirty points by diet alone. I have dropped mine over sixty-five points in sixty days! I am now 140 over 80 and still dropping. The same family member who told me I couldn't do it is 140 over 80 and on Lisinopril blood pressure medication. I wish I had found this diet years ago when I was racing motorcycles. Who knows how fast I could have been? One ingredient in my daily diet is Vitamin B12 which is the only vitamin or supplement Dave takes. It actually helps me focus and think more clearly. I have also lost almost fifteen pounds in sixty days as well, which wasn't part of my goal. My father died of a rare type of Leukemia called Myelofibrosis and I do believe it might have had something to do with all the medications he was on for so many years. Everything from all types of blood pressure medications, cholesterol, gout, diabetes, and the list goes on. With that being said I hate taking any meds including aspirin. I now wonder if I could have gotten him on this diet before his diagnosis which I believe could save lives. If you want to feel energetic, feel healthy, feel smarter, poop better, no mid-day drowsiness, then Dave and Lisa's recipes will make you a better person. I honestly think it can help with any type of depression we are dealing with. Life is short so why not make the best out of it? So when you read my little story in Dave's book, you will see I am a testament to the P53 Diet because it has truly changed my life.

Update: As of Dec 9th, 2023 my BP is 120/80. All just following the P53 Diet & Lifestyle.

Ryan Robinson
Motorcycle Dealership Manager
San Diego, CA

Please check the p53diet.com website for testimonials.

4

Amino Acids

Amino acids play a crucial role in maintaining the health and functionality of the human body, making them essential components of a balanced diet. These organic compounds are the building blocks of proteins, which are fundamental to various physiological processes. There are 20 different amino acids that the body requires for proper functioning, and they can be classified into three categories: essential, non-essential, and conditional.

Essential amino acids are those that the body cannot produce on its own and must be obtained through diet. These include histidine, isoleucine, leucine, lysine, methionine, phenylalanine, threonine, tryptophan, and valine. Non-essential amino acids, on the other hand, can be synthesized by the body, but their availability from external sources can still contribute to overall health. Conditional amino acids are a subset of amino acids that are typically considered non-essential under normal circumstances, as the body can synthesize them internally. However, under certain conditions or states of health, these amino acids become essential, and their dietary intake becomes crucial for maintaining optimal function. The term "conditional" is used to highlight the context-dependent nature of these amino acids.

All types are crucial for the synthesis of proteins, enzymes, hormones, neurotransmitters, and other molecules essential for life.

Proteins are integral components of every cell, tissue, and organ in the body. They contribute to the structural integrity of cells, act as enzymes catalyzing biochemical reactions, transport substances across cell membranes, and play a key role in immune function. The diverse functions of proteins underscore the importance of obtaining an adequate supply of amino acids through diet.

Amino acids also play a vital role in the synthesis of neurotransmitters, which are chemical messengers that transmit signals between nerve cells. For example, tryptophan is a precursor to serotonin, a neurotransmitter that regulates mood and contributes to feelings of well-being. An imbalance in amino acid intake can potentially affect neurotransmitter levels and, consequently, mental health.

We have been taught to understand that amino acids are essential for the maintenance and repair of tissues throughout the body. During physical activity, especially exercise that involves muscle contractions, there is an increased demand for amino acids to support muscle protein synthesis and repair. This is particularly relevant for athletes and individuals engaging in regular physical activity, as insufficient amino acid intake may hinder muscle recovery and growth.

Dietary sources of amino acids are diverse, and they can be obtained from plant-based sources. The P53 Diet plant-based protein sources, such as fruit, vegetables, beans, legumes, grains, nuts, and seeds, can help ensure a sufficient intake of essential amino acids.

Inadequate consumption of amino acids can lead to a range of health issues, including muscle wasting, impaired immune function, and compromised wound healing. Therefore, maintaining a well-balanced diet that provides all essential amino acids in the right proportions is crucial for overall health and well-being.

Amino Acid Groups

Polar Amino Acids (Hydrophilic)

- Asparagine
- Cystine
- Glutamine
- Serine
- Threonine
- Tyrosine

Non-polar Amino Acids (Hydrophobic)

- Alanine
- Glycine
- Isoleucine
- Leucine
- Methionine
- Phenylalanine
- Proline
- Tryptophan
- Valine

Polar Amino Acids (Positively Charged)

- Arginine
- Histidine
- Lysine

Polar Acidic Amino Acids (Negatively Charged)

- Aspartate
- Glutamate

**Hydrophilic* -Seek contact with liquids
**Hydrophobic* – Avoid liquids

Essential Amino Acids

Histidine

Histidine is a crucial amino acid with diverse roles in the body, impacting various metabolic pathways. As one of the essential amino acids, histidine cannot be synthesized by the human body and must be obtained through dietary sources. Its significance lies in its involvement in protein structure, enzyme catalysis, neurotransmission, and the regulation of pH levels.

One fundamental aspect of histidine is its contribution to the structure of proteins. Histidine contains an imidazole ring, making it unique among the amino acids. This imidazole ring is an important structural element in proteins, influencing their folding and stability. Proteins play a vital role in numerous biological processes, serving as enzymes, structural components, transporters, and signaling molecules. Histidine's presence in proteins contributes to the overall functionality and three-dimensional structure of these biomolecules.

Enzymatic activity is another key area where histidine plays a pivotal role. Many enzymes rely on histidine residues for catalytic functions. The imidazole group in histidine can act as a proton donor or acceptor, facilitating various biochemical reactions. One notable example is in the catalytic triad of serine proteases, where histidine participates in the hydrolysis of peptide bonds. Additionally, histidine is often involved in redox reactions and metal ion coordination within enzyme active sites, underscoring its versatility in catalysis.

Histidine's involvement in metabolic pathways extends to its role in buffering and maintaining pH balance. The imidazole group in histidine has a pKa close to physiological pH, allowing it to act as a buffer in cellular environments. This means histidine can donate or accept protons, helping to regulate the acidity of cellular compartments. Maintaining proper pH is crucial for the optimal functioning of enzymes and other cellular processes. Histidine's buffering capacity contributes to the body's ability to resist changes in pH and ensures the stability of biological molecules.

In neurotransmission, histidine plays a vital role as a precursor to histamine. Histamine is a biogenic amine that acts as a neurotransmitter and is involved in various physiological processes, including the immune response and the regulation of gastric acid secretion. Histidine decarboxylase, an enzyme, converts histidine into histamine. The release of histamine in response to certain stimuli has implications for allergic reactions, inflammation, and other immune responses.

Histidine is a precursor to carnosine and anserine, dipeptides with antioxidant properties. Carnosine, found in high concentrations in skeletal muscle, helps buffer intracellular pH during high-intensity exercise and has been implicated in reducing oxidative stress. Anserine, closely related to carnosine, is found in high levels in the brain and may contribute to neurological health.

The metabolic pathways involving histidine are interconnected and illustrate the amino acid's multifaceted roles. From its structural contribution to proteins and enzymatic catalysis to its involvement in neurotransmission and pH regulation, histidine emerges as a linchpin in various biological processes. The intricate interplay between histidine and other molecules highlights the complexity of cellular metabolism and the importance of this amino acid in maintaining physiological balance.

Histidine stands out as an indispensable amino acid with far-reaching implications for the body's metabolic pathways. Its structural role in proteins, involvement in enzymatic catalysis, contribution to pH regulation, and participation in the synthesis of important molecules like histamine, carnosine, and anserine underscore its significance. Understanding the diverse functions of histidine provides valuable insights into the intricate web of biochemical processes that sustain life.

Sources of Histidine:

- **Legumes:**
  - Lentils
  - Chickpeas
  - Black beans
- **Whole Grains:**
  - Quinoa
  - Brown rice
- **Nuts and Seeds:**
  - Sunflower seeds
  - Chia seeds
  - Pumpkin seeds
- **Soy and Soy Products:**
  - Tofu
  - Tempeh
  - Edamame
  - Soybeans
- **Vegetables:**
  - Spinach
  - Peas
  - Root vegetables
  - All green vegetables
  - Pumpkin
- **Fruits:**
  - Bananas
  - Grapes

Isoleucine

Isoleucine, one of the essential amino acids, plays a crucial role in various metabolic pathways essential for maintaining overall health. This amino acid is classified as branched-chain due to its unique structure, making it distinct from others in the amino acid family. Let's delve into the reasons why isoleucine is considered vital and explore its significance in metabolic processes.

First and foremost, isoleucine is indispensable for protein synthesis, a fundamental biological process crucial for the growth, repair, and maintenance of tissues within the body. As an essential component of proteins, isoleucine contributes to the formation of muscle tissue, enzymes, and structural proteins. Its involvement in these processes highlights its significance in sustaining the structural integrity and functionality of various bodily components.

Beyond its role in protein synthesis, isoleucine is a key player in energy regulation. As a branched-chain amino acid (BCAA), isoleucine, along with leucine and valine, is unique in its ability to be directly metabolized in the muscles rather than the liver. This characteristic makes BCAAs, including isoleucine, vital for energy production during exercise and other physically demanding activities. The breakdown of isoleucine releases intermediates that can be readily converted into acetyl-CoA, a key molecule in the citric acid cycle, the primary metabolic pathway for energy production.

This amino acid is intricately linked to glucose metabolism. It participates in the synthesis of glucose through gluconeogenesis, a process crucial for maintaining blood sugar levels during fasting or low-carbohydrate conditions. By providing carbon skeletons that can be converted into glucose, isoleucine contributes to the body's ability to sustain energy production even when glucose availability is limited.

Isoleucine also plays a critical role in the regulation of blood sugar levels by promoting insulin secretion. Insulin, a hormone produced by the pancreas, facilitates the uptake of glucose by cells, thereby lowering blood glucose levels. Isoleucine has been shown to stimulate insulin release, demonstrating its involvement in glucose homeostasis. This insulinotropic effect is particularly significant for individuals with conditions such as diabetes, where maintaining proper blood sugar levels is a key aspect of management.

Additionally, isoleucine has been implicated in immune function. It serves as a precursor for various molecules, including those involved in immune response modulation. The immune system relies on a variety of signaling molecules and proteins, many of which require amino acids like isoleucine for their synthesis. Thus, the availability of isoleucine is essential for supporting immune cells and their functions, contributing to the body's defense against infections and diseases.

Isoleucine is essential for the synthesis of hemoglobin, the protein responsible for transporting oxygen in the blood. Hemoglobin, composed of heme and globin, requires specific amino acids for its formation, and isoleucine is among them. Adequate isoleucine levels are therefore crucial for ensuring the efficient transport of oxygen throughout the body, supporting overall metabolic processes and cellular functions.

The role of isoleucine stands out as a vital amino acid with multifaceted roles in the body's metabolic pathways. From its central involvement in protein synthesis to its contributions to energy regulation, glucose metabolism, immune function, and hemoglobin synthesis, isoleucine's impact is far-reaching. Recognizing the importance of maintaining sufficient isoleucine levels underscores the significance of a balanced and nutrient-rich diet to support overall health and well-being.

Sources of Isoleucine:

- **Legumes:**
  - Lentils
  - Chickpeas
  - Black beans
- **Soy and Soy Products:**
  - Tofu
  - Tempeh
  - Edamame
  - Soybeans
- **Nuts:**
  - Almonds
  - Peanuts
  - Cashews
- **Seeds:**

    - Sunflower seeds
    - Pumpkin seeds
    - Sesame seeds
    - Chis seeds
- **Whole Grains:**
    - Quinoa
    - Brown rice
    - Oats
    - Buckwheat
    - Rye
- **Vegetables:**
    - Spinach
    - Kale
    - Peas
    - Pumpkin
    - Cabbage
- **Fruits:**
    - Avocado
    - Apples
    - Blueberries
    - Cranberries
    - Kiwi

Leucine

Leucine, one of the essential amino acids, plays a crucial role in various metabolic pathways within the human body. As a branched-chain amino acid (BCAA), leucine holds a distinctive position in protein synthesis, energy production, and overall cellular function.

At its core, leucine serves as a building block for proteins, forming the basis of muscle tissue and contributing to the structural integrity of various proteins throughout the body. This amino acid is particularly significant in the context of muscle protein synthesis. Leucine stimulates the mammalian target of the rapamycin (mTOR) pathway, a key signaling pathway that regulates cell growth and protein synthesis. By activating mTOR, leucine promotes the translation of messenger RNA into proteins, fostering the development and repair of muscle tissues.

The role of leucine extends beyond mere protein synthesis. This amino acid actively participates in glucose homeostasis, influencing insulin sensitivity and glucose uptake in skeletal muscles. Studies have shown that leucine can enhance insulin signaling, thereby improving the body's ability to manage blood sugar levels. This metabolic impact is of paramount importance, especially in the context of preventing and managing conditions like diabetes.

Leucine acts as a potent regulator of lipid metabolism. It plays a role in inhibiting protein breakdown during periods of energy deprivation, thus preserving lean body mass. Additionally, leucine has been linked to the promotion of fat loss by modulating key enzymes involved in lipolysis, the process of breaking down fats for energy. This dual role in both protein and lipid metabolism underscores leucine's significance in maintaining a healthy body composition.

The involvement of leucine in metabolic pathways goes beyond its immediate impact on protein and lipid metabolism. It also serves as a precursor for the synthesis of other important molecules, including sterols and other amino acids. The versatility of leucine in contributing to diverse biological processes highlights its indispensability for overall health.

In the realm of energy production, leucine plays a unique role. It can be converted into acetyl-CoA, a key molecule in the citric acid cycle, which is central to the production of adenosine triphosphate (ATP) – the cellular currency for energy. This capacity to contribute to energy production underscores leucine's importance in sustaining vital cellular functions, particularly in tissues with high energy demands, such as skeletal muscles.

Leucine has been implicated in the regulation of gene expression. Through its interaction with mTOR and other signaling pathways, leucine can influence the transcription of genes involved in various cellular processes. This regulatory function adds another layer to its significance in orchestrating a myriad of physiological responses.

The impact of this amino acid on muscle health is particularly noteworthy in the context of aging. Age-related muscle loss, known as sarcopenia, is a significant concern for the elderly, contributing to frailty and decreased quality of life. Leucine supplementation has shown promise in mitigating muscle loss in older adults, highlighting its potential as a therapeutic intervention to promote healthy aging.

While leucine's benefits are apparent, it's important to emphasize the necessity of obtaining it through dietary sources. Since the body cannot produce leucine on its own, it must be acquired through nutrition. For individuals engaged in intense physical activities, such as athletes and bodybuilders, supplementing with leucine has become a common practice to optimize muscle protein synthesis and support recovery.

Leucine is a pivotal player in the intricate web of metabolic pathways within the human body. Its role in protein synthesis, glucose homeostasis, lipid metabolism, energy production, and gene expression showcases its multifaceted contributions to overall health. Whether through dietary intake or supplementation, ensuring an adequate supply of leucine is paramount for maintaining optimal physiological function and promoting longevity.

Sources of Leucine:

- **Legumes:**
    - Lentils
    - Chickpeas
    - Black beans
- **Soy and Soy Products:**
    - Tofu
    - Tempeh
    - Edamame
    - Soybeans
- **Nuts:**

    - Almonds
    - Peanuts
- **Seeds:**
    - Sunflower seeds
    - Pumpkin seeds
    - Hemp seeds
- **Whole Grains:**
    - Quinoa
    - Brown rice
    - Oats
    - Buckwheat
- **Vegetables:**
    - Spinach
    - Kale
    - Peas
- **Fruits:**
    - Avocado

Lysine

Lysine is an essential amino acid, meaning that the human body cannot synthesize it on its own and must obtain it through dietary sources. Its significance lies in its crucial role in various metabolic pathways, making it an essential component for overall health and well-being.

One primary function of lysine is its contribution to protein synthesis. Proteins are fundamental building blocks of the body, serving roles in the structure, function, and regulation of tissues and organs. Lysine, as one of the essential amino acids, participates in the formation of proteins by combining with other amino acids through peptide bonds. This process is vital for the growth, repair, and maintenance of tissues, muscles, and organs.

Beyond its role in protein synthesis, lysine plays a pivotal role in the formation of collagen, a structural protein that provides strength and elasticity to connective tissues such as skin, tendons, and bones.

Collagen is essential for maintaining skin integrity, promoting wound healing, and ensuring the health of joints and cartilage. Lysine contributes to the cross-linking of collagen molecules, enhancing the stability and functionality of this critical protein.

Lysine also plays a significant role in the production of carnitine, a compound essential for the transport of fatty acids into the mitochondria, the powerhouse of cells. This process is crucial for energy production, as it enables the efficient utilization of fats as a fuel source. Carnitine's role in energy metabolism makes lysine important for overall cellular energy balance and contributes to the body's ability to generate and utilize energy effectively.

The regulation of calcium absorption and maintenance of bone health is yet another role for Lysine. It competes with another amino acid, arginine, for absorption in the intestines. This competitive relationship influences the bioavailability of lysine and can impact calcium absorption. Lysine deficiency may result in decreased calcium absorption, potentially leading to bone-related issues. Ensuring an adequate intake of lysine is therefore essential for maintaining proper bone density and preventing conditions such as osteoporosis.

Lysine also exhibits antiviral properties, particularly against the herpes simplex virus (HSV). Research suggests that lysine competes with arginine, an amino acid essential for the replication of HSV, limiting the virus's ability to multiply. While more studies are needed to fully understand the extent of lysine's antiviral effects, its potential role in managing and preventing herpes outbreaks highlights its diverse functions within the body.

This essential amino acid is involved in the synthesis of neurotransmitters, including serotonin and dopamine, which play key roles in mood regulation, sleep, and overall mental well-being. Adequate lysine levels contribute to the balanced production of neurotransmitters, potentially influencing cognitive function and emotional stability.

Despite its importance, lysine deficiency can occur, especially in individuals with limited dietary protein intake or imbalanced diets.

Common symptoms of lysine deficiency may include fatigue, impaired concentration, anemia, and decreased immunity. To prevent deficiency, it is crucial to consume lysine-rich foods from plant-based sources like legumes and nuts.

Lysine stands out as a vital amino acid with multifaceted roles in the body's metabolic processes. From its involvement in protein synthesis and collagen formation to its contribution to energy metabolism, bone health, and antiviral activities, lysine plays a crucial part in maintaining overall health and well-being. Ensuring an adequate intake of lysine through a balanced and varied diet is essential for supporting these diverse functions and promoting optimal physiological functioning.

Sources of Lysine:

- **Legumes:**
    - Lentils
    - Chickpeas
    - Black beans
- **Soy and Soy Products:**
    - Tofu
    - Tempeh
    - Edamame
    - Soy milk
- **Quinoa:**
    - Quinoa is a whole grain that is relatively high in lysine.
- **Nuts and Seeds:**
    - Pumpkin seeds
    - Sunflower Seeds:
    - Pistachios
    - Chia Seeds
    - Almonds
    - Cashews
- **Vegetables:**
    - Green peas contain lysine.

    - Parsley
- **Other:**
    - Watercress

Methionine

Methionine is a crucial amino acid with a fundamental role in various metabolic pathways, contributing to the synthesis of proteins, initiation of translation, and serving as a precursor for essential molecules within the body. As one of the nine essential amino acids, methionine cannot be synthesized by the human body and must be obtained through dietary sources.

First and foremost, methionine plays a pivotal role in protein synthesis, which is integral for the growth, repair, and maintenance of tissues. As the initiating amino acid in the process of protein synthesis, methionine carries a unique responsibility. The initiation of translation, the complex process where the information encoded in mRNA is used to build a protein, begins with the formation of a complex involving methionine. This initial amino acid establishes the starting point for the construction of the polypeptide chain, the backbone of proteins.

Methionine is essential for the formation of S-adenosylmethionine (SAM), a versatile methyl donor crucial for various methylation reactions in the body. Methylation is a biochemical process where a methyl group (CH3) is transferred from SAM to a target molecule. This process is involved in the regulation of gene expression, DNA repair, neurotransmitter synthesis, and the metabolism of hormones and drugs. Consequently, methionine's role in methylation reactions underscores its importance in maintaining the intricate balance of biochemical processes within the body.

Additionally, methionine is a precursor for cysteine, another amino acid with distinct functions. Through a transsulfuration pathway, methionine is converted into cysteine, which is further utilized for the synthesis of glutathione. Glutathione is a powerful antioxidant that helps protect cells from oxidative stress. Oxidative stress, resulting from an imbalance between free radicals and antioxidants in the body, is implicated in various diseases, including cardiovascular diseases, neurodegenerative disorders, and cancer. Thus, methionine indirectly contributes to cellular defense mechanisms through the synthesis of glutathione.

Beyond its role in protein synthesis and the formation of important molecules, methionine is integral to lipid metabolism. It participates in the synthesis of phosphatidylcholine, a crucial component of cell membranes. This underscores the broader impact of methionine on cellular structure and function, influencing the stability and integrity of cell membranes throughout the body.

The significance of methionine extends to its involvement in one-carbon metabolism, a complex network of biochemical reactions essential for the synthesis of nucleotides, the building blocks of DNA and RNA. As a key player in one-carbon metabolism, methionine contributes to the maintenance and replication of genetic material. This is particularly critical during periods of rapid cell division, such as in embryonic development and tissue regeneration.

It is worth noting that while methionine is indispensable for various physiological processes, an imbalance in its intake can have health implications. Excessive methionine consumption has been associated with potential adverse effects, including increased homocysteine levels. Elevated homocysteine is a risk factor for cardiovascular diseases, as it is linked to inflammation and oxidative stress. Therefore, maintaining a balanced intake of methionine through a well-rounded diet is crucial for optimal health.

Methionine stands out as a vital amino acid with multifaceted roles in the body. From serving as the initiator of protein synthesis to contributing to the synthesis of essential molecules like SAM, cysteine, and phosphatidylcholine, methionine is integral to diverse metabolic pathways. Its involvement in one-carbon metabolism and influence on cellular structure further underscore its importance. However, it is essential to approach methionine consumption with balance, as excessive intake may lead to potential health risks. Understanding the intricate roles of methionine sheds light on the complexity of cellular processes and highlights the need for a well-regulated supply of this essential amino acid for overall health and well-being.

Sources of Methionine:

- **Seeds:**
  - Sesame seeds
  - Sunflower seeds
  - Pumpkin seeds
  - Hemp seeds
  - Chia seeds
- **Nuts:**
  - Brazil nuts
  - Walnuts
  - Almonds
- **Whole Grains:**
  - Quinoa
  - Oats
  - Brown rice
- **Legumes:**
  - Lentils
  - Chickpeas
  - Black beans
- **Soy and Soy Products:**
  - Tofu
  - Tempeh
  - Soybeans
- **Vegetables:**
  - Spinach
  - Kale
  - Brussels sprouts
  - Broccoli
  - Onions

  - Garlic
  - Corn
  - Asparagus
- **Fruits:**
  - Watermelon
  - Bananas

Phenylalanine

Phenylalanine is a crucial amino acid that plays a fundamental role in various metabolic pathways within the human body. As one of the essential amino acids, phenylalanine cannot be synthesized by the body and must be obtained through dietary sources. It serves as a precursor for the synthesis of several important molecules, including neurotransmitters and various proteins, making it indispensable for overall health.

One of the primary functions of phenylalanine is its involvement in protein synthesis. Proteins are essential macromolecules that serve as the building blocks of tissues, enzymes, and other vital structures in the body. Phenylalanine contributes to this process by being incorporated into polypeptide chains during translation, a critical step in protein synthesis. Without an adequate supply of phenylalanine, the body's ability to produce necessary proteins would be compromised, leading to detrimental effects on the growth, maintenance, and repair of tissues.

Beyond its role in protein synthesis, phenylalanine is a precursor for the synthesis of other important molecules, including tyrosine. Tyrosine, in turn, serves as a precursor for the synthesis of neurotransmitters such as dopamine, norepinephrine, and epinephrine. These neurotransmitters play crucial roles in the central nervous system, influencing mood, cognition, and overall neurological function. Therefore, phenylalanine indirectly contributes to the regulation of mood, stress response, and various cognitive processes.

Phenylalanine is metabolized in the body through two main pathways: the phenylalanine hydroxylation pathway and the transamination pathway. In the phenylalanine hydroxylation pathway, phenylalanine is converted into tyrosine with the help of the enzyme phenylalanine hydroxylase. This conversion is a vital step in ensuring the availability of tyrosine for neurotransmitter synthesis. Mutations or deficiencies in the phenylalanine hydroxylase enzyme can lead to phenylketonuria (PKU), a metabolic disorder characterized by the accumulation of phenylalanine in the body, which can result in intellectual disabilities if not managed properly.

The transamination pathway involves the conversion of phenylalanine into phenylpyruvate through the action of the enzyme transaminase. Subsequently, phenylpyruvate is further metabolized into other intermediates, ultimately contributing to energy production or being excreted from the body. This pathway highlights the versatility of phenylalanine in participating not only in the synthesis of essential molecules but also in energy metabolism.

Phenylalanine's significance extends beyond its role in the central nervous system and protein synthesis. It is also a precursor for the synthesis of various bioactive compounds, such as phenylethylamine, which is involved in mood regulation, and tyrosine derivatives like melanin, which contributes to skin and hair pigmentation. These diverse roles underscore the importance of phenylalanine in maintaining the overall health and functionality of the body.

In addition to its physiological functions, phenylalanine has garnered attention for its potential therapeutic applications. Research suggests that phenylalanine supplementation may have positive effects on certain health conditions, such as chronic pain and depression. However, it's crucial to note that excessive intake of phenylalanine can lead to adverse effects, and any supplementation should be approached with caution, especially in individuals with certain medical conditions.

From its fundamental involvement in protein synthesis to its contributions to neurotransmitter production and metabolic pathways, phenylalanine plays a central role in maintaining overall health. Understanding its significance sheds light on the intricate web of biochemical processes that govern the functioning of the human body, emphasizing the interconnectedness of various physiological systems.

Sources of Phenylalanine:

- **Legumes:**
  - Lentils
  - Chickpeas
  - Black beans
- **Nuts and Seeds:**
  - Almonds
  - Sunflower seeds
  - Pumpkin seeds
  - Chia seeds
  - Sesame seeds
- **Whole Grains:**
  - Quinoa
  - Brown rice
  - Oats
- **Soy and Soy Products:**
  - Tofu
  - Tempeh
  - Soybeans
- **Vegetables:**
  - Spinach
  - Kale
  - Potatoes
  - Sweet potatoes
  - Olives
- **Fruits:**
  - Strawberries
  - Blueberries
  - Raspberries
  - Bananas

◦ Avocados

Threonine

Threonine is an essential amino acid, playing a crucial role in various metabolic pathways within the human body. As one of the 20 standard amino acids that make up proteins, threonine contributes to the structure and function of proteins, but its significance extends beyond mere structural support. This amino acid is integral to the synthesis of other important biomolecules, participates in metabolic processes, and is vital for overall health.

At a fundamental level, threonine is a building block of proteins, which are essential for the structure and function of cells, tissues, enzymes, and hormones. Proteins are polymers made up of amino acids, and threonine's unique structure contributes to the three-dimensional arrangement of proteins, influencing their stability and function. The hydroxyl group in threonine makes it distinct among amino acids, providing a unique chemical characteristic that contributes to the diversity of protein structures.

Beyond its structural role, threonine is a precursor to various biologically active compounds. One notable derivative is glycine, a non-essential amino acid critical for the synthesis of proteins and other important molecules. The catabolism of threonine yields intermediate metabolites, such as glycine and acetyl-CoA, which further participate in energy production and various biosynthetic pathways. This illustrates threonine's multifaceted role in cellular processes.

Threonine also plays a pivotal role in the synthesis of mucins, which are glycoproteins responsible for the lubrication and protection of mucous membranes. These membranes are found in the digestive, respiratory, and reproductive systems, highlighting the importance of threonine in maintaining the integrity of these vital structures. The incorporation of threonine into mucins contributes to the viscosity and protective properties of mucus, facilitating its role in trapping and eliminating foreign particles and pathogens.

With out a doubt, threonine is a key player in the acetylation process, where acetyl groups are transferred to various molecules. Acetylation is a post-translational modification of proteins that regulates their activity, stability, and localization within cells. Threonine's involvement in acetylation processes highlights its regulatory role in fine-tuning cellular functions and maintaining cellular homeostasis.

Threonine is also crucial for the synthesis of neurotransmitters, such as glycine and serine, which play essential roles in the central nervous system. Glycine acts as an inhibitory neurotransmitter, contributing to the regulation of neuronal excitability, while serine is a precursor to other neurotransmitters like dopamine and norepinephrine. Thus, threonine indirectly influences neurological functions by participating in the synthesis of these neurotransmitters.

In terms of metabolic pathways, threonine is involved in the threonine catabolic pathway, where it is converted into various metabolites that can enter the tricarboxylic acid (TCA) cycle and contribute to energy production. The catabolism of threonine produces intermediates like succinyl-CoA and acetyl-CoA, which can be further metabolized to generate ATP through oxidative phosphorylation. This energy production is crucial for the proper functioning of cells and tissues throughout the body.

Additionally, threonine contributes to the maintenance of a balanced nitrogen pool within the body. The breakdown of threonine results in the release of nitrogen, which can be utilized for the synthesis of other amino acids or nitrogenous compounds. This nitrogen recycling is essential for preventing nitrogen imbalance and ensuring the availability of nitrogen for the synthesis of new biomolecules.

Threonine's significance is further underscored by its essentiality, meaning that the body cannot synthesize it and must obtain it through the diet. Dietary sources rich in threonine include various protein-containing plant-based sources. Ensuring an adequate intake of threonine is crucial for meeting the body's demand for protein synthesis, neurotransmitter production, mucin formation, and energy metabolism.

This essential amino acid's involvement in protein synthesis, mucin formation, neurotransmitter synthesis, acetylation processes, and metabolic pathways highlights its multifaceted contributions to cellular functions and overall health. Understanding the importance of threonine sheds light on the intricate web of metabolic processes that sustain life and underscores the significance of a balanced and nutritious diet to ensure an adequate supply of this essential amino acid.

Sources of Threonine:

- **Legumes:**
  - Lentils
  - Chickpeas
  - Black beans
- **Nuts and Seeds:**
  - Almonds
  - Sunflower seeds
  - Pumpkin seeds
  - Peanuts
  - Chia seeds
- **Whole Grains:**
  - Quinoa
  - Oats
  - Brown rice
  - Wheat
- **Soy and Soy Products:**
  - Tofu
  - Tempeh
  - Soybeans
- **Seeds:**
  - Sesame seeds
  - Chia seeds

- **Fruits:**
    - Avocados
    - Guavas
- **Vegetables:**
    - Spinach
    - Kale
    - Pumpkin
- **Other:**
    - Watercress

Tryptophan

Tryptophan is an essential amino acid that plays a crucial role in various physiological processes within the human body. As one of the nine essential amino acids, the body cannot synthesize tryptophan on its own, making it vital to obtain through dietary sources. Once ingested, tryptophan serves as a precursor for the synthesis of important biomolecules and neurotransmitters, impacting both metabolic and neurological pathways.

One of the primary functions of tryptophan is its involvement in protein synthesis. As an essential building block of proteins, tryptophan contributes to the formation and maintenance of tissues, enzymes, and structural proteins throughout the body. Proteins are fundamental to cellular structure and function, and tryptophan's presence ensures the proper assembly of these biomolecules.

Tryptophan also plays a pivotal role in the formation of niacin, also known as vitamin B3. Niacin is crucial for the synthesis of NAD (nicotinamide adenine dinucleotide) and NADP (nicotinamide adenine dinucleotide phosphate), coenzymes that participate in numerous metabolic reactions. These coenzymes are integral to processes such as glycolysis, the citric acid cycle, and oxidative phosphorylation, which collectively drive energy production within cells.

Another function of tryptophan is a precursor for the synthesis of serotonin, a neurotransmitter with widespread implications for mood regulation, sleep, and appetite. The conversion of tryptophan to serotonin involves a series of enzymatic reactions, and adequate tryptophan levels are essential for maintaining optimal serotonin concentrations in the brain. Serotonin is often referred to as the "feel-good" neurotransmitter, and imbalances in its levels have been linked to various neuropsychiatric disorders, including depression and anxiety.

In addition to serotonin, tryptophan serves as a precursor for the synthesis of melatonin, a hormone that regulates the sleep-wake cycle. Melatonin production is dependent on tryptophan availability, and its rhythmic secretion helps to synchronize circadian rhythms, promoting healthy sleep patterns. Therefore, an adequate intake of tryptophan is essential for maintaining proper sleep-wake cycles and overall circadian rhythm regulation.

Tryptophan's significance extends beyond its role in protein synthesis, niacin formation, and neurotransmitter synthesis. It also participates in the kynurenine pathway, an alternative metabolic route for tryptophan metabolism. In this pathway, tryptophan is converted into kynurenine, which can further be metabolized into various downstream metabolites. The kynurenine pathway has implications for immune function, inflammation, and neurodegenerative diseases.

The immune system benefits from tryptophan through its involvement in the kynurenine pathway. Tryptophan degradation along this pathway results in the production of metabolites that can modulate immune responses. By influencing the balance between pro-inflammatory and anti-inflammatory signals, tryptophan metabolism contributes to immune homeostasis and overall immune function.

The kynurenine pathway has been implicated in the pathophysiology of neurodegenerative diseases. Alterations in tryptophan metabolism along this pathway have been observed in conditions such as Alzheimer's and Parkinson's diseases. Understanding the intricate relationship between tryptophan, the kynurenine pathway, and neurodegenerative processes is a subject of ongoing research, with potential therapeutic implications for these challenging disorders.

Tryptophan is far more than just an essential amino acid involved in protein synthesis. Its multifaceted roles encompass niacin synthesis, neurotransmitter production (specifically serotonin and melatonin), immune modulation, and participation in the kynurenine pathway. A balanced and sufficient intake of tryptophan is crucial for maintaining optimal health, influencing both metabolic and neurological pathways that collectively contribute to the intricate web of physiological processes within the human body.

Sources of Tryptophan:

- **Seeds:**
    - Pumpkin seeds
    - Sunflower seeds
    - Chia seeds
- **Nuts:**
    - Almonds
    - Walnuts
- **Legumes:**
    - Lentils
    - Chickpeas
    - Black beans
- **Whole Grains:**
    - Quinoa
    - Oats
    - Brown rice
- **Soy and Soy Products:**
    - Tofu
    - Tempeh
    - Soybeans
- **Vegetables:**
    - Spinach
    - Kale
    - Asparagus

    - Beets
    - Carrots
    - Celery
    - Mushrooms
    - Peas
    - Pumpkin
    - Parsley
    - Winter squash
- **Fruits:**
    - Bananas contain a small amount of tryptophan.
    - Apples
    - Avocados
    - Oranges
- **Cocoa and Dark Chocolate:**
    - Cocoa powder and dark chocolate can be sources of tryptophan.

Valine

Valine is a crucial amino acid with significant implications for various metabolic pathways in the human body. As one of the nine essential amino acids, valine plays a vital role in protein synthesis, energy production, and overall physiological well-being.

Firstly, valine is essential for the synthesis of proteins, which are the building blocks of tissues, muscles, enzymes, and other biological structures. Proteins are composed of amino acids, and valine contributes to the formation of these complex molecules. In the process of protein synthesis, valine combines with other amino acids through peptide bonds to create polypeptide chains. These chains then fold into specific three-dimensional structures, allowing proteins to carry out their diverse functions within the body.

This amino acid is a branched-chain amino acid (BCAA), along with leucine and isoleucine. BCAAs are unique in their molecular structure, featuring a branched side chain. This structural peculiarity is significant because BCAAs are primarily metabolized in the muscle tissue rather than the liver, unlike other amino acids. Valine, as a BCAA, serves as a major energy source during prolonged exercise or times of increased energy demand. When the body's glucose stores become depleted, valine can be converted into glucose through a process called gluconeogenesis, providing a crucial energy source for various tissues, especially during periods of physical exertion.

Valine plays a powerful role in the regulation of blood sugar levels. The conversion of valine into glucose helps maintain stable blood glucose concentrations, preventing hypoglycemia, a condition characterized by low blood sugar. This is particularly important for individuals engaging in intense physical activities, as the muscles require a constant supply of energy to function optimally.

Additionally, valine contributes to the synthesis of neurotransmitters, which are essential for proper brain function. Neurotransmitters are chemical messengers that transmit signals between nerve cells, facilitating communication within the nervous system. Valine is a precursor to neurotransmitters like gamma-aminobutyric acid (GABA) and glutamate. GABA, an inhibitory neurotransmitter, helps regulate brain activity, promoting a calm and relaxed state. On the other hand, glutamate is an excitatory neurotransmitter involved in cognitive functions such as learning and memory.

Valine's involvement in neurotransmitter synthesis highlights its impact on mood and cognitive function. A deficiency in valine could potentially lead to disruptions in neurotransmitter balance, potentially contributing to conditions like anxiety or cognitive impairment. Ensuring an adequate intake of valine through dietary sources is therefore crucial for maintaining optimal brain health.

Maintaining the nitrogen balance in the body is yet another role for valine. Nitrogen is a fundamental component of amino acids, and its balance is critical for various physiological processes. Valine, like other amino acids, contains nitrogen, and its metabolism helps regulate nitrogen levels in the body. This is important for preventing conditions such as nitrogen imbalances, which can have detrimental effects on overall health.

Being a key player in protein synthesis and serving as an energy source during exercise, regulating blood sugar levels, contributing to neurotransmitter synthesis, and maintaining nitrogen balance, valine is indispensable for overall health and well-being. A balanced and adequate intake of valine through dietary sources is essential to support these critical functions and ensure optimal physiological functioning.

Sources of Valine:

- **Legumes:**
    - Lentils
    - Chickpeas
    - Black beans
- **Nuts:**
    - Almonds
    - Peanuts
    - Cashews
- **Seeds:**
    - Sunflower seeds
    - Pumpkin seeds
    - Hemp seeds
- **Whole Grains:**
    - Quinoa
    - Brown rice
    - Oats
- **Soy and Soy Products:**
    - Tofu
    - Tempeh
    - Edamame
- **Fruits:**
    - Apples
    - Apricots

    - Blueberries
    - Cranberries
    - Oranges
    - Avocados
- **Vegetables:**
    - Broccoli
    - Peas

Conditional Amino Acids

Arginine

Arginine is a crucial amino acid with multifaceted roles in various metabolic pathways within the human body. As one of the 20 standard amino acids that constitute the building blocks of proteins, arginine plays a pivotal role in supporting physiological functions and promoting overall health.

At a fundamental level, arginine is classified as a semi-essential amino acid, meaning the body can synthesize it, but under certain conditions, its intake from external sources becomes essential. This makes dietary sources of arginine, such as nuts, and seeds, vital for maintaining optimal health.

One of the primary functions of arginine is its involvement in protein synthesis. As proteins are integral to nearly every cellular process, the importance of arginine in this regard cannot be overstated. During protein synthesis, ribosomes utilize arginine, along with other amino acids, to construct polypeptide chains according to the instructions encoded in the DNA. This process is fundamental to the growth, repair, and maintenance of tissues throughout the body.

Beyond its role in protein synthesis, arginine is a precursor to nitric oxide (NO), a signaling molecule with profound implications for cardiovascular health. Nitric oxide serves as a vasodilator, meaning it relaxes blood vessels, promoting increased blood flow. This vasodilatory effect is essential for maintaining healthy blood pressure and preventing hypertension. Moreover, adequate nitric oxide levels contribute to the prevention of atherosclerosis, as it inhibits the formation of blood clots and reduces inflammation in the arterial walls.

The many functions of arginine is implicated in the urea cycle, a series of biochemical reactions that occur in the liver, leading to the elimination of ammonia—a toxic byproduct of protein metabolism. Ammonia is converted into urea, which is then excreted in the urine. By participating in the urea cycle, arginine helps maintain nitrogen balance in the body, preventing the toxic buildup of ammonia that could otherwise have detrimental effects on the central nervous system.

Arginine's influence extends to the endocrine system, where it stimulates the release of growth hormone. Growth hormone is essential for the development and growth of bones and tissues, making arginine a key player in the regulation of these processes, particularly during periods of growth such as adolescence.

The immune system also benefits from arginine's presence. It is involved in the production of white blood cells, which play a crucial role in the body's defense against infections and other foreign invaders. Additionally, arginine enhances the function of T-cells, further bolstering the immune response.

Arginine's significance is not limited to these specific pathways; it also participates in the synthesis of creatine, a compound crucial for energy metabolism, especially during short bursts of intense physical activity. This makes arginine particularly relevant for individuals engaged in high-intensity sports or weight training.

In the context of wound healing, arginine's properties as a precursor to nitric oxide contribute to the formation of collagen—a protein vital for the structural integrity of skin, tendons, and other connective tissues. By promoting collagen synthesis, arginine accelerates the healing process, making it an essential component for tissue repair.

While arginine is generally considered beneficial, its metabolism can be influenced by certain health conditions. For example, individuals with arginine deficiency or impaired arginine metabolism may experience compromised immune function, impaired wound healing, and cardiovascular issues. Therefore, maintaining an adequate intake of arginine through a balanced diet or supplementation becomes crucial, particularly for those with specific health concerns.

Despite its numerous benefits, it is important to note that excessive intake of arginine may have adverse effects, especially for individuals with certain health conditions. Overconsumption of arginine-rich foods or supplements can lead to imbalances in the amino acid profile and may exacerbate symptoms in individuals with herpes infections. Therefore, it is essential to strike a balance and consult with healthcare professionals when considering arginine supplementation.

Arginine stands as a versatile and indispensable amino acid, intricately woven into the fabric of various metabolic pathways. From its role in protein synthesis to its contributions to cardiovascular health, immune function, and beyond, arginine emerges as a key player in maintaining overall well-being. Understanding and appreciating the significance of arginine underscores the importance of a balanced and nutrient-rich diet for optimal health and function of the human body.

Sources of Arginine:

- **Legumes:**
  - Lentils
  - Chickpeas
  - Black beans
  - Lima beans
- **Nuts and Seeds:**
  - Almonds
  - Walnuts
  - Sunflower seeds
  - Pumpkin seeds
  - Peanuts
  - Sesame seeds
  - Chia seeds

- **Whole Grains:**
    - Quinoa
    - Oats
    - Brown rice
- **Soy and Soy Products:**
    - Tofu
    - Tempeh
    - Soybeans
- **Cacao (Cocoa) and Dark Chocolate:**
    - Cacao and dark chocolate can contain reasonable amounts of arginine.
- **Grains:**
    - Wheat germ
    - Barley
- **Vegetables:**
    - Spinach
    - Beets
    - Garlic
    - Green Peas
    - Pumpkin

Cysteine

Cysteine is a crucial amino acid that plays a pivotal role in various metabolic pathways within the human body. Its significance lies not only in its structural role in proteins but also in its involvement in antioxidant defense, detoxification processes, and the synthesis of essential biomolecules. Understanding the multifaceted functions of cysteine provides insights into its importance for overall health and well-being.

At the core of cysteine's significance is its unique structure, characterized by a thiol (-SH) group. This thiol group is highly reactive and confers distinctive properties to cysteine, making it a key player in redox reactions. Redox reactions involve the transfer of electrons, and cysteine's thiol group allows it to readily donate or accept electrons, making it an essential component in maintaining cellular redox balance.

One of the primary roles of cysteine is its involvement in the synthesis of glutathione, a potent antioxidant present in almost all cells. Glutathione protects cells from oxidative stress by neutralizing reactive oxygen species (ROS) and free radicals. In this process, cysteine's thiol group acts as the critical site for glutathione's antioxidant activity. This antioxidant defense system helps prevent cellular damage and is crucial for maintaining cellular integrity and function.

Cysteine also plays a vital role in phase II detoxification processes in the liver. These processes involve the conjugation of toxins or drugs with molecules that render them more water-soluble and easily excreted from the body. Glutathione, synthesized from cysteine, participates in the conjugation reactions, highlighting the importance of cysteine in the body's ability to eliminate harmful substances and maintain detoxification pathways.

An essential component for cystine is in the synthesis of metallothioneins, proteins that bind to heavy metals, such as zinc and copper, regulating their levels within cells. This function is critical for preventing metal-induced toxicity and maintaining proper metal homeostasis in various tissues.

Cysteine's significance extends to its involvement in the synthesis of coenzymes and cofactors essential for various metabolic pathways. For instance, cysteine is a precursor for coenzyme A (CoA), a molecule crucial for fatty acid metabolism and energy production. CoA is involved in the citric acid cycle, a central hub of energy metabolism, highlighting cysteine's indirect yet vital role in cellular energy production.

Additionally, cysteine contributes to the structure and function of numerous proteins within the body. Its thiol group is involved in forming disulfide bonds, which are crucial for stabilizing the three-dimensional structure of proteins. This structural role is fundamental for the proper functioning of enzymes, receptors, and other proteins that govern cellular processes.

Cysteine is a precursor for the amino acid taurine, which plays diverse roles in the body, including bile salt formation, cardiovascular function, and neurological regulation. Through its involvement in taurine synthesis, cysteine indirectly influences these physiological processes, underlining its broad impact on overall health.

This conditional amino acid emerges as a cornerstone in various metabolic pathways, with its roles ranging from antioxidant defense and detoxification to the synthesis of essential biomolecules. Its unique thiol group imparts versatility, allowing cysteine to participate in redox reactions, structural protein formation, and the synthesis of critical molecules like glutathione and CoA. Recognizing the importance of cysteine provides valuable insights into the intricate web of metabolic processes that sustain cellular function and contribute to overall health.

Sources of Cystine:

- **Legumes:**
  - Lentils
  - Chickpeas
  - Black beans
- **Nuts and Seeds:**
  - Sunflower seeds
  - Chia seeds
  - Sesame seeds
- **Whole Grains:**
  - Quinoa
  - Oats
  - Brown rice
- **Vegetables:**
  - Garlic
  - Onions
  - Cabbage
  - Broccoli
  - Cauliflower

- Kale
- Brussels sprouts
- Leeks
- Shallots

- **Soy and Soy Products:**
    - Tofu
    - Tempeh
    - Soybeans

Glutamine

Glutamine, a conditionally essential amino acid, plays a crucial role in various metabolic pathways, contributing to the overall health and function of the human body. Its significance extends beyond its classification as a building block for proteins, as it actively participates in energy production, immune system support, and nitrogen balance. This multifaceted amino acid is involved in diverse metabolic processes, making it essential for maintaining physiological homeostasis.

One of Glutamine's primary functions is its role in protein synthesis. As a constituent of proteins, Glutamine aids in the formation and repair of tissues, contributing to the maintenance and growth of muscles. This is particularly important in situations of physical stress, such as intense exercise or injury, where the demand for amino acids, including Glutamine, increases. In these circumstances, supplementing with Glutamine may help support muscle recovery and reduce muscle protein breakdown.

Beyond its role in protein synthesis, Glutamine serves as a key player in energy metabolism. It is a significant substrate for cellular energy production, particularly in rapidly dividing cells such as enterocytes, immune cells, and certain cancer cells. Glutamine undergoes conversion to glutamate and subsequently enters the tricarboxylic acid (TCA) cycle, where it contributes to the generation of ATP, the cellular currency of energy. This makes Glutamine vital for meeting the high energy demands of rapidly proliferating cells, supporting functions like intestinal epithelial renewal and immune cell activation.

Glutamine acts as a critical intermediary in the nitrogen balance within the body. It serves as a primary carrier of ammonia, a byproduct of various metabolic processes, facilitating its safe transport to the liver for conversion into urea. This detoxification process is essential for preventing the accumulation of toxic ammonia levels in the bloodstream, highlighting Glutamine's role in maintaining overall metabolic health.

The immune system also relies heavily on Glutamine for optimal function. Immune cells, such as lymphocytes and macrophages, utilize Glutamine as a key energy source to mount an effective response against pathogens. Additionally, Glutamine supports the production of glutathione, a potent antioxidant that helps protect cells from oxidative stress. By supporting immune cell function and providing antioxidant defense, Glutamine contributes to the body's ability to fend off infections and maintain overall immune resilience.

In times of physiological stress, such as during illness, injury, or intense exercise, the demand for Glutamine often surpasses the body's ability to produce an adequate supply. Under these circumstances, exogenous or supplemental Glutamine becomes crucial to meet the increased requirements and support various metabolic processes. Athletes, individuals recovering from surgery, and those with certain medical conditions may benefit from supplemental Glutamine to enhance recovery, maintain muscle mass, and support overall health.

While Glutamine's importance in metabolic pathways is undeniable, it's essential to note that individual needs may vary, and excessive supplementation should be approached cautiously. The intricate balance of amino acids within the body underscores the importance of a well-rounded diet that includes diverse protein sources to ensure adequate Glutamine intake.

Glutamine is a versatile amino acid with indispensable roles in protein synthesis, energy metabolism, nitrogen balance, and immune function. Its ability to support various metabolic pathways highlights its significance for overall health and underscores the importance of maintaining an appropriate balance through a well-rounded and nutritious diet. Whether in the context of muscle recovery, immune support, or general metabolic health, Glutamine's multifaceted contributions make it a crucial component of the intricate web of metabolic processes that sustain life.

Sources of Glutamine:

- **Legumes:**
    - Lentils
    - Chickpeas
    - Black beans
- **Nuts and Seeds:**
    - Almonds
    - Sunflower seeds
    - Pumpkin seeds
- **Whole Grains:**
    - Quinoa
    - Oats
    - Brown rice
- **Vegetables:**
    - Spinach
    - Cabbage
    - Parsley
    - Asparagus
    - Broccoli
    - Brussels sprouts
    - Kale
- **Soy and Soy Products:**
    - Tofu
    - Tempeh
    - Soybeans
- **Other:**

◦ Watercress

Glycine

Glycine, a simple amino acid with a single hydrogen atom as its side chain, plays a crucial role in various metabolic pathways within the human body. Its significance extends beyond being a building block for proteins; glycine contributes to diverse physiological functions, impacting everything from the central nervous system to the synthesis of important molecules.

First and foremost, glycine is one of the 20 amino acids that form the foundation of proteins. Proteins are essential macromolecules that serve as structural components, enzymes, and signaling molecules within cells. Glycine's unique structure, with its small and non-polar side chain, allows for its incorporation into a wide array of proteins, influencing their overall structure and function.

Beyond protein synthesis, glycine is a key player in the synthesis of various important molecules. One notable example is heme, a component of hemoglobin, the protein responsible for oxygen transport in the blood. Glycine's role in heme synthesis underscores its importance in ensuring proper oxygenation of tissues and organs.

Glycine is also a critical component in the synthesis of creatine, a molecule that plays a crucial role in the production of adenosine triphosphate (ATP), the primary energy currency of cells. Creatine is particularly abundant in tissues with high energy demands, such as muscle tissue. By contributing to creatine synthesis, glycine indirectly supports energy metabolism, making it vital for activities requiring rapid and intense energy production, such as muscle contraction during exercise.

The amino acid glycine is intimately involved in the maintenance of a balanced and healthy central nervous system. It acts as an inhibitory neurotransmitter in the brain and spinal cord, meaning it has a calming effect on neural activity. This function helps regulate mood, sleep, and overall mental well-being. Glycine receptors play a role in various neurological processes, and research suggests that glycine supplementation may have potential therapeutic applications for conditions involving abnormal neural excitability.

Glycine's impact on the central nervous system also extends to its role in the synthesis of glutathione, a powerful antioxidant. Glutathione plays a crucial role in protecting cells from oxidative stress, which is implicated in various diseases and aging processes. Glycine's contribution to glutathione synthesis underscores its importance in cellular defense mechanisms and overall health maintenance.

In addition to the part it plays in neurotransmission and antioxidant defense, glycine is also involved in the regulation of inflammation. It serves as a precursor for the synthesis of serine, which, in turn, contributes to the production of sphingosine-1-phosphate (S1P). S1P is a signaling molecule involved in immune responses and inflammation. By influencing the synthesis of molecules like S1P, glycine participates in the complex network of immune regulation, contributing to the body's ability to respond appropriately to infections and injuries.

Glycine has been studied for its potential benefits in various health conditions. Some research suggests that glycine supplementation may have a positive impact on sleep quality and may help mitigate the negative effects of sleep deprivation. Its role as a neurotransmitter with calming effects on the central nervous system contributes to these potential sleep-related benefits.

The importance of glycine extends far beyond its role as a constituent of proteins. This simple amino acid is a versatile player in various metabolic pathways, impacting everything from the synthesis of proteins and other important molecules to the regulation of neurotransmission, inflammation, and oxidative stress. Its multifaceted contributions make glycine a crucial component for maintaining overall health and well-being.

Sources of Glycine:

- **Legumes:**
    - Soybeans

    - Chickpeas
    - Lentils
- **Nuts and Seeds:**
    - Pumpkin seeds
    - Sunflower seeds
- **Whole Grains:**
    - Quinoa
    - Oats
    - Brown rice
- **Vegetables:**
    - Spinach
    - Kale
    - Cabbage
    - Cauliflower
    - Kale
    - Pumpkin
    - Asparagus
- **Soy and Soy Products:**
    - Tofu
    - Tempeh
    - Edamame
- **Seaweed:**
    - Spirulina
    - Nori
- **Other:**
    - Watercress
    - Bananas
    - Kiwi

Proline

Proline, a non-essential amino acid, plays a crucial role in various metabolic pathways, contributing significantly to the overall health and function of the human body. Its unique structural and functional properties make it indispensable for several physiological processes.

One of the primary functions of proline lies in its role as a major component of collagen, the most abundant protein in the human body. Collagen provides structural support to tissues, tendons, ligaments, and skin, contributing to their strength and integrity. Proline's presence in collagen is particularly significant, as it forms a key structural element that ensures the stability and resilience of connective tissues. This amino acid's contribution to collagen synthesis is pivotal for maintaining healthy skin, promoting wound healing, and supporting overall tissue repair.

Beyond its structural role in collagen, proline participates in the synthesis of other essential proteins. It acts as a precursor for the synthesis of proteins involved in maintaining muscle tissue, supporting immune function, and facilitating enzyme activity. As a component of proteins, proline aids in the proper folding and stabilization of these structures, influencing their functionality and ensuring optimal cellular processes.

Proline also serves as a critical player in cellular protection against oxidative stress. Its unique cyclic structure allows it to act as a potent antioxidant, scavenging free radicals and preventing cellular damage. Oxidative stress, caused by an imbalance between free radicals and antioxidants, is implicated in various diseases and aging processes. Proline's antioxidant properties contribute to the overall defense mechanism of cells, promoting their survival and longevity.

In addition to its role in protein synthesis and antioxidant defense, proline is involved in energy metabolism. It participates in the urea cycle, a series of biochemical reactions that play a central role in the elimination of nitrogen from the body. Through its involvement in this cycle, proline contributes to the removal of excess nitrogen, aiding in the detoxification of ammonia, a waste product of protein metabolism. Maintaining proper nitrogen balance is crucial for preventing the accumulation of toxic substances in the body.

Proline's significance extends to the regulation of gene expression. It has been identified as a key player in modulating the activity of certain transcription factors, influencing the synthesis of specific proteins involved in cell growth, differentiation, and apoptosis. By participating in these regulatory processes, proline contributes to the maintenance of cellular homeostasis and the prevention of abnormal cell proliferation.

Furthermore, proline plays a vital role in the metabolism of neurotransmitters. It serves as a precursor for the synthesis of gamma-aminobutyric acid (GABA), a neurotransmitter with inhibitory effects on the central nervous system. GABA is essential for regulating neuronal excitability and maintaining a balance between excitatory and inhibitory signals in the brain. Proline's involvement in GABA synthesis underscores its importance in neurological function and the maintenance of mental health.

Its involvement in collagen synthesis, antioxidant defense, protein metabolism, nitrogen elimination, gene expression regulation, and neurotransmitter synthesis highlights its indispensability for overall health and well-being. Understanding the intricate ways in which proline contributes to various metabolic pathways provides valuable insights into its therapeutic potential and opens avenues for further research in the fields of medicine and nutrition.

Sources of Proline:

- **Legumes:**
    - Lentils
    - Chickpeas
    - Peanuts
- **Nuts and Seeds:**
    - Almonds
    - Sunflower seeds
- **Whole Grains:**
    - Quinoa
    - Oats

    - Brown rice
- **Vegetables:**
    - Spinach
    - Cabbage
    - Asparagus
    - Broccoli
    - Brussels sprouts
- **Soy and Soy Products:**
    - Tofu
    - Tempeh
    - Soybeans
- **Fruits:**
    - Avocado
    - Watermelon
- **Other:**
    - Bamboo shoots

Serine

Serine is a crucial amino acid that plays a fundamental role in various metabolic pathways within the human body. As one of the 20 standard amino acids that form the building blocks of proteins, serine's significance extends beyond its contribution to protein synthesis. Its unique structural and chemical properties make it an essential player in cellular functions, ranging from DNA synthesis to neurotransmitter regulation. In this exploration, we delve into the multifaceted roles of serine in metabolic pathways, shedding light on its impact on health and well-being.

First and foremost, serine is integral to protein synthesis, a process vital for the growth, maintenance, and repair of tissues in the body. As a constituent of polypeptide chains, serine contributes to the formation of proteins that serve diverse functions, such as enzymes, structural components, and signaling molecules. Its presence in the amino acid sequence determines the protein's structure and function, emphasizing serine's role as a molecular cornerstone in the intricate machinery of life.

Beyond its role in protein synthesis, serine is a key player in the synthesis of other essential biomolecules. One of the most significant pathways involving serine is the biosynthesis of purines and pyrimidines, the building blocks of DNA and RNA. Serine acts as a precursor for glycine, another amino acid crucial for nucleotide synthesis. Through a series of enzymatic reactions, serine contributes carbon units necessary for the de novo production of nucleotides, facilitating DNA replication and cellular proliferation.

Moreover, serine participates in the one-carbon metabolism pathway, a network of interconnected reactions that transfers single-carbon units for various biosynthetic processes. This pathway is crucial for the synthesis of amino acids, nucleotides, and other biomolecules. Serine is a key supplier of one-carbon units through its conversion to glycine, a process catalyzed by the enzyme serine hydroxymethyltransferase. These one-carbon units are essential for the methylation reactions that modify DNA, RNA, proteins, and lipids, influencing gene expression, cellular signaling, and metabolic regulation.

The role of serine extends into the realm of energy metabolism. Serine contributes to the synthesis of phospholipids, essential components of cell membranes. Phosphatidylserine, a phospholipid-containing serine, is particularly abundant in the inner leaflet of the cell membrane and plays a crucial role in maintaining membrane integrity and fluidity. Additionally, serine is involved in the production of sphingolipids, which are important for signaling and structural functions within cells.

In the nervous system, serine serves as a precursor for the synthesis of neurotransmitters, including glycine and D-serine. Glycine is an inhibitory neurotransmitter that regulates neuronal activity, while D-serine acts as a co-agonist for the N-methyl-D-aspartate (NMDA) receptors, which are involved in synaptic plasticity and learning. The availability of serine is thus essential for proper neurotransmission, impacting cognitive function and overall brain health.

The significance of serine in human health is underscored by the fact that alterations in serine metabolism have been linked to various diseases. Deficiencies in enzymes involved in serine biosynthesis or metabolism can lead to serious health conditions. For example, deficiencies in the enzyme 3-phosphoglycerate dehydrogenase (PHGDH), a key player in the serine biosynthetic pathway, have been associated with certain types of cancer. Cancer cells often exhibit an increased demand for serine due to their rapid proliferation, making the serine biosynthetic pathway an attractive target for cancer therapy.

Studies have suggested that disturbances in serine and glycine metabolism may contribute to insulin resistance and glucose intolerance. Understanding the intricate connections between serine metabolism and metabolic disorders holds promise for the development of targeted therapeutic interventions.

Serine emerges as a linchpin in the intricate web of metabolic pathways within the human body. Its roles in protein synthesis, nucleotide biosynthesis, one-carbon metabolism, energy metabolism, and neurotransmission highlight its versatility and indispensability. The delicate balance of serine metabolism is crucial for maintaining cellular function, and its dysregulation can have far-reaching consequences for human health. Continued research into the nuances of serine's involvement in metabolic pathways promises not only to deepen our understanding of fundamental cellular processes but also to uncover new avenues for therapeutic interventions in various diseases.

Sources of Serine:

- **Legumes:**
  - Lentils
  - Chickpeas
  - Black beans
- **Nuts and Seeds:**
  - Sunflower seeds
  - Pumpkin seeds

    - Almonds
    - Pistachios
    - Sesame Seeds
- **Whole Grains:**
    - Quinoa
    - Barley
    - Oats
    - Brown rice
- **Vegetables:**
    - Spinach
    - Cauliflower
    - Asparagus
    - Cabbage
    - Peas
    - Potatoes
    - Sweet potatoes
- **Soy and Soy Products:**
    - Tofu
    - Tempeh
    - Soybeans
- **Seaweed:**
    - Spirulina
    - Nori
- **Fruits:**
    - Watermelon
    - Oranges
    - Bananas

Tyrosine

Tyrosine is a crucial amino acid that plays a vital role in various metabolic pathways within the human body. As one of the 20 standard amino acids, tyrosine is classified as a non-essential amino acid, meaning that the body can synthesize it from another amino acid called phenylalanine. This conversion is facilitated by the enzyme phenylalanine hydroxylase, which is crucial for maintaining adequate tyrosine levels in the body.

One of the primary functions of tyrosine is its role as a precursor for the synthesis of several important neurotransmitters, including dopamine, norepinephrine, and epinephrine. These neurotransmitters are essential for the proper functioning of the central nervous system, influencing mood, cognitive function, and stress response. Tyrosine's involvement in the production of these neurotransmitters makes it a key player in mental health and overall well-being.

In addition to its role in neurotransmitter synthesis, tyrosine is a precursor for the production of thyroid hormones. Thyroid hormones, such as thyroxine (T4) and triiodothyronine (T3), are critical for regulating metabolism and energy balance in the body. Tyrosine is incorporated into the structure of these hormones, highlighting its importance in maintaining proper thyroid function.

Tyrosine is a key component of proteins, and it contributes to the structural integrity of various proteins in the body. Proteins are essential macromolecules involved in numerous physiological processes, including enzyme catalysis, immune response, and cellular repair. Tyrosine's presence in proteins underscores its fundamental role in maintaining the overall structure and function of the human body.

Within the realm of metabolic pathways, tyrosine is involved in the catabolic and anabolic processes that govern energy production and utilization. Through its participation in the citric acid cycle, tyrosine contributes to the breakdown of carbohydrates, fats, and proteins to generate energy in the form of adenosine triphosphate (ATP). This energy is indispensable for powering cellular activities and maintaining the body's vital functions.

This non-essential amino acid is intricately linked to the phenylalanine-tyrosine metabolic pathway. Phenylalanine, an essential amino acid obtained through diet, is converted to tyrosine through the action of phenylalanine hydroxylase. This enzymatic conversion is critical for preventing the accumulation of phenylalanine in the body, which can be toxic. The interconnectedness of these two amino acids highlights the importance of tyrosine in maintaining amino acid balance and preventing metabolic disorders.

Tyrosine extends beyond its functions in the central nervous system, thyroid hormones, and protein structure. It also serves as a precursor for melanin, the pigment responsible for skin, hair, and eye color. Melanin plays a crucial role in protecting the skin from the harmful effects of ultraviolet (UV) radiation by absorbing and dissipating UV light. Tyrosine's involvement in melanin synthesis underscores its significance in both aesthetic and protective aspects of human physiology.

Its involvement in neurotransmitter synthesis, thyroid hormone production, protein structure, and melanin formation highlights its significance in maintaining neurological function, hormonal balance, structural integrity, and skin protection. As a non-essential amino acid, tyrosine's synthesis from phenylalanine adds a layer of complexity to its importance, emphasizing the delicate balance required for optimal health. A deficiency in tyrosine can lead to disruptions in these vital processes, underscoring the necessity of ensuring an adequate dietary intake of this amino acid for overall well-being.

Sources of Tyrosine:

- **Nuts and Seeds:**
    - Almonds
    - Pumpkin seeds
    - Sesame seeds
    - Pine Nuts
    - Pistachios
    - Flaxseeds
- **Legumes:**
    - Lentils
    - Chickpeas
    - Peanuts

    - Spilt Peas
    - Kidney Beans
- **Soy and Soy Products:**
    - Tofu
    - Tempeh
    - Soybeans
- **Whole Grains:**
    - Quinoa
    - Brown rice
    - Oats
- **Vegetables:**
    - Spinach
    - Sweet potatoes
    - Avocado
- **Fruits:**
    - Bananas
    - Watermelon
- **Seaweed:**
    - Spirulina
    - Nori

Non-Essential Amino Acids

Alanine

Alanine is a non-essential amino acid that plays a crucial role in various metabolic pathways within the human body. Its significance lies in its involvement in processes such as energy production, protein synthesis, and the regulation of blood sugar levels. Understanding the importance of alanine requires delving into its functions and contributions to different aspects of metabolism.

One of the primary roles of alanine is its participation in the glucose-alanine cycle, also known as the Cahill cycle. This cycle operates between skeletal muscle and the liver, playing a key role in the transportation of nitrogen from peripheral tissues to the liver. During periods of intense physical activity or stress, muscles produce alanine as a byproduct of glycolysis. This alanine is then transported to the liver, where it undergoes gluconeogenesis, a process that converts it into glucose. The newly synthesized glucose can be released into the bloodstream, providing an additional energy source for the body. This cycle is vital for maintaining blood glucose levels during periods of increased energy demand.

Additionally, alanine contributes to energy production through its involvement in the tricarboxylic acid (TCA) cycle. Alanine can be converted into pyruvate, a key intermediate in the TCA cycle. This conversion allows alanine to serve as a substrate for energy production through aerobic respiration. As a result, alanine plays a role in linking glycolysis, which occurs in the cytoplasm, with the TCA cycle, which takes place in the mitochondria. This interconnectedness highlights the versatility of alanine in supporting energy metabolism.

Furthermore, alanine is a building block for protein synthesis. As one of the 20 amino acids that make up proteins, alanine contributes to the structure and function of various proteins in the body. During protein synthesis, alanine is incorporated into polypeptide chains, where its specific sequence and interactions with other amino acids determine the ultimate structure and function of the protein. Proteins are essential for numerous physiological processes, including enzyme catalysis, structural support, and signaling pathways. Alanine's role as a constituent of proteins underscores its importance in maintaining overall cellular function.

Alanine is particularly notable for its connection to branched-chain amino acids (BCAAs), including leucine, isoleucine, and valine. These BCAAs are essential amino acids that the body cannot synthesize on its own and must obtain from the diet. Alanine can be converted into pyruvate, a precursor for acetyl-CoA, which is a key player in the catabolism of BCAAs. This connection emphasizes the intricate interplay between different amino acids and their contributions to various metabolic pathways.

Moreover, alanine has implications for muscle metabolism and recovery. During periods of intense exercise or fasting, skeletal muscles release alanine into the bloodstream to support energy production, as mentioned earlier. This process helps spare glucose for organs with a high glucose demand, such as the brain. Additionally, alanine can be converted into glutamate, a precursor for glutamine, which is crucial for maintaining acid-base balance and supporting the immune system. The role of alanine in these processes highlights its significance in both energy metabolism and overall physiological homeostasis.

In conclusion, alanine emerges as a multifaceted amino acid with integral roles in the glucose-alanine cycle, energy production, protein synthesis, and the metabolism of branched-chain amino acids. Its contributions to these fundamental processes underscore its importance in maintaining overall metabolic health. As researchers continue to explore the intricate details of cellular metabolism, the significance of alanine is likely to become even more apparent, shedding light on its role in health and disease.

Sources of Alanine:

- **Legumes:**
  - Lentils
  - Chickpeas
  - Black beans
- **Nuts and Seeds:**
  - Almonds
  - Sunflower seeds
- **Whole Grains:**
  - Quinoa
  - Brown rice
  - Oats
- **Vegetables:**
  - Spinach
  - Potatoes

    - Avocado
    - Turnip Greens
- **Fruits:**
    - Oranges
    - Bananas
- **Soy and Soy Products:**
    - Tofu
    - Tempeh
- **Seaweed:**
    - Nori
    - Wakame
- **Whole Grains:**
    - Wheat germ
    - Whole wheat products

Asparagine

Asparagine is a non-essential amino acid, meaning the human body can synthesize it on its own. However, its significance lies in its diverse roles within metabolic pathways, contributing to various physiological functions crucial for the proper functioning of the body.

One of the primary functions of asparagine is its involvement in protein synthesis. Asparagine, along with other amino acids, serves as a building block for the synthesis of proteins. Proteins are essential macromolecules that play a central role in the structure and function of cells. Asparagine's presence in the amino acid pool ensures that the body has an adequate supply of this amino acid to support the continuous process of protein synthesis.

Beyond its role in protein synthesis, asparagine is a key player in the urea cycle. This cycle is responsible for the detoxification of ammonia, a byproduct of protein metabolism that can be toxic to cells. Asparagine combines with ammonia to form asparagine synthetase, a critical enzyme in the urea cycle. This process allows the body to convert ammonia into urea, which is then excreted by the kidneys. Maintaining the proper functioning of the urea cycle is essential for preventing the accumulation of toxic ammonia in the body.

Asparagine also participates in the synthesis of other important biomolecules. It is a precursor for the biosynthesis of aspartate, another amino acid that serves as a building block for nucleotides. Nucleotides are the monomers that makeup DNA and RNA, the genetic material of cells. Thus, asparagine indirectly contributes to the synthesis and maintenance of genetic material, playing a fundamental role in cellular processes such as DNA replication and transcription.

The regulation of cellular osmolarity is yet another role for this amino acid. Osmolarity refers to the concentration of solutes in a solution, and maintaining proper osmolarity is crucial for cell integrity and function. Asparagine, along with other osmolytes, helps regulate osmolarity by balancing water movement across cell membranes. This is particularly important in cells exposed to changing environmental conditions, as osmotic balance is vital for cellular homeostasis.

Recent research has highlighted its significance in supporting the growth of certain cancer cells. Cancer cells often exhibit altered metabolic pathways to sustain their rapid proliferation. Asparagine, being a precursor for protein and nucleotide synthesis, becomes essential for the uncontrolled growth of these cancer cells. Targeting asparagine metabolism has emerged as a potential therapeutic strategy to selectively inhibit the growth of cancer cells while sparing normal cells.

Asparagine has been implicated in the immune response. It is essential for the proper functioning of immune cells, including lymphocytes and macrophages. These cells require asparagine for their proliferation and activation, contributing to the body's ability to mount an effective immune response against pathogens. The link between asparagine metabolism and immune function underscores its importance in maintaining overall health and disease resistance.

Though classified as a non-essential amino acid, asparagine plays a large part in various metabolic pathways. From its involvement in protein synthesis and the urea cycle to its contribution to nucleotide biosynthesis and cellular osmolarity regulation, asparagine is indispensable for the proper functioning of cells and, consequently, the overall well-being of the organism. Understanding the diversetiy of asparagine provides insights into both normal physiological processes and potential therapeutic strategies for conditions such as cancer.

Sources of Asparagine:

- **Legumes:**
  - Lentils
  - Chickpeas
  - Soybeans
- **Nuts and Seeds:**
  - Almonds
  - Sunflower seeds
- **Whole Grains:**
  - Oats
  - Wheat germ
  - Whole wheat products
- **Vegetables:**
  - Asparagus
  - Potatoes
  - Spinach
  - Broccoli
  - Brussels sprouts
- **Fruits:**
  - Avocado
  - Watermelon
  - Oranges
- **Root Vegetables:**
  - Carrots
  - Sweet potatoes
- **Cabbage Family Vegetables:**
  - Cabbage

    - Cauliflower
- **Soy and Soy Products:**
    - Tofu
    - Tempeh

Aspartic Acid

Aspartic acid is a non-essential amino acid, meaning the body can synthesize it on its own. It plays a crucial role in various metabolic pathways, contributing to the overall functioning and well-being of the human body.

One of the primary roles of aspartic acid is its involvement in the urea cycle, a vital process in the elimination of ammonia from the body. As ammonia is a toxic byproduct of amino acid metabolism, the urea cycle helps convert it into urea, which is then excreted through urine. Aspartic acid contributes to this cycle by combining with citrulline to form arginosuccinate, a key intermediate in the urea cycle. This process is essential for maintaining nitrogen balance in the body and preventing the buildup of toxic ammonia.

Furthermore, aspartic acid is a key player in the synthesis of other amino acids. Through transamination reactions, it can donate its amino group to form other amino acids like asparagine, methionine, threonine, and isoleucine. These amino acids are crucial for protein synthesis, neurotransmitter production, and various metabolic functions. Aspartic acid's versatility in participating in these reactions underscores its significance in maintaining the body's overall protein balance and functionality.

Aspartic acid also plays a vital role in the citric acid cycle, also known as the Krebs cycle or tricarboxylic acid (TCA) cycle. This cycle is a central component of cellular respiration, responsible for generating adenosine triphosphate (ATP), the primary energy currency of the cell. Aspartic acid enters the cycle by being converted to oxaloacetate, a precursor for citrate formation. This ensures the smooth progression of the citric acid cycle, contributing to the efficient production of energy through oxidative phosphorylation.

Moreover, aspartic acid is involved in the synthesis of purine and pyrimidine nucleotides, which are the building blocks of DNA and RNA. Aspartic acid contributes its amino group to the formation of inosine monophosphate (IMP), a precursor to both purines and pyrimidines. This underscores its significance in supporting the genetic material of cells and, consequently, the processes of cell division and growth.

The role of aspartic acid extends to the nervous system, where it acts as a neurotransmitter precursor. It serves as a precursor for the synthesis of both asparagine and glutamate, which are neurotransmitters involved in signal transmission between nerve cells. Glutamate, in particular, is a major excitatory neurotransmitter in the central nervous system, playing a crucial role in learning, memory, and overall cognitive function. Aspartic acid's contribution to the synthesis of these neurotransmitters highlights its importance in maintaining proper neurological function.

In addition to its direct involvement in metabolic pathways, aspartic acid has been studied for its potential health benefits. It is considered a non-essential amino acid, meaning that the body can produce it, but its availability from dietary sources is still important. Adequate intake of aspartic acid is essential for supporting the body's various physiological processes, including muscle development, immune function, and overall growth.

This amino acid has a versatile part it plays with a wide range of functions in the human body. From its role in the urea cycle to its involvement in amino acid and neurotransmitter synthesis, aspartic acid is integral to various metabolic pathways. Its contributions to energy production, DNA and RNA synthesis, and neurotransmission underscore its significance in maintaining overall health and well-being. A balanced diet that includes aspartic acid-rich foods is crucial for ensuring the body's optimal function and resilience.

Sources of Aspartic Acid:

- **Legumes:**
  - Lentils
  - Chickpeas
  - Black beans
- **Nuts and Seeds:**
  - Almonds
  - Sunflower seeds
- **Whole Grains:**
  - Oats
  - Quinoa
  - Brown rice
- **Vegetables:**
  - Asparagus
  - Potatoes
  - Avocado
  - Sugar Beets
- **Fruits:**
  - Oranges
  - Bananas
  - Pineapples
- **Soy and Soy Products:**
  - Tofu
  - Tempeh
- **Seaweed:**
  - Nori
  - Wakame
  - Kelp
- **Whole Grains:**
  - Wheat germ
  - Bran
  - Whole wheat products

Glutamic Acid

Glutamic acid is a crucial amino acid that plays a pivotal role in various metabolic pathways within the human body. As one of the 20 standard amino acids, it serves as a building block for proteins, contributing to the structural integrity and function of many essential biological molecules. Its significance extends beyond mere protein synthesis, encompassing key roles in neurotransmission, energy metabolism, and the regulation of acid-base balance.

In the context of protein synthesis, glutamic acid holds a distinctive position as a non-essential amino acid. While the body can synthesize it, its availability from dietary sources ensures an adequate supply for the synthesis of proteins vital for growth, tissue repair, and overall cellular function. Glutamic acid contributes to the formation of polypeptide chains during translation, facilitating the creation of functional proteins that serve as enzymes, structural components, and signaling molecules.

Beyond its contribution to protein synthesis, glutamic acid functions as a neurotransmitter in the central nervous system. In this role, it actively participates in excitatory neurotransmission, influencing neuronal signaling and communication. Glutamate, the ionized form of glutamic acid, is released into synapses, where it binds to receptors on the postsynaptic membrane, initiating a cascade of events that lead to nerve impulse transmission. This excitatory action is fundamental to cognitive processes, learning, and memory.

Glutamic acid is intricately involved in various metabolic pathways that contribute to energy production. Through its conversion to alpha-ketoglutarate, a key intermediate in the citric acid cycle, it becomes an integral part of cellular respiration. This cycle, also known as the Krebs cycle, takes place in the mitochondria and serves as a central hub for the oxidation of acetyl-CoA derived from carbohydrates, fats, and proteins. Glutamic acid's involvement in this cycle highlights its significance in extracting energy from macronutrients.

The metabolic versatility of glutamic acid extends to its role in the synthesis of other important molecules. As a precursor to proline and ornithine, it contributes to the formation of collagen and urea, respectively. Collagen, a structural protein, is essential for the integrity of connective tissues, including skin, cartilage, and bones. Urea, on the other hand, plays a crucial role in the elimination of nitrogenous waste, aiding in the maintenance of acid-base balance and preventing the toxic accumulation of ammonia in the body.

Additionally, glutamic acid participates in the regulation of the acid-base balance within cells. Its ionized form, glutamate, acts as a buffer by accepting or releasing protons, helping to maintain the optimal pH for enzymatic activity and cellular function. This buffering capacity is essential for preventing fluctuations in pH that could disrupt biochemical reactions and compromise cellular homeostasis.

The importance of glutamic acid is further underscored by its association with glutathione, a powerful antioxidant. Glutathione, synthesized from glutamic acid, cysteine, and glycine, plays a crucial role in neutralizing reactive oxygen species (ROS) and protecting cells from oxidative damage. This antioxidant defense system is vital for cellular health and longevity, emphasizing the multifaceted contributions of glutamic acid to overall well-being.

Glutamic acid stands as a vital amino acid with far-reaching implications for human physiology. Its roles in protein synthesis, neurotransmission, energy metabolism, and the regulation of acid-base balance collectively contribute to the intricate web of biochemical processes that sustain life. Recognizing the diverse functions of glutamic acid highlights its indispensability, emphasizing the importance of ensuring an adequate supply through a balanced and nutrient-rich diet.

Sources of Glutamic Acid:

- **Soybeans and Soy Products:**
    - Tofu
    - Tempeh

    - Edamame
- **Legumes:**
    - Lentils
    - Chickpeas
    - Black beans
    - Peas
- **Whole Grains:**
    - Quinoa
    - Brown rice
    - Barley
    - Oats
- **Nuts and Seeds:**
    - Almonds
    - Walnuts
    - Sunflower seeds
    - Chia seeds
- **Vegetables:**
    - Spinach
    - Tomatoes
    - Potatoes
    - Cabbage
- **Seaweed:**
    - Nori
    - Wakame
    - Kelp
- **Whole Grains:**
    - Wheat germ
    - Bran
    - Whole wheat products

5

Toxins

In the fascinating world within the human body, metabolic pathways play a crucial role, ensuring the harmonious balance necessary for optimal health. However, this delicate choreography can be disrupted by the presence of toxins, and insidious intruders that infiltrate the body and interfere with these vital processes. This chapter explores the ways in which toxins impair normal metabolic pathways, drawing upon scientific research to shed light on the mechanisms and consequences of this interference.

Toxins and Metabolic Disruption

Toxins are substances that can cause harm to the body, and their sources are diverse, ranging from environmental pollutants to dietary contaminants. When these toxins enter the body, they can interfere with the finely tuned metabolic pathways that govern energy production, nutrient utilization, and waste elimination. One primary way toxins disrupt metabolism is by affecting enzymes, the molecular catalysts that drive biochemical reactions.

Enzymatic Inhibition

Enzymes are essential for the proper functioning of metabolic pathways, facilitating reactions that convert nutrients into energy and building blocks for cellular processes. Toxins can inhibit enzymes directly by binding to their active sites or indirectly by altering the enzyme's structure. For example, heavy metals like lead and mercury have been shown to bind to enzymes involved in energy production, hindering their ability to carry out their designated tasks.

Mitochondrial Dysfunction

Mitochondria, often referred to as the powerhouses of the cell, are critical for energy metabolism. Toxins can disrupt mitochondrial function, impairing the electron transport chain and reducing the production of adenosine triphosphate (ATP), the cell's primary energy currency. Studies have linked exposure to environmental toxins, such as polychlorinated biphenyls (PCBs) and organophosphate pesticides, to mitochondrial dysfunction and decreased ATP synthesis.

Endocrine Disruption

Toxins can also interfere with the endocrine system, which plays a pivotal role in regulating metabolism. Endocrine-disrupting chemicals (EDCs), such as bisphenol A (BPA) and phthalates, mimic or interfere with hormonal signals, leading to dysregulation of metabolic processes. This disruption can contribute to metabolic disorders, including obesity and insulin resistance.

Oxidative Stress

Toxins often induce oxidative stress, an imbalance between the production of reactive oxygen species (ROS) and the body's ability to neutralize them. Excessive ROS can damage cellular structures, including proteins, lipids, and DNA, further disrupting metabolic pathways. Persistent oxidative stress has been linked to chronic diseases, including cardiovascular disease, neurodegenerative disorders, and metabolic syndrome.

Understanding the impact of toxins on metabolic pathways is crucial for developing strategies to mitigate their harmful effects. By acknowledging the intricate connections between environmental exposures and metabolic disruption, researchers and healthcare professionals can work towards minimizing the prevalence of toxin-induced metabolic disorders and promoting overall well-being. Future studies must continue to explore these intricate relationships, offering insights that pave the way for interventions to safeguard the delicate balance of metabolic processes within the human body.

We have enough scientific research now to know that certain chemicals do not belong in our bodies and that they can cause horrible things to our health. We don't drink gasoline. So why would you allow other food toxins in your body? There are a lot of other chemicals that are allowed to be in our food, and just because they are in smaller amounts, the FDA says it's ok. If drinking a small amount of gasoline won't kill you would you drink it anyway? The right responsible answer is "HECK NO."

Well did you know that some artificial food dyes are made from petroleum, a crude oil product? It's true — more on the food dyes below. I hope you understand the message I am trying to get you to understand. READ THE LABELS and make an effort to understand what these chemicals do to your health. One of the primary sources of toxins that enter our bodies is through the foods we eat, at the top of the list are dairy, meat, fish, and eggs. Applying too much heat to our foods can also create toxins for the body, for instance, if you apply high heat to asparagine an amino acid, and natural sugars (glucose) this forms a cancer-causing substance called "acrylamide."

A common food additive maltodextrin has been linked to Crohn's disease. Maltodextrin is a food additive produced from starch; it acts as a thickener in sauces, and salad dressings and also to help sweeten foods such as powdered drinks, canned fruit, and in desserts. Another sweetener parents use is honey, as you will see in the chapter "Carbohydrates

& Fiber" the toxins that are found in honey include a popular weed killer.

The cooking of certain foods can cause toxins like Advanced Glycation End-Products (AGE's).

AGE can happen when proteins or fat mix with sugar in the blood and can cause heart disease, diabetes, kidney damage and failure, high blood pressure, increased insulin resistance, arthritis, and other ailments. These harmful toxins can build up in the body. Cooking foods at high temperatures like barbecuing, deep frying, and toasting can cause AGE. The body can eliminate these damaging compounds with antioxidants from whole plant foods.

What Is A Carcinogen?

A carcinogen can be any substance, such as radionuclide, or radiation that promotes carcinogenesis. Other non-radioactive carcinogens like dioxins, asbestos, and tobacco smoke are carcinogens as well. There are carcinogens found in the food we eat. Below you will see carcinogens that can be in our food supply. If you buy organic whole plant foods and wash them as I have stated earlier in this book, you can greatly reduce the risk of these carcinogens entering your body. Some carcinogens can mutate genes that can stop the tumor suppressor gene "P53" from doing its job.

Toxins can enter your body in many ways.

- *Absorption* - This means that the toxins will enter the body through the skin by way of shampoo, deodorant, cleaners, laundry soaps, and chemicals placed on our clothing by manufacturing.
- *Consumption* - This means that the toxins have entered our bodies by eating foods or drinking liquids and swallowing pills. The added chemicals in our food supply "ARE KILLING US."

- *Inhalation* - This means that we breathe in carcinogens from air pollutants. Our bodies can breathe in carcinogens by way of cleaners, sprays, paints, etc.

Carcinogenic Compounds:
According to The World Health Organization (WHO) the classifications of carcinogens:

- ***Group 1*** - carcinogenic to humans
- ***Group 2A*** - probably carcinogenic to humans
- ***Group 2B*** - possibly carcinogenic to humans
- ***Group 3*** - not classifiable
- ***Group 4*** - probably not carcinogenic

Food Dyes

Food dyes are in a lot of foods that are targeted to humans. They have been linked to long-term health problems such as cancer and other ailments. These dyes have been banned in Europe and other countries. Now that brings me to the point about food dyes. Food dyes are petroleum-derived products that scientists have linked through research to be harmful to humans. Some of the earlier dyes have been banned due to cancer concerns. This should paint the picture for you. As I used to tell children who came into my restaurant "Anytime you see a color, and a number on a food product put that product back on the shelf."

- ***Annatto*** - This dye is produced from seeds from the achiote tree. There have been reports that this dye might have a link to irritable bowel syndrome, but I have not seen the data to back up these claims. More research is needed.

- ***Blue #1 (E133)*** - Found in beverages, baked goods cereals. Has been shown to cause kidney tumors in mice.
- ***Blue #2 (E132)*** - Found in candies, this dye has been shown to cause brain tumors in mice.
- ***Green #3 (Fast Green) (E143)*** - Found in candies, has been shown to cause tumors in the bladder in male rats as well as tumors in the testes.
- ***Orange #2*** - Banned
- ***Red #1*** - Banned
- ***Red #2 (E123)*** - Banned
- ***Red #3 (E127)*** - Found in candies, baked goods, and maraschino cherries. Researchers have shown a link to thyroid cancer.
- ***Red #4 (E125)*** - Banned
- ***Red #32*** - Banned
- ***Red #40 (E129)*** - Found mainly in cereals and desserts. Scientists have stated that this dye can accelerate immune system tumors as well as trigger allergic reactions and hyperactivity in young children.
- ***Yellow #1, #2, #3, #4*** - Banned
- ***Yellow #5 (E102)*** - Found mainly in baked goods and cereals this dye also triggers hyperactivity and behavioral problems in children.
- Y***ellow #6 (E110)*** - A large South Hampton University study found a link between yellow #6, and sodium benzoate (preservative) to cause hyperactivity in children.

We are now starting to see natural fruit, vegetables, and spices used as food coloring because of health concerns.

Pesticides On Fruit And Vegetables

Pesticides have been shown to have a delayed effect as it relates to health issues. Studies on non-Hodgkin lymphoma and leukemia have found a positive link with exposure to pesticides. There is substantial evidence that has shown a link between organophosphate insecticide and neurobehavioral issues. There have been three pesticides that have been linked to causing cancer;

- ***Glyphosate*** - non-Hodgkin lymphoma
- ***Malathion*** - prostate Cancer and non-Hodgkin lymphoma
- ***Diazinon*** - lung cancer and non-Hodgkin lymphoma

The spraying of pesticides on our fruits and vegetables is causing an array of medical problems. There is a big reason why you want to buy organic fruits and vegetables for your family. That big reason is "NO CHEMICALS" or very small amounts that might get on the fruit or vegetables during transportation. The list below includes fruits and vegetables that were found to contain the most pesticide residues.

- *Strawberries*
- *Spinach*
- *Nectarines*
- *Apples*
- *Peaches*
- *Pears*
- *Grapes*
- *Cherries*
- *Tomatoes*
- *Celery*
- *Potatoes*
- *Bell Peppers*

If you soak your fruit and veggies in warm water and mix in sodium bicarbonate (baking soda) for 15 minutes and then rinse in cold water, this has been shown to remove about 95% of pesticides that are still on the outer skin.

Most Common Toxins Found In Foods We Eat

- ***Acesulfame potassium*** - Is a sweetener that is 200 times sweeter than sugar and is used in over 4,000 food products. This sweetener has been linked to lung and breast tumors in rats.
- ***Acrylamide*** - Has been proven to induce mutations in mammalian cells. It has been concluded that acrylamide is a dangerous genotoxic carcinogen. Acrylamide is formed in foods by high-temperature cooking with the presence of amino acids and sugar. The amino acid asparagine has a greater chance to form acrylamide than other amino acids when heat is applied. Acrylamide can also be formed when fats are heated and oxidized. The three carbon molecules bond with asparagine when heat is applied. Fried foods produce acrylamide. Potatoes chips have one of the highest levels of acrylamide. A metabolic way to detox the body against acrylamide is to eat sulfur-containing foods like garlic, onions, and cruciferous vegetables that have high levels of the amino acid cysteine.
- ***Aflatoxins*** - A dangerous carcinogen produced by molds. When animals are fed food that is contaminated with this mold, it can then enter the food supply via eggs, dairy, and meat. Children can be hit hard by aflatoxins because they can cause liver damage, stunt their growth, and cause a developmental delay.
- ***Aluminum*** - Is a preservative found in packaged foods and deodorants. Scientists have found a link that points to an increased risk of cancer with the aluminum found in the body.

- ***Aspartame*** - Is a sweetener that is 200 times sweeter than sugar. A large study of 125,000 people found a link between aspartame and leukemia, and lymphoma in men.
- ***Azodicarbonamide*** - Found in bread and also used to make yoga mats. Has been known to cause respiratory and skin problems. Azodicarbonamide has also been known to disrupt the immune system.
- ***Benzene*** - Is widely used in the United States. It is used to make resins, dyes, lubricants, pesticides, and more. Benzene has been shown to cause harmful effects on the bone marrow. The Department of Health and Human Services has determined that benzene causes cancer. Sodium benzoate and ascorbic acid could combine to produce benzene.
- ***Brominated vegetable oil (BVO)*** - This is found in soft drinks to help emulsify citrus-flavored soft drinks. BVO has been linked to memory loss, tremors, loss of muscle coordination, fatigue, and headaches.
- ***Carrageenan*** - It is an emulsifier used in ice creams, chocolate products, jellies, and jam to name a few. Scientists have found it to cause sarcomas in rats and mice within 2 years.
- ***Chlorine dioxide*** - This is used to speed up the process of bleaching flour because natural oxidation to flour white takes too much time. Chloride dioxide is toxic according to the United States Environmental Protection Agency and has set maximum levels in food and drinking water. Chloride dioxide has also been used to sanitize fruits such as blueberries, raspberries, and strawberries. Buy organic and wash with baking soda.
- ***BHA/BHT*** - This is a preservative and used in shortenings, and potato chips to extend shelf life. It is an antioxidant that is used to stop fatty or oily foods from oxidation and makes them taste better for a longer time frame. Scientists have proven that high doses can cause cancer in mice and rats.

- ***HCA (heterocyclic amines)*** - When meats are cooked above 360 degrees it has been shown to produce high levels of heterocyclic amines which come from meat muscles. Research has shown us a strong link between people with stomach cancer and meats that were cooked medium-well or well-done. They had more than three times the risk of stomach cancer. Studies have linked HCA to a higher risk of breast cancer, colorectal, and pancreatic cancers. Cooking under 350 has been shown to produce lower levels of HCA's. Broccoli and Brussels sprouts have been shown to partially reduce the risk of cancers.
- ***High fructose corn syrup (HFCS)*** - This is an artificial sugar that is produced from corn syrup. The liver has a hard time processing HFCS. Multiple studies have shown high shown high intakes of HFCS are associated with obesity. This can also lead to diabetes and the risk of other serious diseases.
- ***PAH (polycyclic aromatic hydrocarbons)*** - These are formed when meat is in direct contact with the burnt fuel used to cause the black char on meats. Scientists state that this process can create gene mutations. PAH has also been linked to colon cancer.
- ***Monosodium glutamate (MSG)*** - MSG is a flavor enhancer found mainly in Chinese restaurants that can cause pressure in the chest and, a flushed face. MSG has been shown to over-stimulate the nervous system.
- ***Nitrosamines*** - These are produced from nitrites and secondary amines which occur in the form of proteins. The pH level plays an important role in the creation of nitrosamines. Research found that 90% of nitrosamine compounds are deemed to be carcinogenic and have a link to liver cancer.
- ***Paraben*** - These are the most commonly used preservatives on the surface of potato products and dried meats. They prevent the growth of mold and yeast. It has been found to act like the hormone estrogen in females.

- ***Polysorbate 80*** - Acts as an emulsifier or defoamer that helps with the consistency of products. It is found in a lot of foods like ice cream, shortening, and chewing gum. Found to cause skin and eye irritation. Found to cause cancer in animals.
- ***Polysorbate 60*** - Is a thickener, emulsifier, and stabilizer. It makes chocolate coating not greasy. It is found in foods like doughnuts, salad dressings, cake mixes, and frozen desserts. Also been found to cause cancer in animals.
- ***Potassium bromate*** - It is a maturing agent found in bread to make it rise higher. It is classified as a group 2B carcinogen (possibly carcinogenic to humans) which could cause cancer.
- ***Propyl gallate*** - This is a preservative used to keep fats and oils from spoiling. It is found in ice cream, candy, baked goods, mayonnaise, and many other foods. There is not enough research to draw a conclusion. There is some research that states it has caused cancer in rats.
- ***Recombinant bovine growth hormone (rBGH)*** - This is a genetically engineered bovine growth hormone. This hormone boosts the milk production in dairy cows. To boost milk production higher levels of IGF-1 are needed. High levels of IGF-1 have been linked to a higher risk of getting cancer.
- ***Saccharin*** - Is a sweetener that scientists have found to cause bladder cancer in rats.
- ***Sodium benzoate*** - Sodium benzoate is used as a preservative found in carbonated beverages and salad dressings. Researchers found that when testing multiple drinks that contain sodium benzoate and vitamin C found 2 ppb of benzene. Benzene is a group 1 carcinogen according to International Agency for Research on Cancer.
- ***Sodium nitrate*** - Combined with salvia and secondary amines sodium nitrates can produce nitrosamines. Nitrosamines have been linked to the increased risk of certain cancers.

- ***Sulfites*** - Found in wine and dried fruit. They occur naturally in small amounts in grapes. They are used as a preservative to prevent foods from turning brown. A small percent of the population has some allergic reactions.
- ***Tertiary butylhydroquinone (TBHQ)*** - Is used as an antioxidant in foods. Has been known to help preserve freshness in foods such as chicken nuggets. 5 grams of this stuff can kill you. Just one gram can cause nausea, vomiting, ringing in the ears, delirium, and other health issues. There is no need to put this stuff in food.

Hazards Of Cooking Oils: The Hexane Connection

Cooking oils are a ubiquitous component of modern diets, utilized in a variety of culinary applications. While they play a crucial role in food preparation, recent research has shed light on the potential health hazards associated with their consumption. One concerning aspect is the prevalent use of hexane in the processing of cooking oils, raising questions about the safety of these commonly used kitchen staples.

Hexane in Cooking Oil Processing

Hexane, a hydrocarbon solvent derived from crude oil, is employed in the extraction process of many cooking oils. It is particularly favored for its ability to efficiently extract oil from seeds and plants, making it a cost-effective choice for large-scale commercial oil production. However, the use of hexane has raised health concerns due to its potential toxicity.

Neurotoxicity

Hexane exposure has been linked to neurotoxic effects, primarily affecting the peripheral nervous system. Prolonged exposure or high concentrations of hexane vapors can lead to symptoms such as dizziness, headaches, and in severe cases, peripheral neuropathy characterized by numbness and tingling in the extremities.

Residual Hexane in Cooking Oils

Despite the extraction process being designed to remove most of the hexane, trace amounts can persist in the final cooking oil product. The ingestion of these residual traces raises concerns about potential long-term health effects, especially given the cumulative nature of such exposure over time.

Air Quality Concerns in Processing Plants

The use of hexane in oil extraction poses risks not only to consumers but also to workers in processing plants. Hexane is a volatile organic compound that can contribute to air pollution, affecting the overall air quality in and around these facilities. Workers exposed to hexane vapors may face respiratory issues and other health complications.

Unhealthy Components in Cooking Oils

Apart from the hexane-related concerns, cooking oils themselves can harbor unhealthy components:

Trans Fats and Hydrogenation:

Many commercially available cooking oils undergo hydrogenation to increase shelf life and stability. This process produces trans fats, which are known to elevate levels of bad cholesterol (LDL) and lower good cholesterol (HDL), increasing the risk of heart disease.

Oxidation and Free Radicals:

The exposure of cooking oils to heat and air during processing and cooking can lead to oxidation, resulting in the formation of free radicals. These free radicals contribute to inflammation and oxidative stress in the body, potentially playing a role in the development of chronic diseases.

While cooking oils are a staple in kitchens worldwide, it is imperative to be aware of the potential health risks associated with their consumption. The use of hexane in the processing of these oils introduces an additional layer of concern, given its neurotoxic properties and the challenges in completely eliminating it from the final product.

The Hazards Of Mercury

Mercury is a highly toxic element that can have detrimental effects on the human body when exposure occurs. While mercury exists in various forms, the most common sources of exposure include contaminated fish, dental amalgams, and industrial processes. The impact of mercury on the body depends on the form of mercury, the duration of exposure, and the individual's susceptibility.

One of the primary ways mercury damages the body is through its ability to accumulate in tissues and organs. Methylmercury, a form of organic mercury, tends to accumulate in fish and seafood. When humans consume contaminated fish, the methylmercury is absorbed in the gastrointestinal tract and easily enters the bloodstream. Once in the bloodstream, it can cross the blood-brain barrier, leading to the accumulation of mercury in the brain. The central nervous system is particularly vulnerable to mercury toxicity, and long-term exposure can result in neurological damage.

Neurological effects of mercury poisoning include impaired cognitive function, memory loss, and difficulty concentrating. In children, whose nervous systems are still developing, mercury exposure can lead to developmental delays, learning disabilities, and behavioral problems. Pregnant women are also at risk, as mercury can cross the placenta and affect the developing fetus, leading to cognitive and motor skill deficits.

In addition to its impact on the nervous system, mercury can also damage the cardiovascular system. Elemental mercury vapors, which can be released from dental amalgams, are easily inhaled and absorbed into the bloodstream. Chronic exposure to mercury vapors has been associated with an increased risk of cardiovascular diseases, including hypertension and heart attacks. Mercury may disrupt the normal functioning of blood vessels and contribute to the development of atherosclerosis, a condition characterized by the buildup of plaque in the arteries.

Studies have stated that mercury has been linked to kidney damage. The kidneys play a crucial role in filtering toxins from the bloodstream, and mercury can accumulate in renal tissues, impairing their function over time. This can lead to kidney dysfunction, proteinuria (the presence of excess protein in the urine), and ultimately, renal failure.

The immune system is not spared from the damaging effects of mercury. Prolonged exposure to this toxic element can suppress immune function, making individuals more susceptible to infections and compromising the body's ability to defend itself against foreign invaders.

It is essential to note that different forms of mercury have varying toxicities. While methylmercury is primarily associated with fish consumption, elemental mercury vapors from dental amalgams, and inorganic mercury from industrial sources, can also pose health risks.

The impact of mercury on the body is cumulative, meaning that even low levels of exposure over an extended period can lead to significant health problems.

Mercury poses a serious threat to human health, with the potential to damage the nervous system, cardiovascular system, kidneys, and immune system. Minimizing exposure to mercury by avoiding contaminated fish, choosing alternative dental materials, and promoting strict industrial regulations is crucial for safeguarding public health. Regular monitoring and awareness of the sources of mercury exposure are essential steps in preventing and mitigating the harmful effects of this toxic element on the human body.

The Hazards Of Cadmium

Cadmium is a highly toxic metal that poses significant health risks to the human body when exposed in excessive amounts. It is a naturally occurring element found in the Earth's crust but is most commonly released into the environment through industrial processes, such as mining, smelting, and manufacturing. Once cadmium enters the body, it can accumulate over time and lead to a variety of adverse health effects.

One of the primary routes of cadmium exposure is through the ingestion of contaminated food and water. Cadmium can be absorbed by plants from the soil, and when animals or humans consume these contaminated plants, the metal enters the food chain. Additionally, tobacco plants readily absorb cadmium from the soil, making tobacco products a significant source of exposure for smokers. Inhalation of cadmium-containing dust and fumes in industrial settings is another route of exposure.

Once inside the body, cadmium has a long half-life, meaning it persists for an extended period, particularly in the kidneys, where it has a strong affinity to accumulate. The kidneys are a primary target organ for cadmium toxicity. The metal interferes with the normal functioning of the kidneys and can lead to renal dysfunction. Chronic exposure to cadmium is associated with an increased risk of developing kidney diseases, such as renal tubular dysfunction and glomerular damage.

Cadmium is also known to disrupt the normal functioning of the respiratory system. Inhalation of cadmium-containing particles can lead to lung damage, chronic obstructive pulmonary disease (COPD), and an increased risk of lung cancer. Long-term exposure to cadmium through smoking is a major concern, as it can synergistically enhance the harmful effects of tobacco smoke on the respiratory system.

Studies have shown that elevated cadmium levels in the body are associated with an increased risk of hypertension, atherosclerosis, and cardiovascular disease. The mechanism by which cadmium affects the cardiovascular system is complex and may involve oxidative stress, inflammation, and the disruption of essential metal homeostasis.

In addition to its impact on the kidneys, lungs, and cardiovascular system, cadmium is also known to interfere with the reproductive system. It can disrupt hormone balance and adversely affect reproductive organs, leading to fertility issues. Pregnant women exposed to cadmium may pass the metal to their developing fetuses, potentially causing developmental problems.

Cadmium is a potent carcinogen, and long-term exposure is associated with an increased risk of various cancers. The International Agency for Research on Cancer (IARC) has classified cadmium and cadmium compounds as Group 1 human carcinogens, indicating that there is sufficient evidence to support their carcinogenicity in humans. Cancers linked to cadmium exposure include lung cancer, prostate cancer, and breast cancer.

Cadmium poses a serious threat to human health due to its toxic nature and the wide range of adverse effects it can have on various organ systems. Minimizing exposure to cadmium, particularly through contaminated food, water, and tobacco products, is crucial for preventing the associated health risks.

The Hazards Of Lead

Lead is a toxic metal that, when introduced into the human body, can wreak havoc on various systems and organs. While advancements in science and public health have led to significant reductions in lead exposure over the years, the metal still poses a serious threat to human health. Here's an exploration of how lead damages the body:

1. **Neurological Effects:** One of the most concerning aspects of lead exposure is its impact on the nervous system, particularly in children. Lead interferes with the development and functioning of the brain, leading to cognitive deficits, learning disabilities, and behavioral issues. Even low levels of lead exposure have been linked to decreased IQ and attention-related problems.
2. **Cardiovascular System:** Lead exposure has been associated with an increased risk of hypertension and cardiovascular diseases. The metal can interfere with the production of nitric oxide, a substance that helps regulate blood pressure. Elevated blood pressure, in turn, puts a strain on the heart and can contribute to the development of heart-related conditions.
3. **Renal (Kidney) Damage:** The kidneys are essential for filtering out waste and maintaining the body's balance of fluids

and electrolytes. Lead can accumulate in the kidneys, leading to nephropathy and impaired renal function. Chronic exposure to lead has been linked to an increased risk of kidney disease.

4. **Reproductive System:** Lead exposure can have detrimental effects on both male and female reproductive systems. In males, it can impact sperm production and motility, while in females, it can lead to miscarriages and developmental issues in the fetus. Pregnant women are particularly vulnerable, as lead can cross the placental barrier, affecting the developing baby.
5. **Hematological Effects:** Lead interferes with the production of hemoglobin, the molecule responsible for carrying oxygen in the blood. This can lead to anemia, causing fatigue, weakness, and pale skin. Additionally, lead exposure can disrupt the normal balance of minerals like calcium and iron in the body.
6. **Gastrointestinal Impact:** The gastrointestinal system can also be affected by lead exposure. Ingested lead can be absorbed in the stomach and intestines, leading to abdominal pain, constipation, and nausea. Over time, chronic exposure can contribute to more severe gastrointestinal issues.
7. **Bone Damage:** Lead has an affinity for bones and can accumulate in them over time. It interferes with the normal turnover of bone tissue, leading to decreased bone density and increased fragility. This can result in joint and muscle pain, as well as an increased risk of fractures.
8. **Immunological Consequences:** Lead exposure can compromise the immune system, making individuals more susceptible to infections and illnesses. This is particularly problematic for children, whose developing immune systems can be significantly impacted by exposure to this toxic metal.
9. **Long-lasting Effects:** Perhaps one of the most concerning aspects of lead exposure is its ability to cause long-lasting and sometimes irreversible damage. The effects of lead can persist into

adulthood, impacting overall quality of life and contributing to a range of chronic health conditions.

Lead's damaging effects on the body are widespread and multifaceted. Efforts to reduce exposure and mitigate the consequences of lead toxicity remain critical in safeguarding public health, especially for vulnerable populations such as children and pregnant women. Strict regulations, public awareness campaigns, and ongoing research are essential components of the collective effort to address and minimize the impact of lead on human health.

The Hazards Of Aluminum

Aluminum is a ubiquitous metal found in various natural and man-made environments, and while it is abundant and widely used in everyday products, concerns have been raised about its potential adverse effects on human health. Although aluminum is not inherently toxic, excessive exposure or accumulation in the body can lead to various health issues. It's important to note that the scientific community continues to study the potential health effects of aluminum, and our understanding may evolve with further research. Later in this chapter, I will discuss the damage of aluminum and fluoride as a chemical complex when in the body at the same time.

One primary route of aluminum exposure for humans is through the consumption of food and water. Aluminum can leach into food from aluminum cookware or packaging. Additionally, aluminum compounds are used in water treatment processes, contributing to its presence in drinking water. Aluminum can be found in many different brands of baking powder. While the body can excrete small amounts of aluminum, excessive intake can overwhelm the body's ability to eliminate it efficiently.

One of the main concerns associated with aluminum exposure is its potential link to neurological disorders, including Alzheimer's disease. Some studies have suggested that elevated levels of aluminum in the brain may be associated with the development of neurodegenerative diseases. Aluminum can cross the blood-brain barrier, and once inside the brain, it may contribute to the formation of plaques and neurofibrillary tangles, which are characteristic features of Alzheimer's disease. However, the exact mechanisms and the strength of this association are still subjects of ongoing research, and the role of aluminum in neurological disorders remains complex.

In addition to its potential impact on the brain, aluminum has been linked to other health concerns. High levels of aluminum exposure have been associated with bone disorders, as aluminum can interfere with the formation and function of bone cells. Chronic exposure to elevated aluminum levels may lead to weakened bones and an increased risk of fractures. People with impaired kidney function are particularly vulnerable to aluminum accumulation, as the kidneys play a crucial role in eliminating excess aluminum from the body.

There are concerns about the potential impact of aluminum on the reproductive system. Some studies have suggested that aluminum exposure may have adverse effects on male fertility by affecting sperm quality and function. Aluminum's ability to mimic estrogen, a hormone that regulates various physiological processes, has also raised concerns about its potential role in hormone-related cancers, although the evidence in this area is not conclusive.

The research on the health effects of aluminum is ongoing, it's essential to take precautionary measures to minimize unnecessary exposure.

This includes using aluminum-free cookware, being mindful of aluminum content in processed foods and beverages, and considering alternatives to products containing aluminum, such as antiperspirants that use aluminum-based compounds.

While aluminum is a common and versatile metal, excessive exposure can potentially have adverse effects on various bodily systems. Ongoing research aims to further clarify the relationship between aluminum and health outcomes, but in the meantime, individuals can make informed choices to reduce unnecessary exposure and mitigate potential risks associated with this metal.

The Hazards Of Fluoride

Fluoride is a naturally occurring mineral found in water, soil, and various foods. One of the primary concerns regarding fluoride consumption is its potential impact on the skeletal system. Prolonged exposure to high levels of fluoride has been associated with skeletal fluorosis, a condition characterized by pain and limited mobility in joints. In severe cases, skeletal fluorosis can lead to deformities in the spine and limbs. Long-term exposure to elevated fluoride levels, particularly in areas with naturally occurring high fluoride in drinking water, has been linked to an increased risk of fractures and bone abnormalities.

Furthermore, some studies have suggested a potential connection between high fluoride exposure and disruptions in the endocrine system. The thyroid gland, in particular, has been a focus of research in this regard. Excessive fluoride intake may interfere with thyroid function, potentially leading to conditions such as hypothyroidism. The disruption of thyroid hormones can have widespread effects on the body, impacting metabolism, energy levels, and overall well-being.

Cognitive effects have also been explored in relation to fluoride exposure. Some research has suggested a possible link between high fluoride levels and decreased cognitive function, particularly in children. The developing brain may be more vulnerable to the neurotoxic effects of fluoride, potentially impacting cognitive abilities such as memory and learning. While findings in this area are not conclusive, the potential for cognitive impacts raises concerns, especially considering the widespread exposure to fluoride through various sources.

Fluoride has been shown to accumulate in the pineal gland, a small organ in the brain that produces melatonin, a hormone that regulates sleep-wake cycles. Some studies suggest that fluoride accumulation in the pineal gland may interfere with melatonin production, potentially disrupting sleep patterns. Adequate sleep is crucial for overall health, and any disruption in sleep cycles can have far-reaching consequences on physical and mental well-being.

Excessive exposure to fluoride raises legitimate concerns about its impact on various aspects of human health. The potential risks include skeletal fluorosis, disruptions in the endocrine system, cognitive effects, and interference with sleep patterns. Ongoing research is crucial to better understand the mechanisms and potential long-term effects of fluoride exposure.

Effects of Aluminum And Fluoride Complex

I will attempt to explain the intricate chemistry and consequential health effects resulting from the coexistence of aluminum and fluoride. Both elements are commonly encountered in various industrial, agricultural, and domestic settings, raising concerns about their potential synergistic impact on human health. By examining the chemical interactions between aluminum and fluoride, as well as reviewing relevant scientific literature, this report aims to shed light on the harmful outcomes associated with their combined presence.

Aluminum and fluoride are ubiquitous elements found in nature and are extensively used in various industrial and consumer applications. Aluminum is the third most abundant element in the Earth's crust, while fluoride is commonly encountered in minerals, water sources, and dental products. Despite their individual prevalence, recent studies have raised concerns about the potential health risks associated with simultaneous exposure to aluminum and fluoride.

To understand the harmful consequences of aluminum and fluoride together, it is crucial to examine their chemical interactions. Both elements can form stable complexes, and their behavior is influenced by factors such as pH, concentration, and the presence of other ions. Aluminum readily forms complexes with fluoride ions, leading to the creation of species like AlF3, and AlF4-.

The most significant interaction occurs when fluoride ions complex with aluminum, forming aluminum fluoride (AlF3). This compound has been implicated in various physiological and biochemical processes, particularly in the nervous system. The formation of stable complexes between aluminum and fluoride may enhance the absorption of both elements in the body, intensifying their toxic effects.

Neurological Implications

Numerous studies have explored the impact of aluminum and fluoride exposure on neurological health. The blood-brain barrier (BBB) is a crucial defense mechanism that regulates the passage of substances into the brain. Aluminum has been shown to compromise the integrity of the BBB, allowing it to enter the brain and accumulate in various regions, particularly in the hippocampus and cerebral cortex.

Fluoride, when in the presence of aluminum, may exacerbate these effects. Research suggests that the aluminum-fluoride complex may enhance the transport of aluminum across the BBB, leading to increased neuronal exposure. Once inside the brain, aluminum can interfere with neurotransmitter function, disrupt enzyme activity, and induce oxidative stress, collectively contributing to neurodegenerative disorders such as Alzheimer's disease.

Skeletal Health

The interaction between aluminum and fluoride also raises concerns about skeletal health. Fluoride is well-known for its role in dental health, primarily in preventing tooth decay. However, excessive fluoride intake, especially in the presence of aluminum, may have adverse effects on bone health. Aluminum has been shown to accumulate in bones, disrupting normal bone metabolism and contributing to conditions like osteomalacia and osteoporosis.

The aluminum-fluoride complex can affect bone mineralization and lead to the formation of structurally abnormal bone tissue. Moreover, the joint toxicity of aluminum and fluoride may contribute to an increased risk of fractures and skeletal deformities.

Reproductive and Developmental Effects

The potential reproductive and developmental effects of simultaneous exposure to aluminum and fluoride have been investigated in various animal studies. Both elements have been shown to cross the placental barrier, exposing developing fetuses to their toxic effects. Animal studies suggest that this exposure may lead to developmental abnormalities, including impaired cognitive function, skeletal malformations, and altered behavior.

Aluminum-fluoride interactions may disrupt hormonal balance, affecting the endocrine system and reproductive organs. Female reproductive health, in particular, may be compromised, with studies indicating a possible link between aluminum-fluoride exposure and adverse pregnancy outcomes.

Sources of Aluminum and Fluoride Exposure

Understanding the sources of aluminum and fluoride exposure is essential in mitigating potential health risks. Aluminum is commonly found in food additives, cookware, antacids, and certain medications. Fluoride exposure can occur through drinking water, dental products, and industrial processes. The coexistence of these elements in various consumer products and environmental settings underscores the need for comprehensive risk assessments and regulatory measures.

Given the potential synergistic effects of aluminum and fluoride, regulatory agencies must reevaluate current guidelines for exposure limits. Comprehensive risk assessments should consider the combined impact of these elements, especially in vulnerable populations such as children, pregnant women, and the elderly.

The coexistence of aluminum and fluoride poses a potential threat to human health, with implications for neurological function, skeletal integrity, and reproductive outcomes. The chemistry of aluminum and fluoride interactions reveals a complex interplay that may exacerbate the toxic effects of both elements. As our understanding of these interactions advances, it is imperative to implement regulatory measures and conduct further research to mitigate potential harm and promote public health and safety.

Benzene

Sodium benzoate and ascorbic acid do not directly create benzene. However, when they are combined in the presence of heat and light, a reaction can occur, leading to the formation of trace amounts of benzene. This reaction is a concern in certain beverage products, especially those containing sodium benzoate as a preservative and ascorbic acid (vitamin C).

Yes, the reaction that can lead to the formation of benzene from sodium benzoate and ascorbic acid is more likely to occur at a lower pH. The reaction is influenced by various factors, including acidity. In acidic conditions, such as a low pH environment, the risk of benzene formation may increase. Therefore, controlling the pH is one of the measures taken by the food industry to mitigate the potential formation of benzene in certain products.

Benzene exposure is associated with several health risks. Prolonged or high-level exposure to benzene can lead to serious health issues, including:

- **Bone Marrow Damage:** Benzene exposure can affect the production of blood cells in the bone marrow, leading to conditions like aplastic anemia and leukemia.
- **Immune System Suppression:** Benzene may suppress the immune system, making individuals more susceptible to infections.
- **Reproductive Effects:** Long-term exposure to benzene has been linked to reproductive problems and adverse effects on fetal development during pregnancy.
- **Cancer Risk:** Benzene is classified as a known human carcinogen. Chronic exposure increases the risk of developing cancers, particularly leukemia and other blood-related cancers.

- **Neurological Effects:** Some studies suggest that benzene exposure may have neurological effects, impacting cognitive function and nerve function.

It's important to note that the severity of health effects depends on the level and duration of exposure. Occupational settings with high benzene exposure levels pose greater risks. Regulatory standards aim to limit benzene exposure to protect public health. If you suspect exposure to benzene, it's crucial to seek medical advice promptly.

Below is a list of known human carcinogens according to The National Institute for Occupational Safety and Health (NIOSH).

A

Acetaldehyde
2-Acetylaminofluorene
Acrylamide
Acrylonitrile
Aldrin
4-Aminodiphenyl
Amitrole
Aniline and homologs
o-Anisidine
Arsenic and inorganic arsenic compounds
Arsine
Asbestos
Asphalt fumes

B

Benzene
Benzidine
Benzidine-based dyes

Beryllium
Butadiene
tert-Butyl chromate; class, chromium hexavalent
C
Cadmium dust and fume
Captafol
Captan
Carbon black (exceeding 0.1% PAHs)
Carbon tetrachloride
Chlordane
Chlorinated camphene
Chlorodiphenyl (42% chlorine); class polychlorinated biphenyls
Chlorodiphenyl (54% chlorine); class polychlorinated biphenyls
Chloroform
Chloromethyl methyl ether
bis(Chloromethyl) ether
B-Chloroprene
Chromium, hexavalent
Chromyl chloride; class, chromium hexavalent
Chrysene
Coal tar pitch volatiles; class, coal tar products
Coke oven emissions
D
DDT (dichlorodiphenyltrichloroethane)
Di-2-ethylhexyl phthalate (DEHP)
2,4-Diaminoanisoleo
o-Dianisidine-based dyes
1,2-Dibromo-3-chloropropane (DBCP)
Dichloroacetylene
p-Dichlorobenzene
3,3'-Dichlorobenzidine
Dichloroethyl ether
1,3-Dichloropropene

Dieldrin
Diesel exhaust
Diglycidyl ether (DGE); class, glycidyl ethers
4-Dimethylaminoazobenzene
Dimethyl carbomoyl chloride
1,1-Dimethylhydrazine; class, hydrazines
Dimethyl sulfate
Dinitrotoluene
Dioxane
E-G
Environmental tobacco smoke
Epichlorohydrin
Ethyl acrylate
Ethylene dibromide
Ehtylene dichloride
Ethylene oxide
Ethyleneimine
Ethylene thiourea
Formaldehyde
Gallium arsenide
Gasoline
H-K
Heptachlor
Hexachlorobutadiene
Hexachloroethane
Hexamethyl phosphoric triamide (HMPA)
Hydrazine
Kepone
M
Malonaldehyde
Methoxychlor
Methyl bromide; class, monohalomethanes
Methyl chloride

Methyl iodide; class, monohalomethanes
Methyl hydrazine; class, hydrazines
4,4'-Methylenebis(2-chloroaniline) (MBOCA)
Methylene chloride
4,4-Methylenedianiline (MDA)
N
α-Naphthylamine (alpha-naphthylamine)
β-Naphthylamine (beta-naphthylamine)
Nickel, metal, soluble, insoluble, and inorganic; class, nickel, inorganic
Nickel carbonyl
Nickel sulfide roasting
4-Nitrobiphenyl
p-Nitrochlorobenzene
2-Nitronaphthalene
2-Nitropropane
N-Nitrosodimethylamine
P
Pentachloroethane; class, chloroethanes
N-Phenyl-b-naphthylamine; class, b-naphthalene
Phenyl glycidyl ether; class, glycidyl ethers
Phenylhydrazine; class, hydrazines
Propane Sultone
B-Propiolactone
Propylene dichloride
Proplyene imine
Propylene oxide
R-S
Radon
Rosin core solder, pyrolysis products (containing formaldehyde)
Silica, crystalline cristobalite
Silica, crystalline quartz
Silica, crystalline tripoli

Silica, crystalline tridymite
silica, fused
Soapstone, total dust silicates
T
Tremolite silicates
2,3,7,8-Tetrachlorodibenzo-p-dioxin (TCDD) (dioxin)
1,1,2,2-Tetrachloroethane
Tetrachloroethylene
Titanium dioxide
o-Tolidine-based dyes
o-Tolidine
Toluene diisocyanate (TDI)
Toluene diamine (TDA)
o-Toluidine
p-Toluidine
1,1,2-Trichloroethane; class, chloroethanes
Trichloroethylene
1,2,3-Trichloropropane
U-Z
Uranium, insoluble compounds Uranium, soluble compounds
Vinyl bromide; class, vinyl halides
Vinyl chloride
Vinyl cyclohexene dioxide
Vinylidene chloride (1,1-dichloroethylene); class, vinyl halides)
Welding fumes, total particulates
Wood dust
Zinc chromate; class, chromium hexavalent

This part of the book could be a book all by itself; I wish I could give more details on the toxins. We learned from this chapter, is that not just the added chemicals in our bodies can be carcinogens. When we cook a carbohydrate at a high temperature, we can subject our body to acrylamide which as we now know is a carcinogen. We also know that a drink that has sodium benzoate and ascorbic acid together can produce a group 1 carcinogen called benzene. We learned that heating meats could create both HCA's and PAH's. I will post a lot more detail on the toxins on my website p53diet.com under the members-only section.

Keeping all the bad chemistry out of our bodies should be a top priority. I will keep stressing the importance of buying organic fruit and veggies when you can. Remember you still have to wash with baking soda to remove any possible contaminants. The upcoming chapters will be on the superheroes. My superheroes are the things that give us a healthy life, fruits, and vegetables. You need to plan ahead for your health, it is just like putting a helmet on before you go on a bike ride.

6

The Human Body

Our bodies are made up of about 50 trillion cells. Cells come in different sizes. Our cells are like factories; each cell needs nutrients to process and then create products and waste. The human body is a very complex machine. Our DNA is hit by damage about 19,000 times a day. That damage can cause gene mutations, which can lead to cancer if it is not fixed. The ways we help repair the damage to our DNA is by putting the right phytonutrients in our bodies such as (Apples, Lemons, Strawberries, Broccoli, Celery, Cranberries, Garlic, Persimmons, and Watercress) as an example. Our bodies can heal themselves for the most part just by what we are eating. It is coded in our DNA. Your health depends on putting the right amounts of amino acids in your body and keeping animal products that bring bad chemicals into the body out of your body. I like breaking down the word protein into what it is. A protein is made up of amino acids that code for proteins and enzymes. All proteins are made from twenty different amino acid combinations. We know that there are nine essential amino acids. Please refer back to Chapter 4 *"Amino Acids."*

The human body is made up of organs 72 in men and 76 in women.

There are 13 major organ systems in the human body.

- **Circulatory System** - is responsible for pumping blood to and from the heart and lungs and to the blood vessels.
- **Digestive System** - is responsible for processing food using the salivary glands and also utilizing anas, esophagus, gallbladder, intestines, liver, pancreas, rectum, and stomach.
- **Endocrine System** - is the chemical communication within the body by using hormones.
- **Integumentary System** - is the system for the skin, hair, and nails.
- **Immune System** - is the body's defense system that protects us from disease. The immune system will detect and fight all incoming pathogens.
- **Lymphatic System** - The primary function is to make lymph fluid that contains white blood cells that help the body fight infection. It also removes excess lymph fluid from body tissue and returns it to the blood.
- **Musculoskeletal System** - is the system that makes the body move.
- **Nervous System** - senses changes in the body, then works with the endocrine system to respond to the changes.
- **Reproductive System** - is the system that deals with sexual reproduction.
- **Respiratory System** - is the system for breathing in oxygen and breathing out carbon dioxide.
- **Urinary System** - is the system that gives off waste.

All of these systems are necessary for the body to function correctly. Each system uses amino acids to operate. As our bodies develop, so do the system's requirements for nutrients. Such as Arginine, for example, helps the immune system by manufacturing T cells to help fight bacteria, viruses, cancer tumor cells, and other health-related issues. Arginine also helps the body systems in different ways as we discussed in the chapter *"Amino Acids."* If we want to develop properly, we need to make sure we get the right nutrients NOT TOXINS in our bodies. Eating a whole plant meal helps put all the right amino acids in their bodies and helps keep out most of the food toxins that the animals bring into the body. If you think feeding cheeseburgers, French fries, pizza, and soft drinks is putting the right nutrients into your body think again. These are the things that are making people unhealthy and obese and setting them up for cancers and other diseases later on in life. It also causes the pancreas to release more insulin.

Cells are the building blocks for all living things. As we said, the human body contains about 50 trillion cells. There are two types of cells prokaryotic and eukaryotic cells. Eukaryotic cells contain a nucleus while prokaryotic cells do not. Prokaryotic cells are single-celled organisms, and eukaryotic cells have the ability to be single-cell or multicellular. I won't go into the details of these two types of cells. Our cells take in nutrients from the food we eat by breaking down the food into small parts.

- *Proteins are broken down into amino acids.*
- *Fats break down into fatty acids and glycerol.*
- *Carbohydrates break down into simple sugars.*

Types Of Human Cells

There are 200 different types of cells in the human body; each cell has a different function or forms a kind of tissue. Listed below are some of the types of cells in the human body.

- ***Bone Cells*** – Bones are comprised of a mix of collagen and calcium phosphate minerals. The bone cells come in three primary types. The osteoclasts are the large cells that break down and decompose the bone tissues. They aid in bone resorption which helps regulate the level of blood calcium. Osteoblasts function in groups of connected cells to help regulate bone mineralization and produce a substance called osteoid which helps form the bones. The osteoblasts mature to form osteocytes. Osteocytes help to form the bone and help regulate the calcium.

- ***Cartilage Cells*** – In the early development of life when we were a fetus our initial skeleton was mainly composed of cartilage which is then gradually replaced by bone. Cartilage cells also serve as a cushion between many joints in the bone. Cartilage cells are composed of different minerals and collagen fibers. Cartilage is needed to be flexible.
- ***Endothelial Cells*** – These are the cells that line the lymphatic system walls as well as the lymphatic system walls. The inner walls of the blood vessel walls are composed of endothelial cells, as well as lung, heart, and skin. They also help move fluid, and gases between the blood and tissues in the surrounding area.
- ***Epithelial Cells*** – Our outer layer known as skin, is composed of a layer of epithelial cells called the epidermis. Under the epidermis is a layer of connective tissue called the dermis. Under the dermis is another layer called the hypodermis.
- ***Fat Cells*** – Fat cells are also called adipocytes. The adipocytes contain drops of triglycerides otherwise known as (stored fat). The stored fat can then be used as energy at a later time. After the cells use the stored fat as energy the fat cells then shrink in size. The fat cells also produce hormones needed to regulate blood pressure, blood clotting and cell signaling, and sex hormone metabolism.
- ***Muscle Cells*** - Muscle cells make our bodies move. The cardiac muscle cells form involuntary cardiac muscle in the heart. The skeletal muscle tissue is needed for voluntary muscle movement. Skeletal muscle tissue is attached to the bone. The skeletal muscle cells are covered with connective tissue. Smooth muscle tissue lines the body cavities that form the walls of organs in the body including blood vessels, lung airways, kidneys, intestines, etc. The smooth muscle tissue is an involuntary muscle.

- ***Nerve Cells*** – These are also known as neurons. Neurons are cells that are electric. This is how cells communicate with other cells via connections called synapses. Sensory neurons communicate via light, touch, and sound which affect the sensory organs and send signals to the brain or the spinal cord. The motor neurons receive electrical signals from the brain and the spinal cord to control the muscle contractions.
- ***Neuroglial Cells*** – Also called glia or glial cells. They are non-neuronal cells from the central nervous system and the peripheral nervous system.
- ***Pancreatic Cells*** – Function as an endocrine, and exocrine organ. They produce and secrete the digestive enzymes to the small intestine.
- ***Platelets*** – Platelets have no nucleus and help to stop bleeding by clumping together at the point of the injury.
- ***Red Blood Cells*** – The red blood cells deliver the oxygen to other body tissues.
- ***Sex Cells*** – Sex cells are also called gametes. Sex cells are the sperm in the male and eggs in the female. The sex cells only have half the number of chromosomes, that is because when the sperm (male) fertilizes the egg (female), the number of chromosomes in the offspring must be the same total number as the parents.
- ***Stem Cells*** – Stem cells are referred to as the main cells because other cells such as nerve, liver, cardiac, and blood arise from the stem cells. No other cell in the body has the means to generate a new cell type. Embryonic stem cells come from the embryo between three to five days old. Adult stem cells are found in the bone marrow and fat. New research shows that stem cells can also create new muscle, bone, and heart cells.
- ***White Blood Cells*** – The white blood cells are the body's fighting army. The white blood cells are divided into five main types: eosinophils, neutrophils, basophils, lymphocytes, and monocytes.

The B cells, T cells, and NK cells are a type of lymphocyte. They all help in protecting the body from invading pathogens.

Food Flow

Mouth - The food enters the mouth where it mixes with saliva and starts to break down the food into smaller parts.

Esophagus - The muscles in the esophagus begin the swallowing process. The brain sends signals to start the muscles to push the food down toward the stomach.

Lower Esophageal Sphincter - At the end of the esophagus there is a ring-like muscle called the lower esophageal sphincter, it then relaxes, and the food is then allowed to enter the stomach. It keeps the food in the stomach by closing the sphincter and not letting it back up in the esophagus.

Stomach - Once the food enters the stomach the food is then mixed with digestive juices. Once in the stomach, the stomach muscles, then mix with the food with digestive enzymes. This creates chyme. Chyme then enters the small intestine.

Small Intestine - When the chyme enters the small intestine it is mixed with juices from the liver, pancreas, and the intestine. The walls of the small intestine absorb nutrients and water into the bloodstream. The waste products from the digestive process then move into the large intestine.

Large Intestine - Once in the large intestine water is absorbed and changes the waste into the stool. The stool is then pushed into the rectum.

Rectum - The stool is stored until it is pushed out of the body thru the anus.

Blood Work

When we go to the doctor, we get our blood drawn; we can tell a lot about our health from a blood test. A healthy person's blood should be about 45% red blood cells, 55% plasma, and about 1% white cells. Platelets are a very tiny percentage. What is the chemistry of our blood and why is it so important to test? There are multiple tests that your doctor may want you to take. Below is a list of some of the tests that your doctor may ask for and the normal range for the values.

CBC Test - Stands for "Complete Blood Count"

WBC Count - (white blood count) Is a count of white blood cells in the blood. If the white blood count is elevated it could indicate that there might be an infection somewhere in the body.

Normal Range: 3.80 - 11.00

RBC Count -RBC (red blood cell) erythrocyte count

We have millions of red blood cells in our bodies, and this test measures the number of RBCs in a specific amount of blood. It helps us determine the total number of RBCs and gives us an idea of their lifespan, but it does not indicate where problems originate. If there are irregularities, other tests will be required.

Normal Range: 4.30 - 5.90

Hemoglobin - Hemoglobin (Hgb)

Red blood cells contain hemoglobin, which makes bright blood red. More importantly, hemoglobin delivers oxygen from the lungs to the entire body; then it returns to the lungs with carbon dioxide, which we exhale. Healthy hemoglobin levels vary by gender. Low levels of hemoglobin may indicate anemia.

Normal Range: 13.7 - 17.5

Hematocrit % - Hematocrit (Hct)

Useful for diagnosing anemia, this test determines how much of the total blood volume in the body consists of red blood cells.

Normal Range: 39.0 - 55.0

MCV fl - Mean Corpuscular Volume (MCV)

This test measures the average volume of red blood cells or the average amount of space each red blood cell fills. Irregularities could indicate anemia and/or chronic fatigue syndrome.

Normal Range: 80.0 - 102.0

MCH pg - Mean Corpuscular Hemoglobin (MCH)

This test measures the average amount of hemoglobin in the typical red blood cell. Results that are too high could signal anemia, while those too low may indicate a nutritional deficiency.

Normal Range: 25.0 - 35.0

MCHC g/dl - Stands for Mean Corpuscular Hemoglobin. It is the average concentration of hemoglobin in the red blood.

Normal Range: 31.0 - 37.0

RDW-CV % - This is a test that measures the size and volume of your red blood cells. If the red blood cells are too large, it could indicate a health problem.

Normal Range: 11.0 - 16.0

Platelet Count - These are tiny blood cells to help the body form clots to stop bleeding. If your platelet count is low, it could indicate a wide range of health problems.

Normal Range: 150 - 420

MPV fl - (mean platelet volume) - is a measurement of the average size of platelets in the blood.

Normal Range: 9.4 - 12.4

Neutrophil - is a measurement of the number of neutrophil Granulocytes in the blood. Neutrophils are a type of white blood cells.

Normal Range: 1.90 - 8.00

NRBC - (nucleated red blood cells) -Is a blood cell that has a nucleus. If NRBC is found in the circulation of the blood could indicate severe disease.

Normal Range: 0.00 - 0.12

Neutrophil % - This test measures the percent values in the blood.

Normal Range: 40.0 - 76.0

Immature Granulocytes % - Immature Granulocytes are white blood cells that only are present when there is an infection or an indication of infection in the bone marrow.

Normal Range: 0.0 - 1.0

Lymphocyte % - Measures the percentage of lymphocytes, which are white blood cells that would include B-cells, T-cells, and NK cells. A low percentage could indicate HIV-AIDS or bone marrow failure. A high percentage could indicate a viral infection, leukemia, or lymphoma.

Normal Range: 20.0 - 44.0

Monocyte % - Measures the percentage of monocytes, which are white blood cells that move from the blood into the tissues where they become macrophages.

Normal Range: 5.0 - 13.0

Eosinophil % - Measures the percent of eosinophils which are white blood cells that fight parasitic infections.

Normal Range: 0.0 - 6.0

Basophil % - Measures the percentage of a type of white blood cell basophil, which helps with allergy responses.

Normal Range: 0.0 - 2.0

Lymphocyte - Measures a type of white blood cells made in your bone marrow, some lymphocytes will enter the bloodstream, and the majority of the lymphocytes will go through the lymphatic system to become T-cells while a small amount will stay in the bone marrow where they become B-Cells.

Normal Range: 1.40 - 4.80

Monocyte - Measures a type of white blood cells made in the bone marrow, which circulate in the bloodstream for 1 to 3 days and then move into tissues where they become macrophages and dendritic cells.

Normal Range: 0.10 - 0.80

Eosinophil - Measures a type of white blood cell that helps fight parasitic infection, cancer, and allergic reactions.

Normal Range: 0.00 - 0.50

Basophil - Measures a type of white blood cell that helps with allergy responses.

Normal Range: 0.00 - 1.00

Chemistry Panel (metabolic test) (CMP)
This test looks at the chemistry of the blood.

- ***Albumin*** - measures the protein in the blood. Normal range: 3.9 to 5.0g/dL
- ***Alkaline phosphatase*** - measures levels of this enzyme in the blood (ALP) if the levels are abnormal could indicate a problem with the liver, bones, or gallbladder. Normal range: 44 to 147 IU/L
- ***ALT*** - (alanine aminotransferase) is an enzyme found in the liver. If liver cells are damaged, they release ALT into the bloodstream. If the ALT levels are high, it can indicate that you might have a problem with the liver. Normal range: 8 to 37 IU/L
- ***AST*** - (aspartate aminotransferase) is an enzyme found mainly in the liver as well as in the muscles. If the liver is damaged, it will release this enzyme (AST) high levels of AST in the blood could indicate hepatitis, cirrhosis, mononucleosis as well as other liver diseases and problems with the heart and pancreas. Normal range: Normal range: 10 to 34 IU/L
- ***BUN*** - (blood urea nitrogen) is a test to give info on how the kidneys and the liver are functioning. Normal range: 7 to 20 mg/dL
- ***Calcium*** - 99% of your body's calcium is stored in your bones; the remaining calcium is in the bloodstream. The levels tested will indicate if the calcium is too high or too low. This could mean there are problems like bone disease, thyroid disease, kidney disease, or other ailments. Normal range: 8.5 to 10.9 mg/dL
- ***Chloride*** - This is a type of electrolyte. It helps balance the pH levels in the body. Normal range: 96 to 106 mmol/L
- ***CO2*** - (carbon dioxide) measures the amount of carbon dioxide in the blood. If too high or too low can indicate a potential problem like kidney disease, lung disease, and high blood pressure. Normal range: 20 to 29 mmol/L

- ***Creatinine*** - Is waste from your blood. It comes from the breaking down of proteins and muscles in the body. The kidneys remove it. High levels of creatinine could be a sign of kidney disease. Normal range: 0.8 to 1.4 mg/dL
- ***Glucose*** - This test measures glucose (sugar) levels in the blood. High blood glucose (hyperglycemia) levels can be a sign of diabetes; this can cause blindness, heart disease, kidney failure, and other health-related problems. Low blood glucose (hypoglycemia) levels can lead to brain damage and other health-related issues. Normal range: 100 mg/dL
- ***Potassium*** - This is a type of electrolyte that helps nerves to function and helps muscles contract. It also helps the heartbeat stay regular. It also helps offset sodium as it relates to your blood pressure. Normal range: 3.7 to 5.2 mEq/L
- ***Sodium*** - This is a type of electrolyte. If sodium levels are too high (hypernatremia) it can cause excess thirst, diarrhea, infrequent urination, and vomiting. If the sodium levels are too low (hyponatremia) it can cause confusion, fatigue, muscle twitching, and weakness. Normal range: 136 to 144 mEq/L
- ***Total bilirubin*** - Bilirubin is an orange-yellow pigment found in bile that is made by the liver. When bilirubin levels are high, it is an indication that the red blood cells are breaking down at an unusual rate or that the liver isn't breaking down the waste properly and removing the bilirubin from the blood. This test helps doctors diagnose bile duct and liver issues including cirrhosis, hepatitis, and gallstones. It can also help to diagnose if you have sickle cell disease. Normal range: 0.2 to 1.9 mg/dL
- ***Total Protein*** - This test measures the amount of albumin and globulin proteins in the body. Albumin protein helps to keep fluid from leaking out of the blood vessels. The globulin protein helps the immune system function properly. If the levels of this test are not in the normal range, it could indicate health problems

such as edema (swelling caused by extra fluid in your tissues), fatigue, and kidney or liver disease. Normal range: 6.3 to 7.9 g/dL

••• *Note: Electrolytes are minerals with an electrical charge that helps balance the chemicals in the body related to acids and bases.*

Cholesterol Test

The cholesterol test measures the different kinds of fats in the blood. Cholesterol is produced mostly in the liver. Our bodies need some fat, but too much bad cholesterol (LDL and triglycerides) in the blood is not healthy. Good cholesterol is called HDL, the HDL binds to the LDL and takes it back to the liver to be delivered to bile.

- ***Total Cholesterol*** - This test measures both LDL cholesterol and HDL cholesterol. Normal Range: <200 mg/dL
- ***LDL Cholesterol*** - (low-density lipoprotein) is named as BAD cholesterol, too much LDL can damage your arteries, and lead to heart disease. High LDL levels can also increase your risk of a stroke. Normal Range: <100mg/dL
- ***HDL Cholesterol*** - (high-density lipoprotein) named as GOOD cholesterol. It takes excess cholesterol out of the arteries to the liver where it can be sent to bile to be removed from the body. Normal Range: >60 mg/dL is best to help prevent heart disease.
- ***Triglycerides*** - are also known as lipids. Triglycerides are a type of fat that is found in the blood. Unused calories are converted to triglycerides and stored in your fat cells. When the body needs energy between eating hormones release triglycerides to be used. Fasting Normal Range: <150 mg/dL
- ***Cholesterol ratio*** - This is a ratio that divides HDL cholesterol into your total cholesterol. The lower the ratio indicates a lower risk of heart disease. Normal Range: 3.5 to 1

Other Blood Tests

- ***C - Reactive Protein*** - is a protein found in blood plasma. When levels rise indicates inflammation in the body. Normal Range: <1.0 mg/L
- ***HbA1c/Glycosylated hemoglobin*** - This test measures your blood sugar over weeks or months. Normal Range: <5.7%
- ***Homocysteine*** - This test is to find if there are deficiencies in B12 or folate. A doctor might order this test if the patient has had a heart attack or stroke. Normal Range: 4 to 14 umols/L

The blood is made up of:

- ***Red Blood Cells*** - carry oxygen throughout the body.
- ***White Blood Cells*** - help fight infections and pathogens.
- ***Platelets*** - cells that help stop bleeding when you get a cut.
- ***Plasma*** - is a liquid that carries nutrients, proteins, and hormones throughout the body.

HORMONES

Hormones play a lot of roles in the human body. In short, hormones are chemical messengers. The hormones are made in an organ and then travel through the bloodstream and body fluids to modify and control the functions of organs and tissues. If you have a hormone imbalance, it can cause several problems to your health, like growth development, sexual development, metabolic, and other bodily functions. Not getting the proper phytonutrients can alter the role of the hormone in our bodies.

A List of Some of the Hormones in the Human Body

ADIPONECTIN - is a protein hormone that is involved in regulating glucose levels as well as fatty acid breakdown. Also known as the fat-fighting hormone. It helps muscles use carbohydrates for energy and also helps increase your metabolism. Monounsaturated fats raise levels of Adiponectin which in turn helps to decrease belly fat.

ADRENALINE -This is the flight or fight hormone, which gives the ability to handle dangerous situations. Adrenaline is mainly produced by the adrenal glands and certain neurons. This hormone increases the blood flow to the muscles. This is done by binding to both alpha and beta receptors.

CORTISOL - This hormone is the stress hormone. Cortisol increases respiration blood pressure and muscle tension. Too much cortisol can cause an array of health problems. When the adrenal glands release cortisol, it causes the release of a lot of glucose into the bloodstream to act as instant energy to the large muscles. It will also cause insulin to be released so the glucose will be used and not stored. Scientists have stated for years that the release of cortisol can interfere with learning and memory. High levels of cortisol can cause weight gain, depression, heart disease, and more. The release of cortisol can also decrease bone formation. Cortisol has been shown to weaken the immune system by preventing the proliferation of T-cells. This hormone can also inhibit the formation of collagen.

DOPAMINE - This is the feel-good hormone, it tells the brain that this feels good and to repeat the things that make you feel good. Dopamine functions as a neurotransmitter, which is a chemical released by neurons to send signals to other nerve cells. It releases when having sex and when eating.

ESTROGEN - Produced mainly in the ovaries, is the primary female sex hormone and is responsible for the development and maintenance of the female reproductive system.

GASTRIN – This is a peptide hormone that stimulates the secretion of gastric acid (hydrochloric acid) from the stomach lining.

GHRELIN - This is the hormone in the gut that signals your brain to say you are hungry. People who have higher ghrelin levels tend to eat more, causing weight gain.

GLUCAGON - Produced in the pancreas, this hormone does the opposite of insulin. When blood sugar levels drop, this hormone breaks down the stored glucose and uses it for energy.

GROWTH HORMONE - The growth hormone is produced in your pituitary gland. This hormone is needed to help increase bone and muscle strength in women. Deficiencies in this hormone as a fetus can lead to dwarfism.

IRISIN - A hormone when it is released converts white fat cells into brown fat cells. This hormone is also called the exercise hormone. Research states that higher levels of irisin show a reduced risk of cancer, heart disease, and other age-related diseases.

INSULIN - This is a peptide hormone produced by the pancreas. It is needed to allow the body to use sugar from carbohydrates. It also keeps the blood sugar levels from getting too low or too high. *!!!!! Attention the primary role of insulin is to transport glucose out of the bloodstream and into tissues!!!!!!!!!!* Hopefully, this will help people understand that low-carb diets are bad for you in the long run.

LEPTIN - This hormone is produced in your fat cells and signals to the brain after you have been fed that you are satisfied and can stop eating. This is the opposite of the hormone ghrelin.

MELATONIN - This is a hormone made in the pineal gland and regulates sleep and wakefulness. There is research that states when melatonin is released cancer cell growth is suspended.

OXYTOCIN - This is the hormone that makes us feel closer to each other otherwise known as the bonding hormone. The more we touch, the more the release of this hormone.

PEPTIDE YY - This is the hormone produced in the small intestine and then released into the bloodstream that makes you full after you have eaten.

PROGESTERONE - This is a hormone that is a significant part of the menstrual cycle. This hormone rises after ovulation.

PROLACTIN - This is the hormone that triggers lactation and starts the breastfeeding process.

SEROTONIN - This is the mood hormone. It sends signals between your nerve cells. If levels of serotonin are too low, it can lead to depression. This hormone also helps with learning and memory functions, sleep, and digestion. Most of the serotonin is produced in the gut. A 2007 study showed that low levels of serotonin could lead to anxiety and insomnia.

TESTOSTERONE -This hormone is needed to help with your sex drive, and also helps with muscle strength and bone density.

THYROID HORMONES - The thyroid is responsible for the release of thyroxine (T4) and triiodothyronine (T3) to control your metabolism. There is research that shows some of the dyes can be harmful to thyroid functions.

The hormones listed above are only some of the hormones found in the human body.

Elevated IGF-1 Levels And Weight Gain

Insulin-like Growth Factor 1 (IGF-1) is a crucial hormone that plays a pivotal role in growth and development. While its role in promoting cellular growth and regeneration is well-established, an emerging body of research suggests a potential link between elevated IGF-1 levels and weight gain.

IGF-1, a peptide hormone structurally similar to insulin, is primarily produced in the liver in response to growth hormone stimulation. Its primary function is to stimulate cell growth and division throughout the body. While IGF-1 is essential for normal growth and development, excessive levels have been associated with various health issues, including the intriguing possibility of weight gain.

IGF-1 exerts its effects on metabolism through interaction with the insulin receptor and insulin-like actions. It promotes glucose uptake in peripheral tissues, enhances protein synthesis, and inhibits protein degradation. In the context of weight regulation, these actions could potentially contribute to increased fat deposition and overall weight gain.

Several studies have suggested a direct link between elevated IGF-1 levels and adipogenesis, the process of fat cell formation. IGF-1 promotes the differentiation of preadipocytes into mature adipocytes, leading to an increase in the number of fat cells. This proliferation of adipocytes may contribute to an overall increase in body fat mass.

IGF-1 has been shown to influence appetite regulation through its interaction with the central nervous system. In particular, it modulates the activity of the hypothalamus, a key brain region involved in appetite control. Elevated IGF-1 levels may disrupt the normal signaling pathways that regulate hunger and satiety, potentially leading to increased caloric intake and, consequently, weight gain.

While IGF-1 shares structural similarities with insulin, it also interacts with the insulin receptor. Elevated IGF-1 levels can lead to insulin resistance, a condition in which cells become less responsive to the effects of insulin. Insulin resistance is closely linked to obesity and weight gain, as it impairs the body's ability to regulate blood sugar levels and leads to increased fat storage.

Animal studies have provided valuable insights into the relationship between elevated IGF-1 levels and weight gain. Rodent models with genetically modified IGF-1 expression have exhibited increased adiposity and body weight compared to control animals. These findings suggest a direct influence of IGF-1 on fat accumulation.

Several clinical studies have explored the association between IGF-1 levels and body weight in human populations. Some investigations have reported a positive correlation, indicating that individuals with higher IGF-1 levels tend to have a higher body mass index (BMI) and increased adiposity.

The relationship between IGF-1 and other hormones involved in metabolism, such as leptin and ghrelin, adds another layer of complexity. Leptin, known as the "satiety hormone," regulates energy balance and inhibits hunger. Elevated IGF-1 levels may interfere with the normal functioning of leptin, leading to dysregulated appetite control and increased food intake.

The mechanisms through which IGF-1 influences adipogenesis, appetite regulation, and insulin sensitivity provide a plausible framework for understanding this relationship.

ENZYMES

Enzymes are needed for a healthy digestive system. Enzymes are used in more than 4000 different processes in our bodies. If you have an enzyme deficiency, it can lead to common digestive problems like IBS, bloating, constipation, diarrhea, acid reflux, and heartburn.

Enzymes are proteins that perform chemical functions in the body, like helping with the digestion of food, they help detox the blood, break down toxins, etc.

Classes of Enzymes in the body.

- ***Hydrolase*** - By adding water, this enzyme breaks down large molecules into simple molecules.
- ***Isomerase*** - A class of enzymes that helps facilitate the rearrangements of chemical bonds. Isomerase helps break down carbohydrates.
- ***Kinase*** - This is an enzyme that helps catalyze the transfer of phosphate groups from high energy.
- ***Ligase*** - Catalyze the joining of two large molecules by forming a new chemical bond.

- ***Lyase*** - This is an enzyme that catalyzes the breaking of chemical bonds, other than hydrolysis.
- ***Oxidoreductase*** - Is an enzyme that catalyzes the transfer of electrons from one molecule.
- ***RNA Polymerase*** (RNAP) - Is essential for all life. During the transcription process, it is responsible for the unwinding of the double helix of our DNA.
- ***Transferase*** - This is a class of enzymes that start the process that transferring a specific functional group from one molecule to another.

Food Enzymes

- ***Amylase*** - This is an enzyme that is in our saliva that catalyzes starch into sugars.
- ***Cellulase*** - Is an enzyme that breaks down cellulose molecules into monosaccharides — otherwise known as simple sugars.
- ***Lipase*** - This is an enzyme that catalyzes the hydrolysis of lipids (fats). Lipase plays a vital role in the digestion, transport, and processing of lipids in most living organisms.
- ***Pepsin*** – This is an enzyme that breaks down proteins into polypeptides in the stomach.
- ***Protease*** - Is an enzyme that aids in digesting long-chain proteins into shorter fragments by splitting peptide bonds that link to amino acid residues.

You need enzymes to maintain a healthy life. Cooking raw foods can destroy the enzymes needed. Dangerous chemicals, drugs, and toxins can become inhibitors that block the enzymes from working correctly.

If you have an enzyme deficiency and it goes unattended, it can lead to:

- *Bloating*
- *Chronic Fatigue*
- *Circulatory Problems*
- *Colitis*
- *Crohn's Disease*
- *Diabetes*
- *High Blood Pressure*
- *High Cholesterol*
- *Hypoglycemia*
- *IBS*
- *Weight Gain/Loss*

The best way to ensure that you do not have an enzyme deficiency is to make sure you are getting raw fruit and vegetables daily. Remember that harmful chemicals can act as inhibitors. Meat and dairy have been shown to carry compounds that can act as inhibitors. Notice that the enzymes end with "ase."

The Impact Of Low pH On Human Body Functions

The pH level in the human body plays a critical role in maintaining homeostasis, influencing various biochemical processes essential for life. While the body's internal environment is intricately regulated to sustain a slightly alkaline pH, deviations toward acidity can have detrimental effects on cellular functions. The consequences of low pH in the human body, highlight the impact on physiological processes and the potential health risks associated with acidosis.

The human body maintains a delicate balance between acidity and alkalinity, with a normal pH range of 7.35 to 7.45 in the blood. This narrow range is crucial for enzymatic reactions, cellular communication, and the overall functionality of organs and systems. When this balance is disrupted, and the pH drops below the normal range, a condition known as acidosis occurs, presenting a myriad of adverse effects.

Enzymes, as biological catalysts, play a pivotal role in facilitating chemical reactions within the body. However, these enzymes are highly sensitive to changes in pH. In an acidic environment, enzymes can undergo denaturation, altering their structure and rendering them ineffective. This disruption in enzymatic activity can impede vital metabolic processes, leading to a cascade of physiological dysfunction.

Low pH levels can directly impact the respiratory and cardiovascular systems. In respiratory acidosis, the blood becomes overly acidic due to inadequate removal of carbon dioxide, leading to shallow breathing and impaired oxygen exchange. This not only affects cellular respiration but also places strain on the cardiovascular system, potentially resulting in arrhythmias and compromised heart function.

Acidosis can disrupt the balance of electrolytes, such as potassium, sodium, and calcium, essential for nerve conduction, muscle contraction, and fluid balance. As pH levels decrease, the concentration of hydrogen ions increases, leading to the displacement of essential electrolytes. This imbalance can trigger muscle weakness, and cramps, and, in severe cases, contribute to the development of conditions like rhabdomyolysis.

The skeletal system is intricately linked to the body's acid-base balance. In response to increased acidity, the body may leach calcium from bones to neutralize excess hydrogen ions. Prolonged acidosis can lead to demineralization of bones, increasing the risk of osteoporosis and fractures. This underscores the importance of maintaining optimal pH levels for overall bone health.

The nervous system is highly sensitive to changes in pH, and acidosis can manifest as neurological symptoms ranging from mild confusion to severe impairment. Brain function relies on precise pH levels for neurotransmitter release and signal transmission. Acidosis can disrupt these processes, leading to altered mental status, seizures, and, in extreme cases, coma.

Maintaining the appropriate pH level is essential for the proper functioning of the human body. Deviations towards acidity, resulting in conditions like acidosis, can have widespread and profound effects on enzymatic activity, respiratory and cardiovascular systems, electrolyte balance, bone health, and the nervous system. Understanding the consequences of low pH underscores the importance of lifestyle choices, medical interventions, and ongoing research aimed at preserving the delicate acid-base balance crucial for human health. When you follow the P53 Diet with the recipes on the website a low pH will be hard to achieve.

Metabolic Pathways

Metabolic pathways are sequences of chemical reactions that occur within a cell to regulate and coordinate the complex biochemical processes necessary for life. These pathways involve the conversion of molecules through a series of enzymatic reactions, resulting in the synthesis or breakdown of compounds. Metabolic pathways are crucial for the production of energy, the building and maintenance of cellular structures, and the regulation of various physiological functions.

There are two main types of metabolic pathways:

- **Anabolic Pathways:** These pathways involve the synthesis of complex molecules from simpler ones. Anabolic reactions typically require energy input. Examples include the synthesis of proteins from amino acids, the formation of DNA from nucleotides, and the production of complex carbohydrates.
- **Catabolic Pathways:** These pathways involve the breakdown of complex molecules into simpler ones, releasing energy in the process. Catabolic reactions are often associated with the generation of ATP (adenosine triphosphate), which serves as a primary energy currency in cells. Examples include the breakdown of glucose in cellular respiration and the degradation of fatty acids in lipid metabolism.

Metabolic pathways are interconnected and regulated to maintain the balance of cellular processes and respond to changing environmental conditions. Enzymes play a crucial role in catalyzing the specific reactions within these pathways, and the overall coordination of these pathways allows cells to adapt to varying energy demands, nutrient availability, and other factors.

The Role of Hydrogen

The human body utilizes hydrogen atoms in various essential ways, playing a crucial role in fundamental physiological processes. At the molecular level, hydrogen is a key component of many biomolecules, contributing to the structure and function of proteins, nucleic acids, and other vital compounds.

One primary role of hydrogen in the body is as a constituent of water (H2O). Water is the universal solvent and a fundamental component of all bodily fluids, including blood, lymph, and intracellular fluids. Hydrogen's presence in water is essential for the maintenance of proper cellular hydration, nutrient transport, and temperature regulation. Additionally, water participates in various biochemical reactions, influencing metabolic processes that are vital for sustaining life.

Hydrogen atoms also form an integral part of organic molecules, particularly in macromolecules like proteins and nucleic acids. Proteins, which serve as the building blocks of tissues and enzymes, consist of amino acids, each containing hydrogen in their chemical structure. The precise arrangement of hydrogen atoms within amino acids contributes to the three-dimensional structure and function of proteins, influencing cellular processes such as signaling, transport, and catalysis.

In nucleic acids, the genetic material of cells, hydrogen bonding is crucial. The double helix structure of DNA relies on hydrogen bonds between complementary base pairs (adenine-thymine and guanine-cytosine). This hydrogen bonding stability is paramount for the accurate transmission of genetic information during cellular replication and division.

Beyond these structural roles, hydrogen atoms participate in cellular respiration, a process crucial for generating energy. In the mitochondria, often referred to as the powerhouse of the cell, hydrogen atoms play a central role in the electron transport chain. During the breakdown of glucose, hydrogen atoms are stripped from molecules and carried by coenzymes such as NADH and FADH2. These hydrogen carriers donate electrons to the electron transport chain, ultimately facilitating the production of adenosine triphosphate (ATP), the cell's primary energy currency.

Hydrogen's involvement in cellular respiration extends to the synthesis of ATP through oxidative phosphorylation. The movement of hydrogen ions across the inner mitochondrial membrane generates a proton gradient, and as these protons flow back into the mitochondrial matrix through ATP synthase, ATP is synthesized. This process underscores the indispensable role of hydrogen atoms in energy production, sustaining the various activities of cells and tissues.

Hydrogen atoms also contribute to maintaining the body's acid-base balance. The pH of bodily fluids is tightly regulated to ensure optimal enzymatic activity and overall cellular function. Hydrogen ions (H+) play a central role in this regulation. For example, in the blood, the bicarbonate ion (HCO3-) acts as a buffer, helping to neutralize excess hydrogen ions and prevent abrupt changes in pH that could be detrimental to cellular function.

In the nervous system, hydrogen ions are involved in neurotransmission. The movement of hydrogen ions across cell membranes influences the excitability of neurons, contributing to the generation and transmission of electrical impulses. This intricate interplay of hydrogen ions is essential for proper cognitive function and communication within the nervous system.

Hydrogen atoms are also crucial in the detoxification processes of the liver. The liver utilizes hydrogen to chemically modify and neutralize various toxins, making them more water-soluble and easier to eliminate from the body. This phase of detoxification, often involving enzymes like cytochrome P450, highlights the versatile role of hydrogen in maintaining the body's homeostasis and protecting it from harmful substances.

The body's utilization of hydrogen atoms extends across a spectrum of vital functions, from the structural integrity of biomolecules to the generation of energy, maintenance of pH balance, and detoxification. Understanding the many roles of hydrogen in the human body provides insights into the intricacies of physiological processes and underscores its significance in sustaining life.

Electricity in the Human Body

Electricity plays a crucial role in the functioning of the human body, orchestrating a complex symphony of signals that control various physiological processes. At its core, the generation and transmission of electrical signals in the human body are driven by the activity of specialized cells called neurons.

Neurons are the primary components of the nervous system, which includes the brain, spinal cord, and peripheral nerves. These cells are equipped with a unique property known as excitability. Excitability allows neurons to generate electrical impulses or action potentials in response to stimuli. These stimuli can be sensory inputs, chemical signals, or electrical signals from other neurons.

The basic unit of the nervous system is the neuron, and it comprises a cell body, dendrites, and an axon. When a neuron receives a stimulus, ion channels on its cell membrane open, allowing ions such as sodium and potassium to flow in and out of the cell. This creates a shift in the electrical charge across the cell membrane, resulting in a rapid change in voltage known as an action potential.

The action potential travels along the axon of the neuron, acting like a wave of electrical activity. At the end of the axon, the electrical signal triggers the release of neurotransmitters into the synapse, a small gap between the axon of one neuron and the dendrite of another. These neurotransmitters bind to receptors on the receiving neuron, transmitting the electrical signal from one neuron to the next.

This process of electrical transmission allows for the rapid communication and coordination of various bodily functions, including movement, sensation, and thought. In essence, electricity in the human body is the language of the nervous system, enabling the intricate and dynamic communication network that governs our physiological processes.

Krebs Cycle

The Krebs cycle takes place in the mitochondria of eukaryotic cells and is a crucial part of aerobic respiration. It involves a series of chemical reactions that result in the complete oxidation of acetyl coenzyme A (acetyl-CoA), a molecule derived from the breakdown of carbohydrates, fats, and proteins.

Key Steps of the Krebs Cycle:

- **Acetyl-CoA Formation:**
- The Krebs cycle begins when a two-carbon acetyl group combines with a four-carbon molecule called oxaloacetate, forming citrate. This reaction is catalyzed by the enzyme citrate synthase.
- **Decarboxylation Reactions:**
- Citrate undergoes a series of reactions involving isomerization and decarboxylation, leading to the release of two molecules of carbon dioxide. These steps are catalyzed by enzymes such as aconitase, isocitrate dehydrogenase, and alpha-ketoglutarate dehydrogenase.
- **Generation of Reduced Coenzymes:**
- As the cycle progresses, high-energy electrons are transferred to carrier molecules, NAD+ (nicotinamide adenine dinucleotide) and FAD (flavin adenine dinucleotide). These reduced

coenzymes, NADH and FADH2, carry the electrons to the electron transport chain for ATP synthesis.

- **ATP Synthesis:**
- GTP (guanosine triphosphate), which is structurally similar to ATP, is produced during the substrate-level phosphorylation step in the conversion of succinyl-CoA to succinate. One molecule of GTP can later be converted to ATP.
- **Regeneration of Oxaloacetate:**
- After completing the series of reactions, oxaloacetate is regenerated, allowing the cycle to continue. The final product of the Krebs cycle is not only energy-rich molecules but also a precursor for the next round of the cycle.

Importance of the Krebs Cycle:

- **Energy Production:**
- The primary role of the Krebs cycle is to generate energy in the form of ATP. High-energy electrons extracted during the cycle are used in the electron transport chain to produce ATP through oxidative phosphorylation.
- **Carbon Skeletons for Biosynthesis:**
- The intermediates of the Krebs cycle serve as precursors for the biosynthesis of various molecules. For instance, oxaloacetate can be used in gluconeogenesis to produce glucose, while other intermediates contribute to the synthesis of amino acids.
- **Reduction of Coenzymes:**
- The reduced coenzymes (NADH and FADH2) produced in the Krebs cycle play a crucial role in delivering high-energy electrons to the electron transport chain. This electron transfer ultimately leads to the production of a significant amount of ATP in the mitochondria.

Regulation of the Krebs Cycle:

Several factors regulate the Krebs cycle to ensure its efficiency and coordination with other metabolic pathways. The cycle is influenced by the availability of substrates, the concentration of products, and the presence of allosteric effectors. Enzymes within the cycle are also subject to feedback inhibition to prevent unnecessary energy expenditure.

In summary, the Krebs cycle is a pivotal component of cellular respiration, providing both energy and precursor molecules for various cellular processes. Its intricate series of reactions highlight the interconnectedness of metabolic pathways, emphasizing the remarkable efficiency with which cells extract energy from nutrients to sustain life.

Gluconeogenesis

Gluconeogenesis, a critical metabolic pathway in the human body, plays a pivotal role in maintaining blood glucose levels and ensuring a constant energy supply, especially during periods of fasting or low carbohydrate intake. The term "gluconeogenesis" literally means the synthesis (genesis) of new (neo) glucose. This intricate biochemical process enables the generation of glucose from non-carbohydrate precursors, such as amino acids, lactate, and glycerol.

Importance of Glucose:

- Glucose serves as a primary energy source for various tissues, particularly the brain and red blood cells. Maintaining glucose levels within a narrow range is crucial for sustaining normal physiological functions.

- **Location of Gluconeogenesis:**
    - Gluconeogenesis primarily occurs in the liver, and to a lesser extent, in the kidneys. These organs contain the necessary enzymes and substrates to carry out the sequence of reactions involved in gluconeogenesis.
- **Precursors for Gluconeogenesis:**
    - The precursors for gluconeogenesis include lactate, pyruvate, glycerol, and certain amino acids. These substrates enter the gluconeogenic pathway after being converted into intermediates such as oxaloacetate or phosphoenolpyruvate.

The Biochemical Steps of Gluconeogenesis:

- **Pyruvate Carboxylation:**
    - The process begins with the carboxylation of pyruvate to form oxaloacetate, catalyzed by the enzyme pyruvate carboxylase. This reaction occurs in the mitochondria.
- **Transport of Oxaloacetate:**
    - Due to the impermeability of the mitochondrial membrane to oxaloacetate, it is converted to malate, which can cross the membrane. Malate is then reconverted to oxaloacetate in the cytoplasm.
- **Phosphoenolpyruvate Formation:**
    - Oxaloacetate is further decarboxylated and phosphorylated to form phosphoenolpyruvate (PEP) by the enzyme PEP carboxykinase.
- **Conversion of Fructose-1,6-bisphosphate:**
    - Fructose-1,6-bisphosphatase catalyzes the hydrolysis of fructose-1,6-bisphosphate to fructose-6-phosphate, an irreversible step that bypasses glycolysis.

- **Formation of Glucose-6-phosphate:**
  - Gluconeogenesis continues with the conversion of fructose-6-phosphate to glucose-6-phosphate by glucose-6-phosphatase, another irreversible step.
- **Glucose Release:**
  - The final step involves the dephosphorylation of glucose-6-phosphate to release glucose, which can then be transported out of the cell to contribute to blood glucose levels.

Regulation of Gluconeogenesis:

- **Substrate Availability:**
  - Gluconeogenesis is influenced by the availability of precursors. High levels of lactate, pyruvate, glycerol, or certain amino acids can stimulate gluconeogenesis.
- **Hormonal Regulation:**
  - Hormones play a crucial role in regulating gluconeogenesis. Glucagon, released in response to low blood glucose, promotes gluconeogenesis, while insulin inhibits this pathway, favoring glycolysis.
- **Allosteric Regulation:**
  - Several enzymes involved in gluconeogenesis are regulated by allosteric effectors. For instance, fructose-1,6-bisphosphatase is inhibited by AMP and activated by ATP, reflecting the cell's energy status.
- **Transcriptional Control:**
  - Transcription factors, such as FOXO and CREB, modulate the expression of genes involved in gluconeogenesis in response to various signals, including hormonal cues.

Physiological Significance:

- **Fasting and Starvation:**
    - Gluconeogenesis is especially vital during fasting or starvation when glycogen stores are depleted. It helps maintain blood glucose levels to sustain energy-demanding processes.
- **Low-Carbohydrate Diets:**
    - When dietary carbohydrates are limited, gluconeogenesis becomes essential for providing glucose to meet the body's energy needs.
- **Tissue-Specific Needs:**
    - Certain tissues, like the brain, are highly dependent on glucose. Gluconeogenesis ensures a constant supply of glucose even when dietary sources are scarce.

Gluconeogenesis is a finely orchestrated biochemical pathway that allows the body to generate glucose from non-carbohydrate precursors. This intricate process is essential for maintaining glucose homeostasis, supporting energy-demanding tissues, and adapting to varying nutritional conditions. Its regulation by hormones, substrates, and allosteric effectors highlights its dynamic nature, illustrating the sophisticated mechanisms our body employs to ensure a constant and adequate energy supply. The study of gluconeogenesis not only deepens our understanding of fundamental biochemistry but also holds significant implications for addressing metabolic disorders.

Cellular Signal Transduction Processing And Nutrition

Cellular signal transduction is a complex and intricate process that allows cells to communicate with each other and respond to external stimuli. Nutrients play a crucial role in regulating and influencing this intricate signaling network, ensuring proper cellular function and maintaining overall organismal homeostasis.

At the heart of cellular signal transduction are signaling molecules, receptors, and intracellular signaling pathways. These pathways are responsible for transmitting information from the cell surface to the nucleus, where gene expression is regulated. Nutrients, including vitamins, minerals, and various organic compounds, serve as essential components in this process, influencing the efficiency and accuracy of signal transduction.

One key aspect of nutrient involvement in signal transduction is their role as co-factors and coenzymes. Many signaling molecules, such as kinases and phosphatases, require specific cofactors or coenzymes to function properly. For instance, certain vitamins like B vitamins function as coenzymes in phosphorylation reactions, a common mechanism in signal transduction. These reactions involve the addition or removal of phosphate groups, which can activate or deactivate proteins in the signaling cascade.

Additionally, minerals like calcium and magnesium play pivotal roles in signal transduction. Calcium ions, for example, act as secondary messengers, relaying signals within the cell. They bind to proteins like calmodulin, initiating a cascade of events that ultimately lead to a cellular response. Magnesium, on the other hand, influences the activity of various enzymes involved in phosphorylation and dephosphorylation reactions, affecting the overall signaling process.

Nutrients can directly influence the expression of genes involved in signal transduction. Certain vitamins, such as vitamin D, have been shown to modulate gene expression, including genes related to immune responses and inflammation. By regulating gene expression, nutrients can impact the production and activity of signaling molecules, receptors, and other components of the signaling pathways.

Omega-3 fatty acids, essential components of cell membranes, also play a role in signal transduction. They can affect the lipid composition of cell membranes, influencing the structure and function of membrane-bound receptors and signaling molecules. This, in turn, can impact the initiation and propagation of signaling cascades.

Nutrients in cellular signal transduction extend beyond direct involvement in biochemical reactions. They also contribute to the overall health and integrity of cells, ensuring that cellular membranes are functioning optimally.

It's important to note that deficiencies or imbalances in nutrients can have profound effects on cellular signal transduction. For example, vitamin deficiencies can impair the activity of enzymes involved in phosphorylation reactions, disrupting the normal flow of signals. Similarly, alterations in mineral concentrations can lead to aberrant signaling events.

Unlocking The Secrets Of Telomeres

In the amazing world of cellular biology, telomeres emerge as tiny but pivotal players, holding the key to the cellular aging process. These protective caps, situated at the ends of our chromosomes, bear the responsibility of preserving genetic information and maintaining the stability of our cells. As we explore the fascinating realm of telomeres, we uncover the mysteries surrounding their function and the groundbreaking research that sheds light on ways to enhance telomere length.

Imagine chromosomes as the instruction manuals for building and maintaining the human body. Telomeres function as the protective caps at the end of these manuals, preventing the fraying and deterioration of essential genetic information during cell division. With each round of cell division, telomeres naturally undergo shortening, serving as a cellular countdown clock.

When telomeres become critically short, cells can no longer divide, leading to cellular senescence or apoptosis (programmed cell death). This process is a fundamental aspect of aging and contributes to the development of age-related diseases. Understanding the dynamics of telomeres opens a gateway to unraveling the mysteries of aging at the cellular level.

In the quest to extend the lifespan of cells, scientists have identified a remarkable enzyme called telomerase. Telomerase has the unique ability to add DNA to the ends of chromosomes, counteracting the natural shortening of telomeres that occurs with each cell division. While telomerase is active in certain cells, such as embryonic cells and certain immune cells, its activity is typically suppressed in most somatic cells after birth.

Research has shown that the reactivation of telomerase could potentially slow down or even reverse cellular aging. The research provides compelling evidence for the role of telomerase in cellular rejuvenation and suggests its potential as a target for anti-aging interventions.

As we navigate the realms of telomeres and aging, it becomes evident that lifestyle factors play a crucial role in influencing telomere length. Several studies have explored the impact of various lifestyle choices on telomeres, offering insights into how our daily habits may influence cellular aging.

- **Nutrition:** A study published in the *"Advances in Nutrition" in 2019 stated* " The growing number of articles published on diet and TL over recent years confirms the increasing interest in dietary anti-aging properties. Given that there is an existing link between oxidative stress and telomere attrition, it is plausible that consuming antioxidant-rich foods, for which edible plants are particularly well suited, may have important health benefits by helping to counteract telomere attrition."
- **Physical Activity:** Regular exercise has been linked to telomere maintenance and lengthening. A study published in the journal *"Preventive Medicine"* in 2017 showed that individuals who engaged in moderate to vigorous physical activity had longer telomeres compared to their sedentary counterparts. Exercise is thought to enhance the activity of telomerase and reduce oxidative stress, promoting telomere health.
- **Stress Management:** Chronic stress and its associated hormonal changes have been implicated in telomere shortening. Mind-body practices, such as meditation and yoga, have shown promise in mitigating the effects of stress on telomeres.

The Blood-Brain Barrier (BBB)

The blood-brain barrier (BBB) is a highly specialized and intricate system that regulates the passage of substances between the bloodstream and the brain. It plays a crucial role in maintaining the stability of the brain's internal environment, protecting it from potentially harmful substances while allowing essential nutrients to enter. Understanding the mechanisms of the BBB and the influence of nutrition on its function is essential for comprehending brain health and addressing various neurological conditions.

The BBB is formed by a layer of endothelial cells lining the capillaries in the brain. These cells are tightly packed together, creating a physical barrier that restricts the movement of molecules. Additionally, there are specialized structures known as tight junctions that further seal the gaps between these cells, preventing the free passage of substances. This selective permeability is essential for maintaining the delicate balance required for optimal brain function.

Nutrition plays a pivotal role in supporting the integrity and function of the blood-brain barrier. The composition of the diet can influence the structure of the BBB, impacting its ability to protect the brain from potentially harmful agents. Several nutrients have been identified as crucial for maintaining BBB integrity, and deficiencies in these nutrients can compromise the barrier's function.

1. **Omega-3 Fatty Acids:** Omega-3 fatty acids, particularly docosahexaenoic acid (DHA), are essential for brain health and the maintenance of the BBB. These fatty acids contribute to the fluidity of cell membranes, including those of the endothelial cells forming the BBB. Sources of omega-3 fatty acids include flaxseeds and walnuts.
2. **Antioxidants:** Antioxidants such as vitamins C and E play a vital role in protecting the BBB from oxidative stress. Oxidative stress can damage the endothelial cells and compromise the integrity of the barrier. Fruits, vegetables, and nuts are excellent sources of antioxidants that contribute to BBB health.
3. **Vitamin B Complex:** B vitamins, including B6, B9 (folate), and B12, are essential for the synthesis of molecules involved in maintaining the BBB. Deficiencies in these vitamins can lead to structural abnormalities in the barrier. Foods such as leafy greens, and legumes, are rich in B vitamins.
4. **Curcumin:** Curcumin, a compound found in turmeric, has anti-inflammatory and antioxidant properties that may help

protect the BBB. It has been studied for its potential to enhance BBB function and mitigate the effects of neuroinflammation.

5. **Polyphenols:** Polyphenols found in green tea, berries, and dark chocolate have been associated with improved BBB function. These compounds possess anti-inflammatory properties and may contribute to the maintenance of barrier integrity.

While proper nutrition is crucial for supporting the blood-brain barrier, it's important to note that other lifestyle factors, such as exercise and adequate hydration, also play roles in maintaining BBB health. Additionally, certain diseases and conditions can impact the BBB, highlighting the need for a holistic approach to brain health like the P53 Diet.

The blood-brain barrier serves as a vital guardian for the brain, regulating the passage of substances and maintaining a stable internal environment. Nutrition plays a fundamental role in supporting the structure and function of the BBB, emphasizing the importance of a well-balanced diet for optimal brain health. As research continues to uncover the intricate details of the BBB, the connection between nutrition and brain function becomes increasingly apparent, paving the way for new insights into neurological health.

Oxidative Stress

Oxidative stress is a physiological imbalance between the production of reactive oxygen species (ROS) and the body's ability to detoxify them, resulting in potential damage to biomolecules such as lipids, proteins, and nucleic acids. ROS, including free radicals and non-radical species, are natural byproducts of cellular metabolism and play crucial roles in various signaling pathways. However, when their production exceeds the cellular antioxidant capacity, oxidative stress occurs.

One major source of ROS production is the electron transport chain (ETC), a fundamental process in cellular respiration that takes place in the inner mitochondrial membrane. The ETC consists of a series of protein complexes, including NADH dehydrogenase (complex I), succinate dehydrogenase (complex II), cytochrome b-c1 complex (complex III), cytochrome c, and cytochrome c oxidase (complex IV). Electrons from donors, such as NADH and succinate, move through these complexes, ultimately reducing molecular oxygen to water.

During this electron transfer, some electrons leak prematurely, leading to the formation of superoxide radicals ($O2^{\bullet -}$) primarily at complexes I and III. Superoxide radicals can further generate other ROS, creating a cascade of reactive species. The process is regulated by the redox potential of electron carriers within the complexes and the presence of specific antioxidant enzymes.

Mitochondrial antioxidants, like superoxide dismutase (SOD), catalase, and glutathione peroxidase, help neutralize superoxide radicals and other ROS. However, when ROS production overwhelms these defenses, oxidative stress ensues. This phenomenon has been implicated in numerous pathological conditions, including neurodegenerative diseases, cardiovascular disorders, and cancer.

Beyond the mitochondria, other cellular components, such as peroxisomes, endoplasmic reticulum, and plasma membrane, also contribute to ROS production. Enzymatic and non-enzymatic antioxidants in the cytoplasm and extracellular space further counterbalance this oxidative load.

Oxidative stress induces damage through several mechanisms. Lipid peroxidation, initiated by ROS attacking unsaturated fatty acids in cell membranes, results in the generation of lipid peroxides and other toxic byproducts. Protein oxidation, involving modifications to amino acid residues, can impair protein structure and function. DNA damage can occur through direct attack by ROS or indirectly through oxidative stress-induced inflammation.

Chronic oxidative stress is implicated in aging and age-related diseases. It can modulate signal transduction pathways, leading to altered gene expression and promoting inflammation. Additionally, ROS can activate stress-responsive kinases, such as mitogen-activated protein kinases (MAPKs) and nuclear factor-kappa B (NF-κB), amplifying the inflammatory response.

Oxidative stress can induce mutations in cells through various mechanisms. Reactive oxygen species (ROS), which are generated during oxidative stress, can directly damage DNA. Here's how it typically happens:

- **DNA Base Modifications**: ROS can interact with DNA and cause modifications to its bases. For example, guanine, one of the DNA bases, is particularly susceptible to oxidative damage. This can result in the formation of modified bases like 8-oxoguanine.
- **Single-Strand Breaks (SSBs):** ROS can cause breaks in the sugar-phosphate backbone of DNA, resulting in single-strand breaks. Repair processes may introduce errors or mutations during the repair of these breaks.
- **Double-Strand Breaks (DSBs):** Prolonged or severe oxidative stress can lead to double-strand breaks in the DNA molecule. Incorrect repair of these breaks may introduce mutations.
- **Indirect Effects:** ROS can also indirectly contribute to mutagenesis by activating signaling pathways that influence cellular processes like proliferation and apoptosis. Dysregulation of these

processes can favor the survival and proliferation of cells with genetic mutations.

Accumulation of mutations in critical genes can lead to uncontrolled cell growth, a hallmark of cancer. It's important to note that while oxidative stress is a natural part of cellular processes, excessive and prolonged oxidative stress, as seen in conditions like exposure to certain environmental toxins, can increase the risk of mutagenesis and contribute to various diseases, including cancer.

Oxidative stress is a complex physiological phenomenon arising from the imbalance between ROS production and antioxidant defenses. The electron transport chain, a vital component of cellular respiration, plays a central role in ROS generation. Mitochondrial and cellular antioxidant systems work together to mitigate the detrimental effects of oxidative stress, but when overwhelmed, it contributes to the pathogenesis of various diseases. Understanding these processes is crucial for developing therapeutic strategies to manage oxidative stress and its associated disorders. Numerous studies have stated the importance of antioxidant-rich diets, including fruits and vegetables, in mitigating oxidative stress-related diseases.

Hair Growth Biochemistry Process

The chemistry of hair growth involves intricate cellular processes within the hair follicles.

Here's a concise overview:

- **Hair Follicle Structure:**
    - The hair follicle is a complex structure located in the skin.
    - The base of the follicle contains dermal papilla, a cluster of cells with blood vessels that nourish the growing hair.

- **Cell Proliferation and Differentiation:**
    - Hair growth begins with the proliferation of cells in the hair matrix, an actively dividing region in the hair bulb.
    - These cells differentiate into keratinocytes, the primary component of hair.
- **Keratin Synthesis:**
    - Keratinocytes produce keratin, a fibrous protein that forms the structural basis of hair.
    - Keratinization involves the hardening of cells as they move upwards through the hair follicle.
- **Melanin Production:**
    - Melanocytes, located in the hair bulb, produce melanin—the pigment responsible for hair color.
    - Two types of melanin, eumelanin (brown/black) and pheomelanin (red/yellow), contribute to various hair colors.
- **Hormonal Regulation:**
    - Androgens, particularly testosterone and dihydrotestosterone (DHT), influence hair growth.
    - Androgens bind to receptors on hair follicles, affecting the duration of the hair growth cycle.
- **Anagen, Catagen, and Telogen Phases:**
    - **Anagen (Growth):** The active phase where cells in the hair bulb divide rapidly, leading to hair elongation.
    - **Catagen (Transition):** A short phase involving the cessation of cell division and the detachment of the hair from the blood supply.
    - **Telogen (Rest):** The resting phase is when the hair is shed, and the follicle remains inactive before re-entering the anagen phase.
- **Blood Supply and Oxygenation:**
    - Adequate blood supply is essential for hair growth.

    - Blood vessels around the follicle deliver oxygen and nutrients, sustaining the metabolic processes required for hair formation.
- **Signal Transduction Pathways:**
    - Signaling pathways like Wnt/β-catenin play a crucial role in activating hair follicle stem cells, influencing the hair growth cycle.
- **Nutrient Supply and Oxidative Stress:**
    - Proper nutrition, including vitamins (e.g., vitamin C, B7, B6, B12, B9, E, A, D) and minerals (e.g., copper, iron, magnesium, selenium, zinc), supports healthy hair growth.
    - Oxidative stress, caused by free radicals, can negatively impact hair health.
- **Environmental Factors:**
    - External factors like UV radiation and pollutants can affect hair growth and quality.

Understanding these chemical processes provides insight into potential targets for interventions addressing hair loss or promoting hair health. Ongoing research aims to unravel more details of the intricate chemistry governing hair growth.

Heme vs Non-Heme

Heme iron and non-heme iron are two forms of dietary iron, and their differences lie in their chemical structures and sources. Iron is an essential mineral that plays a crucial role in various physiological processes, such as oxygen transport, energy production, and DNA synthesis. Understanding the distinctions between heme and non-heme iron is vital as they are absorbed and utilized differently by the human body.

Heme iron is found in animal-based foods, particularly in red meats, poultry, and fish. It is a component of hemoglobin, the protein in red blood cells responsible for transporting oxygen from the lungs to tissues throughout the body. The heme structure consists of a central iron atom bound to a porphyrin molecule, giving it a distinctive red color. This unique structure contributes to the characteristic color of red meat.

On the other hand, non-heme iron is present in both plant and animal-based foods but is more abundant in plant sources. It is not part of a hemoglobin structure but is typically bound to compounds like phytates and polyphenols. Unlike heme iron, non-heme iron is not inherently red in color. Plant-based sources of non-heme iron include beans, lentils, tofu, and spinach.

One significant difference between the two forms of iron is their bioavailability or the extent to which the body can absorb and utilize them. Heme iron has higher bioavailability than non-heme iron. The presence of heme iron in animal tissues allows for more efficient absorption in the small intestine. The body can absorb approximately 15-35% of heme iron, compared to only 2-20% of non-heme iron.

Several factors contribute to the enhanced absorption of heme iron. Heme iron is less affected by other dietary components that can inhibit or enhance iron absorption. For instance, substances like calcium and tannins, which are present in certain plant foods, can reduce the absorption of non-heme iron. On the contrary, heme iron is less influenced by these inhibitors and is more readily absorbed even in the presence of other dietary components.

Additionally, the body has specific mechanisms to regulate the absorption of heme iron based on its iron status. When iron stores are low, the absorption of heme iron increases, and when iron stores are sufficient, absorption decreases. This regulatory mechanism helps prevent excessive iron absorption and potential toxicity.

The differences in absorption efficiency also have implications for individuals with different dietary patterns. While individuals who consume a diet rich in animal products may have a higher intake of heme iron, those following a vegetarian or plant-based diet may rely more on non-heme iron sources. To enhance non-heme iron absorption from plant-based foods, it is recommended to consume vitamin C-rich foods alongside iron-containing meals.

Heme iron and non-heme iron differ in their sources, chemical structures, and bioavailability. Heme iron, predominantly found in animal-based foods, has a higher absorption rate due to its unique structure and is less influenced by other dietary components. Non-heme iron, present in both plant and animal-based foods but more abundant in plant sources, has lower bioavailability and can be affected by various dietary factors. Understanding these differences is crucial for individuals to optimize their iron intake based on their dietary preferences and nutritional needs.

Studies have suggested a potential link between heme iron consumption and an increased risk of cancer, research in this area is still ongoing.

One proposed mechanism for the association between heme iron and cancer involves the production of N-nitroso compounds (NOCs) in the digestive tract. These compounds are formed when nitrates and nitrites, which are commonly present in processed meats, react with amines and amides. Heme iron can enhance the formation of NOCs, and some NOCs have been identified as potential carcinogens.

Additionally, heme iron may contribute to oxidative stress and inflammation. The absorption of heme iron in the intestine is a complex process that involves the conversion of ferric iron (Fe^{3+}) to ferrous iron (Fe^{2+}). This conversion can generate reactive oxygen species (ROS), which are molecules that can cause damage to cells and DNA. Chronic oxidative stress and inflammation are known to be involved in the development of various diseases, including cancer as I stated earlier in this chapter.

The gut microbiota may play a role in the relationship between heme iron and cancer. Some studies suggest that certain bacteria in the gut can convert heme iron into potentially harmful metabolites. These metabolites may have pro-carcinogenic effects, contributing to the overall risk of cancer.

It's crucial to highlight that the evidence regarding heme iron and cancer is not uniform, and not all studies support a clear association. Additionally, other factors, such as an individual's overall diet, lifestyle, and genetic predisposition, can significantly influence cancer risk.

It is also stated the type of meat, cooking methods, and overall dietary choices may influence the impact of heme iron on cancer risk. For instance, processed and well-cooked meats may have different effects compared to lean, unprocessed meats.

While there is some evidence suggesting a potential link between heme iron and an increased risk of cancer, the relationship is complex and not fully understood. Ongoing research aims to provide a more comprehensive understanding of the mechanisms involved and the factors that may modulate this association. In the meantime, individuals are encouraged to maintain a balanced and varied diet, taking into account overall dietary patterns and lifestyle choices for optimal health.

Pharmaceutical Pills can Inhibit Normal Pathways

Pharmaceutical pills, while often designed to address specific health issues, can sometimes have unintended consequences on normal metabolic pathways within the body. The complexity of human physiology means that medications can interact with various biochemical processes, leading to alterations in normal metabolic functions. Understanding how pharmaceuticals can influence metabolic pathways is essential.

One common way in which pharmaceutical pills can impact metabolic pathways is through enzyme inhibition. Enzymes play a crucial role in catalyzing biochemical reactions, and many medications are designed to target specific enzymes associated with disease processes. However, these medications may also inhibit enzymes that are vital for normal metabolic functions.

For example, statins, a class of drugs commonly prescribed to lower cholesterol levels, function by inhibiting the enzyme HMG-CoA reductase. While this is effective in reducing cholesterol synthesis, it also disrupts the normal production of other essential molecules derived from the same pathway, such as coenzyme Q10. Coenzyme Q10 is involved in mitochondrial function and energy production within cells, and its depletion due to statin use has been associated with side effects like muscle pain and fatigue.

Another way pharmaceutical pills can impact metabolic pathways is by altering nutrient absorption. Some medications may interfere with the absorption of essential nutrients, leading to nutritional deficiencies that can disrupt normal metabolic processes. Proton pump inhibitors (PPIs), commonly prescribed for acid reflux, reduce stomach acid production. While effective in managing acid-related conditions, long-term

PPI use has been linked to decreased absorption of certain nutrients like calcium, magnesium, and vitamin B12. Deficiencies in these nutrients can impact bone health, neurological function, and overall metabolic balance.

In addition to nutrient absorption, pharmaceutical pills can influence metabolism through changes in hormone levels. Hormones act as chemical messengers that regulate various physiological processes, including metabolism. Some medications, such as corticosteroids used for inflammation or certain contraceptives, can disrupt the normal balance of hormones in the body. For instance, corticosteroids can lead to insulin resistance, affecting glucose metabolism and potentially contributing to conditions like diabetes.

Furthermore, pharmaceuticals may affect metabolic pathways by influencing the gut microbiota. The gut microbiota, a complex community of microorganisms in the digestive tract, plays a crucial role in nutrient metabolism and overall health. Antibiotics can indiscriminately target both harmful and beneficial bacteria in the gut. This disruption can impact the normal metabolic activities of the microbiota, potentially leading to gastrointestinal issues and alterations in nutrient metabolism.

It's important to note that the impact of pharmaceutical pills on metabolic pathways can vary widely depending on the specific medication, dosage, and individual factors. Genetic variations among individuals can also contribute to different responses to medications, influencing how drugs are metabolized and their potential side effects.

Pharmaceutical pills can influence normal functioning metabolic pathways through various mechanisms, including enzyme inhibition, nutrient absorption interference, hormonal changes, and alterations in the gut microbiota. Understanding these potential impacts is essential.

Detrimental Effects of Antibiotics on the Human Body

The widespread and often indiscriminate use of antibiotics has raised concerns about their potential detrimental effects on the human body. While antibiotics play a crucial role in treating bacterial infections, their impact on the body's delicate balance extends beyond the intended targets, leading to a myriad of side effects and potential long-term consequences.

One of the most significant ways antibiotics can damage the human body is by disrupting the delicate balance of the microbiome. The human body is home to trillions of microorganisms, collectively known as the microbiome, which play a crucial role in maintaining various bodily functions. Antibiotics, designed to target and eliminate harmful bacteria, can also decimate beneficial bacteria in the process. This disruption can lead to an imbalance in the microbiome, paving the way for opportunistic pathogens to thrive and cause further complications.

The overuse and misuse of antibiotics contribute to the development of antibiotic-resistant bacteria, posing a severe threat to public health. When antibiotics are used frequently, bacteria have a higher chance of developing resistance mechanisms, rendering these drugs ineffective. As a result, common infections become more challenging to treat, leading to prolonged illness, increased healthcare costs, and, in some cases, life-threatening complications. Antibiotic resistance is a global health crisis that demands a concerted effort to preserve the effectiveness of these crucial medications.

The microbiome plays a vital role in supporting the immune system, and its disruption by antibiotics can compromise the body's ability to defend against infections. Some studies suggest that alterations in the gut microbiota can lead to immune dysregulation, increasing susceptibility to various diseases. This weakened immune response may not only hinder the body's ability to fight off infections but also contribute to the development of autoimmune disorders and other immune-related conditions.

A common side effect of antibiotic use is gastrointestinal distress, including symptoms such as nausea, diarrhea, and abdominal pain. These symptoms occur due to the disruption of the balance between beneficial and harmful bacteria in the gut. The depletion of beneficial bacteria can create an environment conducive to the overgrowth of harmful bacteria, leading to inflammation and gastrointestinal discomfort.

Emerging research suggests that the impact of antibiotics on the microbiome may extend to long-term effects on metabolism. Altered gut bacteria composition has been associated with metabolic disturbances, including obesity and insulin resistance.

The disruption of the microbiome, increased antibiotic resistance, compromised immune function, gastrointestinal distress, and potential long-term effects on metabolism highlight the importance of understanding the damaging effects antibiotics have on the human body.

The Immune System

I remember when I was a kid, there were very few kids that were sick. Now go forward 40 or 50 years, and it seems that there are so many kids sick nowadays. I know what you are thinking, that I wasn't alive 40 or 50 years ago, but I was. The immune system is a very complex machine. Today it seems people react every time a person coughs the response is pouring chemicals down their throat. When in fact they are doing more harm to them. The immune system needs to learn how to handle pathogens. (See memory cells below). A chemical that can cause an immune reaction is known as an antigen. The response can either be an innate response or an adaptive response as described below. I can't cover everything about the immune system, but I can give you a brief overview. I will cover later in this book more on which whole plant foods help keep your immune system healthy. Young children and the elderly immune systems are more susceptible to pathogens.

The immune system is a very complex system that is divided into two main strategy types:

1. Adaptive Immunity (Acquired) - The adaptive immune is composed of B cells and T cells. The adaptive immune can remember the specific pathogen that has been encountered before. This immune is not passed down through DNA. Adaptive is developed during a person's lifetime. Adaptive immunity has memory. The adaptive immune response is slow for 1 to 2 weeks and fights only specific infections.

2. Innate Immunity - This is the first response to a foreign invader to our bodies that we were born with. Let's say you get a cut on your arm that allows bacteria to enter the body that will then activate the effector cells to release cytokines. Cytokines are a type of small proteins that aid in cell signaling. Cytokines are produced by a wide range of cells including immune cells like B and T lymphocytes, mast cells, and macrophages. The innate immune is composed of mast cells, natural killers (NK), macrophages, dendritic cells, basophils, eosinophils, neutrophils granulocytes. The innate immune system has no memory. The innate response is rapid and fights any foreign invaders.

When a pathogen attacks our body, the army inside begins its attack by the release of neutrophils at the point where the pathogens have entered the body. They try to engulf the pathogen and then destroy it. If the pathogen gets by the neutrophils, the macrophages are then signaled to help kill the pathogen. The macrophages will also send out signals to ask for help from other cells. Dendritic cells are out always seeking to find pathogens to destroy. The primary role of the immune system is to protect our cells from pathogens like bacteria, fungi, parasites, viruses, and toxins that have entered the body. According to experts, children do not have a fully developed immune system until they are

7 - 8 years old. You need proper nutrition to build a healthy immune system that includes vitamins A, C, and E and essential fatty acids. You should make sure that you get a daily dose of vitamin D. The best way of getting Vitamin D is outdoors in the sunlight. According to research having low levels of vitamin D has been associated with an increased risk of some autoimmune diseases like multiple sclerosis. Get outside more. When I was young, I wanted to play outside all day that's what we did. Nowadays parents have to beg and bribe kids to get them to play outside. Research has shown us that Omega 3 fatty acids play a role in helping our immune system. This research shows that people with low Omega 3 fatty acids have been associated with autoimmune disease.

Minerals such as copper, germanium, iron, manganese, magnesium, selenium, sulfur, and zinc are needed for a healthy immune. You need to have a healthy balance of zinc in your body. Zinc deficiencies can suppress the functions of the T-cells. Good sources of zinc include cashews, spinach, lentils, pumpkin seeds, quinoa, and garbanzo beans. Iron deficiencies have been shown to impair responses to antibodies. Garlic is another excellent choice for building your immune system.

Research also indicates that dairy brings toxins into your body that are harmful to your health. It is better for you to get these vitamins and minerals from whole plant foods. We also know that sugar has been shown to reduce white blood cell count. We know that processed foods can weaken the immune system. There has been research that shows that people who have taken beta-glucan (Yeast) and then exercise, show a boost in immunoglobulin A (IgA). Beta-glucan is the fiber found in yeast. IgA is an antibody that plays a crucial role in membranes that are in wet areas such as the eyes, nose, and mouth. In these studies, people have been shown to strengthen their immune system with yeast beta-glucans. People with Crohn's Disease should not eat yeast, based on the results of other studies.

Lymphoma is a type of cancer that is from having abnormal growth of B and T lymphocytes. There are two main types of lymphoma, Hodgkin's, and Non-Hodgkin's lymphoma. Doctors can tell the difference between Hodgkin's, and Non-Hodgkin's by examining the cancer cell under a microscope. They are looking for a specific type of abnormal cell called Reed-Sternberg cell if found it is classified as Hodgkin's Lymphoma. Meaning they are mainly derived from B lymphocytes. These cells have not gone through hyper-mutation to express their antibody. Hodgkin's Lymphoma has a strong incidence rate among males. It also has the ability to affect children. It is the 5th leading cancer in children. The exact cause of lymphoma is not yet known. Some of the risk factors include hepatitis B, and hepatitis C, inherited immunodeficiency. Other risk factors include chemicals like pesticides, herbicides, and benzene. See the chapter "Toxins" for a list and the harm they cause. Remember to wash fruit and veggies in warm water with sodium bicarbonate (baking soda) for 15 minutes then rinse with cold water. This process has been shown to remove a lot of unwanted pesticides from fruit and vegetables.

What are the Components of the Immune System?

- ***Mast Cells*** - Mast cells are associated with wound healing and defense against pathogens. They release a chemical alarm that alerts the body's other immune cells that the body is being invaded.
- ***Lymphocytes*** - Lymphocytes are a type of white blood cell found in the vertebrate immune system. B Cells, T Cells, and Natural Killers (NK) are lymphocytes found in the lymph node. Lymphocytes have a large nucleus and can be easily identified. They make antibodies that will attack bacteria and toxins in the body.
- ***Leukocytes*** - These are a type of white blood cell that identifies and then destroys pathogens.

- ***T Cells (lymphocytes)*** - T Cells are a type of white blood cell that is developed from stem cells and then mature in the thymus only about 2 percent of T cells make it to maturity. The rest of the rejected T cells are rejected because they might attack us.
- ***B Cells (lymphocytes)*** - These are a type of white blood cells that are produced in the bone marrow. B cells mature in the bone marrow. B cells are part of the adaptive immune system. B cells secrete antibodies
- ***Effector Cells*** - When activated produce antibodies that target a specific antigen. Effector cells are like a factory making an antibody just for a certain pathogen.
- ***NK Cells (lymphocytes)*** - Natural Killers (NK) cells don't attack the pathogens directly; they attack cells that have become infected and cause apoptosis of those cells. These cells are critical to the innate immune system.
- ***Pathogens*** - Pathogens are disease-causing organisms.
- ***Helper T Cells*** - A type of T cell mainly in the adaptive immune system helps other cell activity by releasing cytokines.
- ***Cytotoxic T-cells*** - They express T-cell receptors that can recognize a specific antigen.
- ***Monocytes*** - These are a type of white blood cell that travels in the blood then into tissue and then transfers into macrophages and dendritic cells.
- ***Cytokines*** - Cytokines are a type of small proteins that aid in cell signaling. Cytokines are produced by a wide range of cells including immune cells like B and T lymphocytes, mast cells, and macrophages.
- ***Macrophages*** - These are a type of white blood cell that engulfs and then digests cells and foreign substances that are not the body's healthy cells.
- ***Phagocytes*** - Engulf pathogens and then the enzymes inside break down the pathogens and discharge the remains.

- ***Basophils (granulocyte)*** - Basophils are a less common granulocyte type of white blood cells. Basophils produce histamine serotonin and heparin (Heparin is a blood-thinning substance to help prevent blood clots). Basophils are also thought to produce antibodies called immunoglobulin E (IgE). These can be higher than normal due to Crohn's disease, asthma, sinusitis, myelofibrosis, chickenpox, eczema, collagen vascular disease, and low progesterone.
- ***Neutrophils (granulocyte)*** - Are a white blood cell type that is the most abundant of white blood cells and is the first line of defense against inflammation caused by pathogens. These can be higher than normal due to stress, arthritis, rheumatic fever, myelogenous leukemia, infection, acute kidney failure, thyroiditis, and eclampsia.
- ***Eosinophils (granulocyte)*** - A type of white blood cell that controls mechanisms associated with allergy and asthma. They are developed in the bone marrow and then migrate into the bloodstream. If the eosinophil count is high, it could mean collagen vascular disease.
- ***The Lymph Node*** - This is a small bean-shaped organ that is part of the lymphatic system. The lymph node also stores a clear fluid called "lymph" which travels throughout the body carrying lymphocytes to help fight bacteria and toxins.
- ***Pathogens*** - A pathogen can be described as a microorganism such as a bacterium, fungus, prion, protozoa, or virus. Pathogens can commandeer valuable nutrients, enter tissue, colonize, and produce toxins. Pathogens cause great harm to our bodies.
- ***Dendritic Cells*** - These are a special type of macrophage. Dendritic cells are found in tissues that are exposed to the external environment like the skin and epithelial lining of the nose. These cell types are antigen-presenting cells. Dendritic cells engulf microbes and other kinds of invaders.

- ***Antibodies*** - These are also known as immunoglobulin (lg) and are a Y-shape protein. These antibodies are secreted and produced mostly by plasma cells. They detect an antigen and then respond by producing the antibodies that are specific to that antigen. The antibodies bind to those antigens and then activate a defense response that leads to the destruction of the pathogen. Some of the activated B cells stay in service as memory B cells. Our bodies contain millions of antibodies.
- ***Antigens*** - These are any foreign molecule that interacts with cells of the immune system and could invoke an immune response. Antigens are proteins, but they can also be carbohydrates, lipids, or nucleus acids.
- ***Parasites*** - A parasite is an infectious organism that relies on a host to obtain nutrients from the tissue and blood.
- ***Auto Immune Disorder*** - Our cells can also be attacked by rogue invaders from the inside of the body in the form of autoimmune disorders. This is where the immune system mistakenly attacks cells and organs inside the body because they thought they were foreign invaders. The immune system also fights against the body's cells that have changed due to illness or cancer. Keeping our inside army ready at all times to fight off attacks is a critical role. Rheumatoid Arthritis, Multiple Sclerosis, Pernicious Anemia, and Diabetes (Type 1) are examples of autoimmune diseases.
- ***Immunodeficiency*** - There are two types of immunodeficiency "Primary" and "Secondary." Primary immunodeficiency is a genetic condition otherwise known as germline. B lymphocyte deficiencies T lymphocyte deficiencies combined with B and T cell deficiencies or phagocyte deficiencies are primary. Secondary immunodeficiency happens due to medical conditions like cancer, or medication.
- ***Memory Cells*** - This system keeps a list of what is bad for our bodies so it can be called quickly if invaders strike again. These

are called memory cells. After the 1st attack, the memory cells remember the attack, and if there is a second attack, the immune system can respond quickly and in a more powerful way.

The reason I have listed parts of the immune system and what their roles are is to help you understand what is needed to make you healthy. These cells listed above all need nutrients to do their job. When there are deficiencies in the body, these cells cannot function properly and will not be at full strength to stop an attack from pathogens. When you eat animal products, you are also ingesting toxins into your body that the immune system will try to fight. Toxins are known to wreak havoc on the body's immune system. Studies have shown that consuming a high-fat diet can lead to your immune system decreasing the function of T lymphocytes.

Be responsible and think about what you are putting in your mouth. I want everyone to understand that putting harmful chemicals in your body can be very dangerous. I just read about two dozen babies in France being born without hands and arms. Also, some animals during this same timeframe were born with missing limbs. They have not found the exact cause of these mutations. The reason I point this out is that some of the chemicals in processed foods are harmful to humans in larger quantities, that's like saying it is okay to drink just a little gasoline. Keeping the immune system healthy gives you a higher chance of fighting off pathogens. Eat whole plant foods such as garlic, onions, and cabbage to name a few.

I could write a whole book about the human body, but this book I want to keep focused on the role of proper nutrition and how some chemicals in food cause the body harm. Having a lack of the proper nutrients in our bodies can start us down a very unhealthy path. We know through science that our bodies need the right amount of amino acids to code for proteins and enzymes to help protect and help our bodies without the high risk of diseases and cancer. After talking with parents while shopping for their families, most of those parents had no idea how harmful some ingredients are in processed foods these days. The reason I have taken the time to list the hormones, enzymes, blood work values, and the type of cells is to stress the importance of putting proper nutrition in your body. Everything listed above needs the proper nutrients to function.

7

Carbohydrates & Fiber

Carbohydrates play a crucial role in supporting proper brain function, and understanding the distinction between good and bad carbohydrates is essential for maintaining overall health. The brain, a highly metabolically active organ, relies heavily on glucose as its primary energy source, which is derived from carbohydrates. Here's an exploration of why carbohydrates are necessary for optimal brain function and a breakdown of the differences between good and bad carbohydrates.

To comprehend the significance of carbohydrates for the brain, one must first understand the body's energy metabolism. Carbohydrates are broken down into glucose during digestion, and glucose serves as the primary fuel for the brain. Unlike other organs, the brain has limited energy stores and cannot store glucose for long periods. Therefore, a continuous and sufficient supply of glucose is essential to support cognitive functions such as concentration, memory, and overall mental alertness.

Good Carbohydrates

Good carbohydrates, also known as complex carbohydrates, are composed of long chains of sugar molecules that take longer to break down. These carbohydrates are found in whole, unprocessed foods such as fruits, vegetables, legumes, and whole grains. The gradual release of glucose from complex carbohydrates provides a steady and sustained supply of energy to the brain, preventing spikes and crashes in blood sugar levels. This stable energy supply is crucial for maintaining focus and preventing fatigue, supporting optimal brain performance throughout the day.

Bad Carbohydrates

On the other hand, bad carbohydrates, often referred to as simple carbohydrates or refined carbohydrates, undergo processing that removes essential nutrients and dietary fiber. Examples of bad carbohydrates include sugary snacks, pastries, sodas, and white bread. These carbohydrates are quickly digested and lead to rapid spikes in blood sugar levels, followed by crashes. The erratic energy supply associated with bad carbohydrates can result in feelings of lethargy, difficulty concentrating, and mood swings.

Consuming a diet rich in good carbohydrates provides not only the necessary energy for the brain but also essential vitamins, minerals, and fiber. Whole grains, fruits, and vegetables contain nutrients such as B vitamins, which are crucial for brain health. Additionally, dietary fiber supports digestion and helps regulate blood sugar levels, contributing to overall metabolic health.

In contrast, a diet high in bad carbohydrates has been linked to various health issues, including obesity, type 2 diabetes, and cardiovascular disease. The rapid fluctuations in blood sugar levels associated with the consumption of refined carbohydrates can contribute to insulin resistance and inflammation, negatively impacting not only the body but also the brain.

Carbohydrates are essential for proper brain function, serving as the primary energy source for this metabolically active organ. Choosing good carbohydrates over bad ones is crucial for maintaining stable blood sugar levels, supporting cognitive function, and promoting overall health. Incorporating whole, unprocessed foods into the diet, such as fruits, vegetables, and whole grains, provides the brain with the necessary nutrients and sustained energy it needs to function optimally. Understanding the role of carbohydrates and making informed dietary choices can contribute to long-term brain health and well-being.

Keto Fog

Keto fog, often referred to as "keto brain fog," is a term used to describe a temporary cognitive state that some people may experience when transitioning to a ketogenic diet. The ketogenic diet is characterized by a significant reduction in carbohydrate intake, leading the body to enter a state of ketosis, where it primarily burns fat for energy.

The brain, accustomed to using glucose derived from carbohydrates as its primary fuel source, undergoes an adaptation period during the switch to ketones. This transition can result in symptoms collectively known as keto fog. Common manifestations include difficulty concentrating, mental fatigue, and a sense of clouded cognition.

The lack of carbohydrates, which are a quick and readily available source of energy, can contribute to these symptoms. While the brain is capable of utilizing ketones for fuel, the adjustment period may lead to a temporary decline in cognitive function.

Not so Sweet

Sweet is not so sweet! According to the USDA, the consumption of sugar has been steadily climbing to the tune of an average of 70 pounds of sugar per year per person in America. With those rates of consumption of sugar, it shouldn't shock anyone how obese people are these days. With type 2 diabetes on the rise, heart disease and cancer rates increasing and starting at younger ages now; we need to get a handle on this runaway train of ill health.

Some people think that consuming honey is healthy. This approach is very wrong. Researchers have found that honey can contain pesticides as well as glyphosate found in weed killers. A study done by Boston University showed that 59% of the honey that was sampled showed it contained higher levels of glyphosate.

In another study, honey was found to contain spore-forming microorganisms that can survive in honey at low temperatures. This study also found that honey was contaminated with Clostridium Botulinum. This 2012 study found that 25% of the honey products in the United States contained spores of Clostridium botulinum. Honey should not be a choice of sweeteners; this is due to the toxins found in honey. Researchers have stated that honey has also been found to contain things like antifreeze, motor oil, and other toxins.

Research done by Dr. Robert H. Lustig, M.D. Professor of Pediatrics Division of Endocrinology at the University of California, San Francisco has stated that the consumption of sugar has a very damaging effect. He has done excellent research on obesity in children and points to fructose as the problem. Fructose does not suppress the hunger hormone ghrelin. Not suppressing this hormone tells the brain I am still hungry. Acute fructose does not stimulate insulin or leptin. Not stimulating leptin means that there is no signal that tells the brain we are full. Therefore, we keep eating. We all should know by now the problems associated with High Fructose Corn Syrup (HFCS). I would encourage all parents to take the time to look up Dr. Lustig's work on sugar and fructose. The metabolic pathways Dr. Lustig describes show the damage from fructose on children and the problems with obesity in the U.S. and around the world. Dr. Lustig stated that one of the problems with fructose is that it is seven times more likely than glucose to form Advanced Glycation End-Products (AGE's). Researchers have stated that the fructose found in fruit is NOT THE SAME as fructose found in industrial fructose like HFCS. Studies have shown that the industrial fructose has been shown to cause liver damage. Scientists have concluded that fruit fructose does not cause liver damage, this is linked to the fiber in the fruit, as well as the antioxidants and other needed phytochemicals. The fructose found in soft drinks is very damaging to our health. Please note that fruit is GREAT for you.

One of the top products on the sugar consumption chart is soda pop and energy drinks. Most 12oz cans of soda pop contain about 10 tsp of refined sugar. Each teaspoon of sugar equals 4 grams; each gram of sugar is close to 4 calories, so one teaspoon of sugar equals 16 calories.

16 calories x 10 teaspoons of refined sugar = 160 calories in a 12oz can of soda.

Researchers have seen an increase in the consumption of sugary drinks. The average calorie intake from sugary drinks is around 226 calories per day for teens. This equals an estimated 10% of daily values of calories, which is equal to 1 or 2 cans of soda each day. The point I am trying to make here is the fact of how much sugar intake comes from soft drinks. Some people drink up to 4 cans of soda a day; this is bad for them. A recent study claimed that people who drank between two and six drinks with added sugar including soft drinks, fruit fruits, energy drinks, and sports drinks were 6% more likely to die during the course of the study. The people in this study who drank up to two sugar-sweetened drinks per day were 14% more likely to die during the course of the study. There have been multiple studies done on obesity and its relationship to consuming sugary drinks. Scientists have stated that the intake of sugary drinks increases the risk of obesity, diabetes, heart disease, and gout. We know that an increase in sugar also increases the amount of insulin that is released from the pancreas. When the pancreas slows down the production of insulin over time and can't produce enough insulin to keep blood glucose at normal levels, that is referred to as type 2 diabetes and when the pancreas stops producing insulin that is referred to as type 1 diabetes. Type 1 diabetes usually occurs in children and young adults. When glucose enters the bloodstream insulin is released, and insulin is needed to aid glucose to enter the cell to be used as energy for the cell.

Glucose and fructose are not the same. Glucose is a six-member ring, and fructose is a five-member ring. Glucose is an aldohexose. The glucose carbon atom is attached to a hydrogen atom by a single bond, and the oxygen atom is a double bond. Fructose is a ketohexose. The fructose carbon atom is only attached to the oxygen atom by a single bond.

Sugar is referred to as a simple sugar. Monosaccharides and disaccharides are known as sugars or simple carbohydrates.

Carbohydrates are divided into four groups:

- **Monosaccharides** - Simple sugar made up of 1 sugar. Examples are glucose, fructose, galactose, mannose, and ribose all are hexoses meaning they contain six carbon atoms.
- **Disaccharides** - 2 monosaccharides linked together is a disaccharide; table sugar is sucrose which is made up of 1 unit of fructose and 1 of glucose. Examples of lactose (milk sugar) are composed of glucose and galactose. Sucrose is a disaccharide as well as isomaltulose and trehalulose which are composed of fructose and glucose.
- **Oligosaccharides** - 3 to 10 monosaccharides linked together. Examples are raffinose, stachyose, and verbascose which are found in beans, cabbage, lentils, and whole grains.
- **Polysaccharides** - These are long chains of monosaccharides. Examples are starch (potatoes, pasta, rice), modified starches, glycogen, cellulose, and maltodextrins.

Processed sugar and its impact on oxidative stress have become subjects of growing concern in the field of nutrition and health. As our modern diets increasingly include high amounts of processed foods, which are laden with refined sugars, the implications for our well-being are coming under closer scrutiny. Oxidative stress, a physiological imbalance between the production of free radicals and the body's ability to counteract their harmful effects, is implicated in numerous chronic diseases. Emerging evidence suggests a strong link between the consumption of processed sugar and the promotion of oxidative stress within the body.

Processed sugars, particularly refined sugars like sucrose and high-fructose corn syrup (HFCS), are prevalent in a wide range of food products, from sugary snacks to sweetened beverages. Unlike natural sugars found in fruits and vegetables, the refined sugars used in processed foods undergo extensive processing that removes fiber, vitamins, and minerals, leaving behind empty calories. This refined nature makes them easily digestible, causing a rapid spike in blood glucose levels.

The connection between processed sugar consumption and oxidative stress lies in the metabolic processes triggered by excessive sugar intake. When the body metabolizes sugar, it generates reactive oxygen species (ROS) as byproducts. While the body has mechanisms to neutralize these free radicals under normal circumstances, excessive sugar consumption can overwhelm these defense mechanisms, leading to an accumulation of ROS. This imbalance can result in oxidative stress, causing damage to proteins, lipids, and DNA.

One significant contributor to oxidative stress associated with processed sugar is the increased production of advanced glycation end-products (AGEs). These are compounds formed when sugars bind to proteins or lipids without the controlling action of enzymes. AGEs can induce oxidative stress by promoting the generation of free radicals and triggering inflammatory responses. Over time, this can contribute to the development and progression of chronic diseases, including diabetes, cardiovascular diseases, and neurodegenerative disorders.

The impact of processed sugar on oxidative stress extends beyond its direct effects on cellular processes. High sugar consumption is often linked to obesity, insulin resistance, and metabolic syndrome – conditions that further exacerbate oxidative stress. Adipose tissue in obese individuals, for example, can produce inflammatory substances that contribute to oxidative stress. Additionally, insulin resistance, a common outcome of excessive sugar intake, may impair the body's ability to regulate oxidative stress effectively.

Scientific studies have provided compelling evidence supporting the association between processed sugar and oxidative stress. For instance, research has demonstrated increased markers of oxidative stress in individuals with high-sugar diets compared to those with lower sugar intake. Animal studies have also shown that diets rich in sugars can induce oxidative stress in various tissues, emphasizing the systemic impact of sugar consumption on redox balance.

The link between processed sugar and oxidative stress underscores the importance of dietary choices in maintaining optimal health. Reducing the intake of processed sugars, opting for whole and minimally processed foods, and emphasizing a balanced diet rich in antioxidants are essential steps in mitigating the adverse effects of sugar-induced oxidative stress. As our understanding of these connections continues to evolve, promoting awareness and making informed dietary choices become crucial elements in preventing and managing oxidative stress-related health issues.

Fiber

In the pursuit of a healthy lifestyle, dietary choices play a pivotal role. Among the various components that constitute a balanced diet, dietary fiber stands out as a crucial element that significantly contributes to overall well-being. Fiber, found in plant-based foods, is renowned for its numerous health benefits, ranging from digestive health to disease prevention.

Fiber is technically a carbohydrate that the body can't digest. Other carbohydrates are broken down into simple sugars. There are two types of fiber:

- **Soluble fiber** - Soluble fiber dissolves in water. This type of fiber has been proven to help lower glucose levels in the body. It also helps lower blood cholesterol levels. Examples of Soluble fiber include apples, berries, pectin in fruit, flax seeds, chia seeds, beans, peas, and Brussels sprouts.
- **Insoluble fiber** - Insoluble fiber does not dissolve in water. It also helps prevent constipation and keeps you regular by assisting foods in moving through your system. Examples of insoluble fiber: are brown rice, wheat, carrots, cucumbers, tomatoes, and legumes.

Dietary fiber refers to the indigestible parts of plant foods, such as fruits, vegetables, whole grains, legumes, and nuts. Unlike other components of food that are broken down and absorbed by the body, fiber remains largely intact as it passes through the digestive system. It is classified into two main types: soluble and insoluble.

Soluble fiber dissolves in water, forming a gel-like substance that helps regulate blood sugar levels and lower cholesterol. Sources of soluble fiber include oats, beans, fruits, and vegetables. On the other hand, insoluble fiber adds bulk to the stool, promoting regular bowel movements and preventing constipation. Whole grains, nuts, and the skins of fruits and vegetables are rich sources of insoluble fiber. Insoluble fiber, on the other hand, adds bulk to the stool, preventing constipation and promoting a healthy digestive system.

Dietary fiber plays a significant role in weight management and obesity prevention. Foods rich in fiber are often less energy-dense, meaning they provide fewer calories for the same weight compared to low-fiber foods. Additionally, high-fiber foods tend to be more filling, promoting a sense of satiety and reducing overall calorie intake. This can be particularly advantageous for those looking to maintain a healthy weight or lose excess pounds.

Numerous studies have linked a high-fiber diet to a reduced risk of cardiovascular diseases. Soluble fiber helps lower levels of LDL (low-density lipoprotein) cholesterol, often referred to as "bad" cholesterol, by binding to it and aiding in its elimination from the body. The overall effect is a healthier lipid profile, which is essential for cardiovascular health and the prevention of conditions like heart disease and stroke.

In addition to digestive and cardiovascular benefits, dietary fiber has been associated with a lower risk of various chronic diseases. Adequate fiber intake has been linked to a reduced risk of certain cancers, particularly colorectal cancer. The antioxidant properties of fiber-rich foods may also contribute to the prevention of chronic diseases by neutralizing harmful free radicals in the body.

One large-scale 2016 study stated that high intakes of fiber reduced the risk of breast cancer. When teenage girls ate more foods that were high in fiber, they lowered their chance of getting breast cancer as young adults. Fiber can also make you full when you eat, which will prevent you from overeating.

The best sources of fiber include broccoli, black beans, hummus, lentils, parsnips, pears, pistachios, prunes, and raspberries to name a few. Later in this book, I will show you how to plan your meals to make sure you get a balance of fiber and other nutrients daily.

When you go shopping in the grocery stores it is hard to read the labels to figure out what all this means, later in this book I will explain how to read the labels as well as what all those items on the label say. Just remember that most of the items mentioned above are sugars.

Sugar has also been known to cause systemic inflammation like joint pain. I think we all have had a sugar high a couple of times in our lives. This adds instant energy and then burnout. After we have felt the burnout a couple of times, we try not to feel it again.

The brain needs carbohydrates. Researchers have stated in multiple studies that children with a low carbohydrate diet also had lower IQs than children with a higher carbohydrate diet. In the chapter on *"Animal Products,"* I explain the difference between human breast milk and bovine milk. Well, one of the significant differences in human milk is that there are a lot more carbohydrates compared to cow's milk. This is because baby humans need more carbohydrates than baby cows. Young human brains need extra carbohydrates to develop.

If you are eating a lot of simple carbohydrates as defined in the chapter "SAD" you can create a quick rise in your insulin levels, which can cause a sharp drop in blood sugar (glucose). Then the low blood sugar levels signal that the body needs more energy by telling you to eat more. This can cause weight gain when insulin levels are high; the excess insulin wants to store fat.

We need to remember that all carbohydrates are broken down into simple sugars, then absorbed into the blood and cause the release of insulin. When a person has cancer the insulin receptors on the outside cell bind to the glucose and allow the glucose to enter the cell, when the cell is a cancer cell, it has more insulin receptors that can give more fuel (glucose) for that cancer cell to grow.

Fruits contain high amounts of dietary fiber as well as fructose, that will not cause alarming changes in the blood sugar level. Most fruits are listed as a "low glycemic index food." Natural sugars that are found in fruit are healthier than added sugars found in processed foods according to the American Heart Association.

What are the glycemic index and glycemic load?

A glycemic index (GI) tells us how fast the food you have eaten affects your blood glucose in 2 or 3 hours after eating. The GI uses a scale of 1 to 100 to rank the sugars in foods. The rankings are separated into three groups:

- LOW = 1 - 55
- MEDIUM = 56 - 69
- HIGH = 70 - 100

The processed foods that fall into the HIGH group should be removed from your diet. The glycemic index is focused on the quality of the carbohydrates in foods.

The glycemic load (GL) is a formula that is based on the glycemic index to tell us how much sugar is in our serving. Once you have the glycemic index of food, you then multiply it by the number of carbohydrates in your serving then divide it by 100.

Example 48 x 19(grams of carbohydrates) = 912/100 = 9.12 glycemic load.

Glycemic load scale

- LOW= 10 or less
- MEDIUM= 11 to 19
- HIGH = 20 or more

You also need to keep track of your portion size to get the right number from the glycemic index list; otherwise, it will throw off the glycemic load number.

Controlling your sugar is a task most find challenging. If you introduce good healthy whole plant foods into your diet early on, you will grow up not craving the sugar fix. That means saying no to all the sugary treats. You have to look closely at the labels to find all the hidden sugars. Scientists have found links between sugar and high LDL levels, high triglycerides, and lower HDL levels. A study published in the Journal of the American Medical Association (JAMA) states that people in the study who consumed the least amount of sugar had the lowest triglycerides levels and the highest HDL (good) cholesterol. Sugars can act like alcohol on the liver which can damage the liver. The risk of heart and kidney disease is high because high sugar levels can create high uric acid levels.

The bottom line is the human body needs sugar; the young brain needs carbohydrates to grow. But when you are consuming too much sugar, you become overweight and obese. People these days are not getting the right amount of exercise. When the body doesn't move it is not using the fuel for the cells, so it is stored as fat. It is a sad cycle of events that can lead to significant health problems for you. Keep a balance of natural sugar in the body with the right amount of exercise to burn the fat. I saw a TV commercial begging parents to get their kids outside and exercise for 30 minutes a day. When I was young, we played outside all the time even if it was raining or snowing. Our parents had to yell at us to get us to come inside. Your health depends on you making the right health decisions! Remember that the brain needs good-quality carbohydrates to function properly.

8

Fats & Proteins

Fats

Fats are described as evil in our society. According to the Centers for Disease Control (CDC) 65.2 of Americans are overweight or obese. This is based on a BMI (Body Mass Index) calculation. BMI is a calculation to see if you are overweight or obese. To get your BMI number:

1. Convert your height to inches.
2. Take the number in inches and multiply by the same number(example 72 x 72 = 5,184)
3. Multiply your weight by 703lbs(example 185 lbs x 703 = 130,055)
4. Then divide the two numbers 130,055/5,184 = 25.08 this is your BMI number. Now match the 25.08 to the chart.

BMI Chart

- Below 18.5 = Underweight
- 18.5 - 24.9 = Normal
- 25 - 29.9 = Overweight
- 30.0 + = Obese

As we can see this 25.08 number means that the person is just a little overweight.

This obesity thing is out of control, look at what is happening to our health. The reason I bring the BMI calculation up is that I want you to use this as a tool to check how you are doing as it pertains to being overweight. Check your BMI every two months. The problem with today's obese society is that there are too many bad foods and not enough plant-based foods in our bodies. As stated in earlier chapters obesity is the cause of an array of serious medical issues. In a recent study, it stated that a high-fat diet can lead to a decreased function of the T lymphocytes. A lot of people in the dieting community think that a low carb high-fat diet is the way to go. This is nonsense.

In the previous chapters, I have explained the sources that people on these types of diets are using to get high fat, and those sources like dairy and meats are NOT healthy sources. We know through science that, yes you can have weight loss, but the types of fat sources are a big problem. Your body can have weight loss from these types of diets, but in this process, you are exposing your body to oxidation, cancer, and many other issues. You can achieve the ideal weight just by eating a plant-based diet. It might not happen as quickly as you want, but it will happen. I have been doing this for years now, and I am healthier than I have ever been. These stupid diets that try to trick the body are unhealthy. Please do not expose any overweight or obese person to eating a low-carb high-fat diet unless for other medical reasons that your doctor states, meet their specific needs. Fat is one of the three macronutrients along with proteins and carbohydrates. Both children and adults need fats in their diets. Let's take a look at what a fat cell is.

Fat cells (adipocytes) are fat tissue that is found throughout the body. Fat contains 9 calories per gram. Fat cells can be small, or large. Fat is broken down into fatty acids and triglycerides. Triglycerides are formed when glycerol and fatty acids have a covalent bond with the three carbon atoms in glycerol via the carbonyl group. When these covalent bonds are broken down energy is released. Fats are needed for energy and in the brain.

Stored fat is most commonly found just below the dermis in the subcutaneous layer. Fat is sometimes stored in the liver as well as some small amounts in muscle. Males and females will store fat in different places in the body. Fats also carry toxins into the body; when your child consumes animal proteins, they are also ingesting toxins into their body as we know from the chapter *"Animal Products"* dairy and meat bring unwanted chemicals into our body. Some of these chemicals are very harmful.

Fat cells are programmed to store excess blood sugar as fat that can be used if needed. The fat cell is like a balloon that holds a droplet of fat. In the fat cell is a cytoplasm that takes up about 15% of the volume of the cell. There is also a small nucleus and a large droplet of fat. This will take up 85% of the fat cell volume. The most common type of fat found in the blood is triglycerides as stated in an earlier chapter. Triglycerides and cholesterol are both lipids (fat). Cholesterol is needed in the body in controlled amounts to produce hormones. There are three main types of lipoproteins 1. Low-density lipoproteins, also known as LDL (bad cholesterol). 2. High-density lipoproteins also known as HDL (good cholesterol). 3. Very Low-Density Lipoproteins also known as VLDL, there is no simple way to measure VLDL. VLDL is estimated as a percentage of the triglycerides value. Other types of lipoproteins that help transport fat to the cells are chylomicrons. Chylomicrons are made up of triglycerides and small amounts of protein and are the least dense of the lipoproteins. Another lipoprotein is Intermediate Density Lipoprotein (IDL). This lipoprotein is formed from the degradation of the Very Low-Density Lipoprotein (VLDL) as well as the High-Density Lipoprotein (HDL). Their role is to help fats and cholesterol to be transported in the water-based solution of the bloodstream. IDL will slowly be converted into LDL.

There are two kinds of fat cells in the body:

- **Brown Fat** - While brown fat is mainly found in newborn babies. Brown fat cells are smaller than white fat cells. The brown fat is significant for the newborn by making heat otherwise known as thermogenesis. Adults have very little brown fat or none at all.
- **White Fat** - White fat is the one that is needed for our metabolism by creating energy and also acts as a protective cushion for some organs.

Fat is broken down in the small intestine by the lipase enzymes into fatty acids and glycerol. Glucose is used as the source of energy for the body, and since only 5% of glycerol can be converted into glucose, the rest is stored as body fat.

Fatty Acids Defined:

- ***Saturated Fats*** - No carbon-to-carbon double bonds. Researchers have stated in an array of studies that saturated fats can lead to a host of medical problems.
- ***Unsaturated Fats*** - These types of fats are liquid at room temperature, they help improve HDL levels. HDL binds to LDL to be removed from the body. They also promote nutrient absorption.
- ***Monounsaturated*** - Contains one carbon-to-carbon double bond. Monounsaturated fats are found in plants like olives, avocados, and nuts and can lower the LDL in the body. Research shows that they can also reduce the risk of cancer and well as reduce the risk of inflammation.
- ***Polyunsaturated*** - Contains two or more carbon-to-carbon double bonds. Polyunsaturated fats are liquid at room temperature.

They are split into omega-3 and omega-6 fatty acids. These are essential fatty acids.

- ***Omega-3*** - Alpha-Linolenic Acid (ALA) - Eicosapentaenoic acid (EPA) is an omega-3 fatty acid that has 20 carbon atoms with five double bonds. EPA is needed for your mental. EPA is useful in other parts of the human genome like weight management, maintaining a healthy heart, and helping is discomfort in the joints. Docosahexaenoic acid (DHA) is an omega-3 fatty acid that has 22 carbon atoms with six double bonds. DHA is essential to the development of the young brain and helps with visual development.
- ***Omega-6*** - Linoleic Acid (LA) - Omega-6 plays a crucial role in the development of the brain and also promotes skin and hair growth.
- ***Trans Fats*** - Trans fats contain carbon-to-carbon double bonds in the form of trans instead of cis form. These are formed using a process called hydrogenation. They can also be found in small amounts in dairy and meat. Trans fats can raise LDL levels. As we know LDL is the bad cholesterol.

Despite some research reports that state saturated fats are not bad for you, I am still waiting for more research that isn't paid for by the industry. Meanwhile, if your kids consume a lot of unhealthy fat in their diet, their chance of becoming overweight and obese will be high. I know from my own experience the things I did to get my overall health in check. One of the things I did was decrease the number of saturated fats in my diet while keeping the proper amounts of unsaturated (omega-3 and omega-6 balance).

Proteins

What are proteins? Proteins are chains of amino acids. A protein has one or more long polypeptides. The polypeptide is a long chain of peptides covalently bonded together meaning that peptides have fewer than 50 amino acids. Polypeptides are formed during the process of translation where amino acids are coded for on the codons on the mRNA (messenger ribonucleic acid). The incoming tRNA (transfer ribonucleic acid) carries an amino acid to be used during the production of a protein at the ribosome. Transfer RNA is needed in the translation process of making a protein. Each codon in the mRNA codes for a specific amino acid in a particular protein. After amino acids are used to make proteins, the protein is then folded into a specific shape depending on the kind of protein it is. Most enzymes but not all are proteins. Some allergies happen because of a protein that has been folded the wrong way; the immune system can't produce antibodies for it because it does not understand the protein structure.

The main question I get all the time from people who know my lifestyle is "What do you do for protein?". That answer is pretty simple for me "fruit, vegetables, nuts, seeds legumes, and whole grains." We have been convinced that we need to get a lot of proteins in our daily diet and that the only real way to get proteins is through animals. This is so wrong! The other myth is that you need animal protein to build and maintain muscles. This is wrong as well. There are a lot of pro athletes and professional bodybuilders that are plant-based. Most of these pro athletes have stated that they perform better once they switch to a plant-based diet. I get all the protein I need, and I am not oxidizing on the inside and mutating genes, and I don't take any animal proteins. There has been a lot of research these days that has stated getting too much protein can harm you and your children. Recent studies show that having too much protein in the body can damage the liver and the kidneys. How much protein does a child need each day to grow and develop?

Remember proteins are a chain of amino acids that are bonded together. The big misconception is that you need animal proteins to get complete proteins. The term "complete protein" means that you are getting all essential amino acids from one source. But people fail to tell you that your body also ingests terrible chemicals that are harmful to you. So how can you get the right amount of amino acids in your body daily? You can manage this by combining foods that will get all the essential amino acids in their bodies all at the same time. You can achieve this if you give yourself plant-based proteins. Plant protein is by far the healthiest way to get the essential amino acids. A diet that is rich in leafy greens, fruit, legumes, and whole grains is the best way to achieve a healthy start. This is not hard to do I do it every day.

I make this fruit smoothie every week I combine three tablespoons of hemp powder with two tablespoons of flaxseed powder, with pineapple, cranberries, strawberries, and raspberries all of which are frozen, and then I add a freshly cut-up orange. I will add distilled bottled water that is more alkaline about 7.4pH. The body needs to be more alkaline than acidic. The three tablespoons of hemp powder that I add to my fruit smoothie each day contains all 20 amino acids including the nine essential amino acids (histidine, leucine, lysine, methionine, phenylalanine, threonine, tryptophan, and valine). Hemp powder also contains the essential fatty acids needed such as omega-3 and omega-6 at a 3:1 ratio. You can even get a hard-to-get gamma-linolenic acid (GLA). Research has stated that GLA helps people with obesity, ADHD, and a list of other health-related issues.

The takeaway you should get from the proteins is the fact that you need proteins daily to stay healthy. We also know that we need the right amount of proteins; otherwise, we can damage our bodies. We also know through science that we can achieve the right amount of proteins without the need for animal proteins. In earlier chapters, I stated that science had shown us how harmful animal proteins are to humans. In a later chapter, I will discuss how to get the right amount of proteins (amino acids) in your body.

The breaking down of proteins begins in the mouth. Your teeth chew to break down the food into small particles. Then the oral mucosa releases digestive juices. The salivary glands then secrete saliva that helps break down food into smaller pieces. The food is mixed with these juices to form a bolus. The smooth muscles of the digestive system contract in a peristaltic wave to help the bolus move down the digestive tract. Once in the stomach, the bolus is mixed with gastric juices (hydrochloric acid) from the lining of the stomach. The hydrochloric acid converts pepsinogen to pepsin. Pepsin is an enzyme that breaks down proteins into polypeptides in the stomach. The stomach lining also releases the enzyme protease. Protease is an enzyme that aids in digesting long-chain proteins into shorter fragments by splitting peptide bonds that link to amino acid residues. Once in the small intestine, two more enzymes are released trypsin from the pancreas, and peptidase to help break down proteins into amino acids that then enter the bloodstream to be used in other locations in the body.

Plant-Based Protein Replacements:
Black Beans
Chia Seeds
Chickpeas
Edamame
Flaxseed
Hemp Seeds/Powder
Green Peas
Kidney Beans
Leafy Greens
Lentils
Nuts
Pinto Beans
Quinoa
Seitan

Sunflower Butter
Sunflower Seeds
Tempeh
Tofu
Unsweetened Cocoa Powder

Remember that research studies have shown that too much protein can cause weight gain.

9

Animal Products

When I was 50 pounds overweight, the thing I loved to eat the most was ice cream. When I was driving to Portland, Oregon from Boise, Idaho to watch the Portland Trailblazers play, I would stop a couple of times along the way for gas and ice cream. This was my thing, and I just loved the taste of ice cream. Even while I was doing my research back then, I still was eating meat and dairy. Again, when I was researching, I heard both sides of the argument about whether dairy was good or bad for you. I can't believe that humans drink the breast milk of another species! That is so weird. Being raised that this was ok, really freaked me out.

The more I researched, the more I started seeing a pattern about some of the research on dairy. I noticed this pattern and it made me start thinking about the tobacco industry's tactics back in the day and how their messaging campaigns were meant to confuse the public about the health risks of smoking tobacco. Nowadays almost everyone is aware of the dangers of smoking; it is even printed on the side of the package of cigarettes. This made me start to rethink my eating habits. I had just gone through a divorce, and other unpleasant issues in my life and I thought this was a great time to regain my health. I am a very stubborn and passionate man when I am convinced about something I jump in with both feet. With all this excitement I had a game plan. I was going to start with cutting out all dairy and see what the difference would be. I decided to no longer consume any dairy products. That also meant that my trips to Portland would only be stops for gas, and now healthy treats. With my new plan underway, I was all excited. I was still eating meat at this point, but not that much at all. About three weeks into eating this way leaving out dairy, I started feeling a lot better.

Let me make something very clear; during this time, I was still eating fruits and veggies. I remember mountain biking on this same trail in Eagle, Idaho that I always ride on, and now without dairy in my body I have so much more energy, and I could breathe better. Before when I was climbing up this trail called "Twisted Sister" I would get out of breath. Now I was climbing it was a lot easier. I have always been very active, playing baseball and basketball. Before I cut out dairy, playing baseball was hard. I was running slowly, and I was out of breath quickly. Now after I stopped all dairy I could run faster, I started losing weight I could breathe so much better I was feeling great. I told myself I was never going back to the way I was. It was a couple more months after this that I started applying what I was reading in my research and I cut all animal protein for my diet. I now focus on eating healthy by making what I put in my mouth is what my body needs. I started focusing not on proteins so much, but on putting the right amino acids in my body daily. My world has changed for the better. I still eat ice cream the non-dairy type with a low sugar count. There are types of non-dairy ice cream at the grocery stores that are made from cashew milk, coconut milk, and soy milk, some of these are very good in taste and are healthy for you and the kids.

Back when I was eating animal proteins my cholesterol was over 277. Now my direct LDL cholesterol levels are under 100. I sleep so much better now. I am amazed that by cutting out animal proteins I can feel this way. I do have to take a supplement; I take vitamin B12 because I no longer eat animal proteins and the body needs vitamin B12. Vitamin

B12 used to be in the water supply, but nowadays we add chemicals to our drinking water that kill the B12 bacteria. I remember after ditching the dairy that wonderful feeling when I was going up "Twisted Sister" and hardly breaking a sweat. Now "Twisted Sister" seems so easy. What a difference in eating right can make. With this being said there are a lot of pro athletes that now do not eat any animal proteins and the results for them are amazing they say. Dairy does not do a body good. Those parents who have their kids in sports try cutting out all animal proteins in their diet and see the difference it can make. If you do make this switch, please be sure they get a daily dose of B12. They will also need to make sure they have the right amounts of amino acids in their bodies as I stated earlier in this book proteins are just amino acids that have been folded in a certain way. Later in this book, I will present ways to eat a healthy lifestyle and a daily plan to get the proper amino acids in your body.

Now let me get down to what are some of the major causes of ill health. It is what you eat, along with unhealthy lifestyle choices. When I was younger, my parents used to tell me to drink my milk by doing it I would have strong bones due to all the calcium in milk. I believed that statement for so long because why would someone lie about that? Well, I know the truth about that now thanks to all the research that has been done through the years. What about what my parents told me about how milk builds strong bones? Well, a study done by Harvard University titled The Harvard Nurse's Health Study says otherwise in this study they followed 72,000 women for 18 years and showed that no protective effect of increased milk consumption on fracture risk. This study showed that the women who consumed the most milk were more likely to suffer from a hip fracture than those who avoided milk consumption. Around the world, studies have shown us that countries with the lowest dairy consumption, like Africa and Asia, have the lowest rates of osteoporosis. The Inuit people have the highest rate of calcium on the planet they consume animal rich diet; they also have the highest rate of osteoporosis on earth. As parents, we need to take an intense look at the evidence science presents to us and ask ourselves "Do we want to be unhealthy and possibly get cancer?" Research has shown us that when young consume animal proteins as part of their regular diet, they have a higher risk of starting puberty and an earlier age. Too much calcium is not a good thing. WAKE UP, PEOPLE.

The Pitfalls of Dairy

Here are some of the things that the scientists are saying.

- **Aging** - Dairy has been known to cause inflammation and skin breakdown. The skin cells take 120 days to create new skin cells try leaving out dairy for 120 days and see how it can make a difference.
- **Asthma** - There have been multiple studies that have shown that dairy has been a trigger for asthma and other mucous-forming respiratory conditions. Many doctors and scientists have stated that dairy products are the leading cause of food allergies. Many cases of sinus infections and asthma have been managed or eliminated by removing all dairy products from their diets.
- **Autism** - Autism seems to be increasing these days. Scientists have linked BCM-7 from dairy cows to Autism in children. The people in one study seemed to aggravate the disorder when cow's milk was reintroduced back into their diet. They measured the peptides found in the urine and found increased levels of the peptides.
- **Prostate Cancer** - Research has found that dairy is one of the leading causes of Prostate cancer. One study done by Harvard Medical points to too much calcium being linked to advanced prostate cancer by suppressing vitamin D. In the 1980s a study was done with 27,000 Seventh Day Adventists in California the

study linked positively to milk consumption in prostate cancer mortality. An EPIC study showed that increasing dairy consumption by 35g per day also increased the risk of prostate cancer by 32%. Too much dairy calcium was found to be associated with this risk increase. Calcium from other food sources, however, was not associated with the increased risk. Other studies have been done on dairy products and their link to prostate cancer and found similar results.

- **Breast Cancer** - Research has found that dairy and IGF-1 levels play a critical role in women who get breast cancer. In these studies, it showed that increased IGF-1 levels increased the growth of cancer cells. There have also been reports that Soya has been linked to breast cancer, but the research that I have seen states that the isoflavones in soy can mimic estrogen and bind to estrogen receptors. In the human body, there are two types of estrogen receptors alpha and beta. The alpha receptor is the one that creates the problem. The beta receptor has been known to have a reverse effect. The soy isoflavones bind mainly to the beta estrogen receptor. Studies conducted with women in Asia countries that have the highest dairy consumption also have the highest cases of breast cancer. The soy consumption in Asia countries is high, but the women with the highest dairy consumption had the greatest risk of getting breast cancer.
- **Crohn's Disease** - Crohn's disease usually starts to develop between the ages of 16 - 30. Research has stated that one of the proposed factors is environmentally caused by an infectious bacterium called Mycobacterium Avium Paratuberculosis (MAP). This infection comes from livestock. It is also present in pasteurized milk. This MAP infection was reported in a 1991-2007 USDA Survey to be 68.1 %. This infection can survive the pasteurization of milk. There are multiple studies done to date that expose dairy as a contributing factor to Crohn's Disease. I will

cover this topic in my upcoming books that are targeted at adult women and men.

- **Multiple Sclerosis (MS)** - This is an autoimmune disorder which means the body attacks its own tissue. MS is scarring of the brain and the spinal cord the multiple means the multiple places it can happen. A study published in the Lancet in 1990 showed that the group that had less than 20mg of low-saturated fat diet at the early stages of MS, 95% of them had survived and were physically active for 30 years.
- **Diabetes** - Multiple studies have found evidence that when an infant child has been exposed to cow's milk (formula), it might trigger Type 1 diabetes. Other studies also have shown that when the mother is breastfeeding her child, if she was exposed to bovine casein that also increases the risk of her child getting Type 1 diabetes.
- **Allergies** - According to a Finnish study that stated a diet that is rich in saturated fats can lead to allergies. Another study states that the most common food allergy is that of cow's milk. Cow's Milk allergy can also lead to asthma, colic, eczema as well and ear infections in young children.
- **Colic** - Dairy has been linked to colic in infants. About 28% of infants suffer from colic in the 1st month.
- **Sudden Infant Syndrome** - A 2007 study states that bovine BCM-7 is a possible cause of sudden infant death syndrome.
- **Migraines**- Scientists have suggested that fluctuating hormones can cause migraines. Foods can trigger the migraine and dairy is one of the most common food products to be a factor. Fried and fatty foods were also factors.
- **Chronic Inflammation** - Dairy is known for being acid-forming. It is a highly inflammatory food second only to gluten. Inflammation is the cause of multiple health problems in the human body.
- **Chronic Digestive Problems** - Studies have shown that dairy can inflame the gut lining. It has been stated to be a factor in leaky gut

syndrome. This, in turn, can lead to autoimmune disease. Once dairy has been removed from people's diets, most stomach issues seem to go away.

- **Skin Problems** - Research has shown how dairy has been a factor in acne.
- **Child Constipation** - Dairy and anal fissures have been linked to constipation.
- **Obesity/Overweight** - Dairy has long been one of the causes of overweight and obese people because of the saturated fats that dairy brings into our bodies. People that overweight and obese can have many health-related problems. Saturated fats in your diet can come from milk, cheese, and other dairy products. A large-scale study of over 12,000 people showed that the people who drank the most milk also gained the most weight.

What is in Dairy?

What is the difference between bovine (cow) milk and human milk?

Well, let's start by stating the obvious *"Cow's milk is meant for baby cows"* and *"Human milk is meant for baby humans."* This is not too hard to figure out. Cow's milk is designed to meet the needs of a young calf. A young calf that is meant to add more weight than a baby human in the same timeframe needs more protein whereas human milk has more carbohydrates than cow's milk with fewer proteins. The fat in human milk is slightly higher than the cow's milk. If you have more milk proteins means that species has a faster growth rate. The fatty acid composition of 100g of whole cow's milk shows 2.5g of saturated fat, 1.0g of monounsaturated fat, and 0.1g of polyunsaturated fat. The human fatty acid breakdown of 100g of human milk has 1.8g of saturated fat, 1.6g of monounsaturated fat, and 0.5g of polyunsaturated fat. The unsaturated fat of human milk plays a vital role in the development of the human brain in young children. Infants need omega-3 and omega-6 to develop. Cow's milk does not contain the longer chain of these acids. Cow's milk also contains about 3.5 times the amount of calcium and twice the amount of sodium. Cow's milk has very little iron in it. Children under the age of 12 months need a good rich supply of iron. Cow's milk is also low in vitamin C, and vitamin D. This is why human milk, has the right amount of nutrients for human growth and cow's milk has the proper nutrients for a calf's growth.

- **Casein** - Casein is a protein that is found in dairy milk. The A1 and A2 proteins found in casein have caused quite a stir lately. I will discuss this in more detail in the next paragraph. Casein is 87% of the dairy cow's protein, and studies have shown us the link that casein promotes the cancer process.
- **IGF-1** - Stands for Insulin-like growth factor 1 which is a 70 amino acid polypeptide hormone that is produced primarily in the liver. IGF-1 in cows is exactly the same as human IGF-1, and the amino acids are in the same location in the chain as humans. The reason that dairy cows have higher IGF-1 levels is that cows have been injected with recombinant bovine somatotropin (rBST) to increase their milk production. This bovine hormone is not healthy for humans. There have been studies showing the link between high IGF-1 levels and a high risk of lung and prostate cancer. See the chapter *"The Human Body"* for more information on IGF-1 titled *"Elevated IGF-1 Levels and Weight Gain."*
- **Toxins** - Dairy brings toxins into a young child's body through the digestion of dairy. In the forms of pesticides and other chemicals that the dairy cows might have digested. These neurotoxins found in dairy can have a long-lasting effect. There have been studies that state that Polychlorinated Biphenyl (PCB) found in dairy products has been linked to Parkinson's Disease. See the chapter "Toxins" for more information on toxins.

A1 vs. A2 beta-casein arguments state that the A2 beta-casein protein is better for you than the A1 beta-casein protein. Regular milk contains both the A1 and A2 proteins. The A1 beta-casein protein is found in certain breeds of dairy cows that originated from Northern Europe. The A1 breeds are Ayrshire, British Shorthorn, Friesian and Holstein. The A2 beta-casein protein has a high level of A2 protein. The A2 breeds are Charolais, Guernsey, Jersey, and Limousin they originated from the South of France and the Channel Islands. There is only one amino acid difference between the A1 protein and the A2 protein. The claim is based on an A2 marketing program that states it is healthier than milk with the A1 proteins. Casein is broken down into casomorphins (BCM-7) when digested. Bovine casomorphins have been linked to multiple health-related issues in children and adults. Scientists have discovered that cow's BCM-7 has an opioid-like effect on the brain. Other studies showed that when human infants digest cow's milk and then convert to BCM-7, it shows a delay in psychomotor development and muscle tone. Human casomorphin has seven amino acids, Tyr-Pro-Phe-Val-Glu-Pro-Ile, while bovine casomorphins have a two amino acid difference. The bovine casomorphin has seven amino acids as well, Tyr-Pro-Phe-Pro-Gly-Pro-Ile. Bovine casomorphins act like morphine. The morphine-like effect on humans has been shown to interfere with opioid and serotonin receptors.

The 2011 study on the casomorphins from the stomach juices of humans found no difference between A1 milk and A2 milk. The early study showed that these tests were done on the digestion juices of pigs and cows. The bottom line here is cow's milk is meant for cows, and human breast milk is meant for infant humans. It's not hard to figure this one out. I know it is hard to try to keep dairy out of your diet. Dairy seems to be in everything. If you look around these days, you see a lot of non-dairy options. That should tell you that if there are so many non-dairy options a lot of people are starting to figure out how bad dairy is to your body.

The tide is changing regarding health concerns with dairy, one day while visiting my favorite coffee shop, Piccolo Caffe located in beautiful downtown Camas, Washington a very energetic and friendly gal Allie Janelle and I were talking about how many people have requested a dairy alternative over the last 4-to 5 years, she was telling me that there has been 50 to 60 percent change in the people that patron the coffee shop that have switched to alternative dairy products such as oat, soy, and almond milk. She posted a question to all her Facebook friends with the question of why people have switched to dairy alternatives. Listed below are some of the responses:

"Had to switch due to developing an allergy"

"Milk gives me migraines"

"It seems unnatural"

"Naturopath said I have an auto-immune disorder and milk and gluten make it worse"

"Didn't want my daughter getting 2nd hand hormones from cows' milk.."

"Milk gives me really bad heartburn and stomach issues"

"I'm allergic to dairy"

"I developed an allergic reaction to the casein in cows milk. It causes inflammation in my sinuses."

"I feel lighter and less sick when I stick to plant milk"

"Dairy upsets my stomach"

"I have used a variety of milk alternatives in an effort to discontinue cows milk because of digestive issues"

"I have not had cow milk in 16 years. I would never ever go back. It caused me to have acne and gastric issues."

As you can surmise from these statements people are starting to understand how they have been misled for many years on the damaging effects of dairy. Remember as I stated earlier, cow's milk is for baby cows, and human milk is meant for baby humans. Have you ever heard of giving baby calfs human milk? Sounds weird, doesn't it? I wonder what health issues would be in store for the baby calf getting more carbohydrates than proteins from drinking human breast milk.

There are great tasting and healthy choices that replace dairy, just make sure they don't contain any harmful food additives. Dairy is not needed for you to be healthy.

Meat, Eggs And Fish

When I was a young man both my parents worked to make enough money for my four other siblings and myself to have the things we needed in life. We did not have a lot of money, so when it came to buying food, my parents didn't have the extra money to buy a lot of meat. As I remember we only had a meat meal about once a week. With what I know now, I am thankful to my parents for not serving us meat too often. Most people these days are aware of the medical problems that come with eating meat. Some people have switched from eating red meat to eating chicken these days. Research has shown us how all animal proteins can harm our bodies. The misconception that has been out there for a long time is that we need animal proteins as the only real way to get proteins in our bodies. Which is not correct, I don't eat any animal proteins, and yet I get the right amount of amino acids that my body needs daily. As I stated in a previous chapter, proteins are amino acids that have been coded through RNA with transcription and translation processes and then folded in a certain way to be recognized by cell receptors as needed by the cells. The question is can you get the amino acids you need daily to maintain a healthy body? The answer is an overwhelming "YES." You do not need animal proteins to be healthy and develop. I eat each day, without any animal proteins in my body. My bloodwork is the healthiest it has ever been. It is so easy for us to stop at the local fast food place and get a fast meal. These meals lack the nutrients required for our bodies to be healthy and carry toxins that are harmful to them. Let's look at what the latest research says about the problems with humans eating animal proteins. The Department of Agriculture (USDA) states in a report that contaminated animal flesh causes 70% of food poisoning. Animal proteins can raise the risk of poisoning you by eating the bacteria that is contained in the animal's flesh. A study done by Consumer Report stated that 97% of raw chicken in grocery stores in the United States was contaminated with bacteria that could make you sick. A study done by Harvard University stated that one serving a day of red meat during the adolescent years was associated with a 22% higher risk of developing pre-menopausal breast cancer.

By now we have all heard about how processed meats are very unhealthy for our bodies, but yet everyday parents pack their kid's lunches with these harmful animal products. I don't understand why parents continue sending their children off to school knowing that processed meats have been linked to causing cancer. When I ask parents what scares you the most about your children's health? The thought of their children getting cancer was at the top of the list, but yet these were some of the parents that said a typical school lunch for their children including processed meats. I had a hard time trying to figure out if one of a parent's biggest fears was their child getting cancer, and yet they send them to school each day with foods that scientists have stated can cause cancer, why would parents do it?

A 20-year Harvard University study found that a 3-ounce serving of unprocessed meat a day was associated with a 13% greater chance of dying during the study. The study also found that a daily serving of processed meat, like hot dogs, bacon, lunch meats, etc. was associated with a 21% increased risk.

Antibiotics in Animal Agriculture

The use of antibiotics in animal agriculture poses a significant threat to human health, creating a cascade of harmful effects that extend from the farm to the dinner table. Antibiotics are routinely administered to livestock to promote growth and prevent disease in crowded and unsanitary conditions. However, the overuse of these drugs has dire consequences for human consumers.

Firstly, the widespread use of antibiotics in animals contributes to the emergence of antibiotic-resistant bacteria. These resistant strains can be transferred to humans through the consumption of contaminated meat, leading to infections that are difficult to treat. The use of antibiotics and hormones in animals has created a high risk to young children and adults, but again young children's immune systems are not fully developed.

Even if the bacteria themselves are killed during cooking, residues may persist, entering the human body and potentially disrupting the delicate balance of the microbiome. This disruption can compromise immune function and pave the way for the development of various health issues. Yet another reason to have a plant-based diet.

Meat was thought to be the only way for people to get the proper nutrients in their diets such as iron. This, of course, is not true. There are whole plant sources to achieve the iron requirements for us.

The best way for you to get the proper amount of iron is in non-animal foods such as broccoli, dark leafy greens, tofu, whole grains, legumes, nuts, dark chocolate, cocoa powder, dried fruit, and blackstrap molasses to name a few.

Meats

- **Red Meat** - Red meat has been linked in a lot of studies to be a significant factor in the probable cause of colon cancer. According to the World Health Organization and The International Agency for Research on Cancer (IARC) has classified red meat as a group 2 carcinogen, something that probably causes cancer. A study done by Karolinska Institute in Stockholm, Sweden stated that eating more than 100g of unprocessed meat a day increased the risk of advanced prostate cancer by 19% and bowel cancer by 17%. The risk of death from heart disease increased by 15% and breast cancer by 11%. One of the factors is that when you cook meats at high temperatures, it produces a carcinogen called heterocyclic amines (HCA). HCA's are formed from cooking the muscle of meats in beef, pork, poultry, and fish. When the muscles are cooked at a high temperature the amino acids, and a chemical in the muscle tissue called creatine react to heat creating heterocyclic amines. Research has shown that if you add garlic, fresh lemon juice, or olive oil you can cut the levels of HCA by as much as 50%. The National Cancer Institute has discovered through research a link between the consumption of cooked meats and stomach cancer. In other studies, breast cancer, colon cancer, and pancreatic cancer were associated with high consumption of meats that were cooked well. This included fried and barbecue meats. Red meats contain saturated fats.
- **Chicken** - Chicken is one of the top causes of saturated fats in our diet. Saturated fats can lead to multiple health problems. According to the FDA chicken that is sold in grocery stores across America is fed with inorganic arsenic. Arsenic is harmful to humans. Studies have shown that arsenic can be damaging to a developing brain. Arsenic is said to be about four times as poisonous as mercury. It builds up in the body over time. Cooking chicken at high temperatures also produces (HCA's). The FDA has shown

that their research has that arsenic has been added to chicken feed and ultimately ends up in the meat. Arsenic is a carcinogen. Poop from chickens has been fed to beef operations and is found in the tissue of the cows that people consume. The FDA has stated that farmers feed their cattle about 1 to 2 million tons of this chicken feces each year. This was back in 2009. I don't know if this is still happening today. Some are suggesting that an E.coli outbreak in the romaine lettuce from the Yuma, Arizona area may have been caused by a cattle operation that is next to a water canal where water is then used to water the lettuce.

- **Pork** - Pork has been given a Group 2 classification from the IARC as probably causes cancer. Pigs are home to parasites just like other animal species people eat.
- *Taenia solium* which is called the pork tapeworm grows to 9 plus feet long. This tapeworm can cause loss of appetite and tissue infection.
- *Trichinella* worm is found in undercooked meat of animals. It can be found in certain wild carnivorous animals such as bears or cougars and omnivorous such as pigs or wild boars.

Pork has an abundance of sulfur in the connective tissue of pigs which helps contribute to osteoporosis. Processed pork such as bacon has been classified as a Group 1 carcinogen that can cause cancer.

- **Turkey** - While turkey might be one of the less harmful meats, it still adds unnecessary cholesterol to the body. With any animal protein, you still have the risk of the turkey carrying pathogens into your child's body.
- **Processed Meats** - Hot Dogs, bacon, sausages, salami, ham, beef jerky, lunch meats like bologna. The World Health Organization and The International Agency for Research on Cancer (IARC) have classified processed meats as a probable carcinogen that can cause cancer. Processed meats have been linked in multiple studies

with an increased risk of death. Other studies have shown that the consumption of processed meats has been linked to increased risk of Heart Disease and Diabetes. The World Health Organization has stated that eating 50g of bacon a day can increase the risk of dying from heart disease by 24% and increase the risk of diabetes by 32% it also increases the risk of dying from cancer by 8%.

Eggs

A study done by Harvard University stated that a high intake of choline found in eggs was found to be associated with a higher risk of getting prostate cancer, they found it also increased the risk of dying from it. This study found one of the direct causes might be the choline in the eggs. Granted this does happen overnight. In the Harvard study, it stated that men who ate the most choline had a 70% increased risk of getting and dying from prostate cancer. A separate study came to the same conclusions, they found that men who ate 2.5 eggs or more per week had an 81% increased risk of prostate cancer. Choline is needed in the body, but too much seems to have a negative effect. Eggs have also been shown to increase the risk of women getting breast cancer; the study stated that women who eat more than five eggs a week have an increased risk of breast cancer.

While people are going both ways on the egg issue, most of the non-industry funded research points to the animal proteins in eggs are not the best source for proteins for children or adults. Because of the cholesterol and the increase of choline and the fact that eggs can bring pathogens into our bodies making it tough on the immune system to fight off the pathogens. The safest route to take for you to obtain proteins is still eating fruits, vegetables, legumes, and whole grains. I have studied nutrition and the effects it has on the body for about 17 years now. I have been my own research subject or guinea pig, and I know what the facts have been on my health. There are good doctors and bad doctors, good policemen and bad policemen, good teachers and bad teachers. Your role is to ask a lot of questions to protect your health. Ask for research reports from doctors that state some things are healthy. I had doctors say that processed meats aren't that bad, even when the World Health Organization lists processed meats as a carcinogen.

Research has shown us that high cholesterol plays a role in the development of certain cancers such as breast, colorectal, and prostate cancers. Studies have stated that the higher the egg intake, the higher the risk of breast cancer. Studies show that women with higher LDL have a link to higher breast cancer cell proliferation. They have found that oxidative cholesterol metabolite in the bloodstream called 27-Hydroxycholesterol (27-HC) has been shown to act like estrogen and cause breast cancer cell proliferation. This also has had the same proliferation in prostate cancer cells.

Fish

In the United States seafood is one of the leading causes of food poisoning.

I grew up hearing that fish was very good for you and that it helps make your skin healthy. While researching, I was beginning to see the truth about fish. Fish contain a variety of toxins, such as Polychlorinated Biphenyl (PCB), bacteria, and heavy metals such as methyl mercury. Methylmercury (MeHg) is acquired from bigger fish consuming smaller fish that consumed yet smaller fish in the food chain. The older the fish, the chances of more methyl-mercury are higher. The methyl mercury toxin is not soluble, so it builds up in the adipose tissue. We know that methyl-mercury can bioaccumulate in humans causing an array of medical problems such as shrunken brain disorder, kidney damage, cancer, and behavioral problems in children. Studies have shown that pregnant women should avoid certain types of fish that contain high amounts of mercury. Methylmercury is excreted into the breast milk. When you eat fish that contains mercury, it is then stored in the fat and stays in your body for many years. Scientists have stated that high levels of mercury have been shown to reduce motor skill coordination. See the chapter *"Toxins"* for information on mercury. The fish that contain the highest amounts of methylmercury are:

The Highest Levels of Methyl Mercury

- Tilefish
- Swordfish
- Shark
- King Mackerel
- Tuna
- Orange Roughy
- Marlin
- Spanish Mackerel
- Grouper
- Bluefish
- Sablefish
- Chilean Bass
- White Croaker
- Halibut

The Lowest Levels of Methyl Mercury

- Scallop
- Clams
- Shrimp
- Oyster
- Sardines
- Tilapia
- Salmon
- Anchovies

- Catfish
- Squid

Most people I talk to about fish only hear that fish contain healthy omega-3, and they don't hear about the levels of toxins that they contain. Young children and the elderly are the ones most at risk of the toxins in fish. You can get the required omega-3, and omega-6 your body need. You can achieve this by eating chia seeds, brussels sprouts, flax seeds, hemp seeds, and walnuts. Research has shown that salmon contains minimal amounts of methylmercury if you do choose to eat fish, ocean-caught salmon is better than farmed-raised salmon according to the researchers. No animal products of any kind are allowed in the P53 Diet. As you can see now, animal products bring unwanted health concerns to your body.

10

Cancer & Other Ailments

Cancer is a formidable adversary, not only for the individual diagnosed but also for their entire family. The repercussions extend across various facets of life, creating a complex web of challenges that are both emotionally and practically demanding.

Financial strain is one of the most palpable impacts of cancer on a family. The costs associated with medical treatments, medications, and frequent hospital visits can quickly escalate, burdening families with significant financial responsibilities. Even with insurance, out-of-pocket expenses, coupled with potential loss of income due to caregiving responsibilities, can lead to substantial economic distress. Families often find themselves navigating a delicate balance between securing the best possible care for their loved one and managing the financial strain that comes with it.

Emotionally, the toll of cancer is profound. The psychological impact is not limited to the patient alone but ripples through every family member. Fear, anxiety, and grief become constant companions as the family grapples with the uncertainty of the disease. Witnessing a loved one battle cancer can evoke a range of emotions, from helplessness to frustration, and the emotional strain can strain even the strongest familial bonds.

The professional realm is not immune to the ripple effect of cancer. A family member's cancer diagnosis often necessitates adjustments to work schedules, leaves of absence, or even a complete career shift for the caregiver. Balancing the demands of caregiving with professional responsibilities can lead to stress and job insecurity. The emotional toll from witnessing a loved one's suffering can further impact job performance, creating a challenging dynamic for the working member of the family.

Friendships, a source of support and comfort, can also be affected. While some friends may rally around the family during challenging times, others may find it difficult to cope with the emotional intensity of the situation. This divergence in responses can lead to strained relationships, making an already arduous journey even lonelier. The dynamic changes within social circles can result in a sense of isolation for the family, compounding the emotional challenges they face.

Hair loss is a visible manifestation of the toll cancer treatments take on the body. For many individuals undergoing chemotherapy, the loss of hair is a stark reminder of the battle against the disease. While the physical aspect of hair loss can be addressed with wigs or scarves, the emotional impact is profound. It alters one's self-image and can contribute to a sense of vulnerability, affecting not only the patient but also those close to them who witness these physical changes.

Energy loss is another significant variable in the cancer equation. Cancer treatments, particularly chemotherapy and radiation, often leave individuals fatigued and physically weakened. This depletion of energy has cascading effects on daily life, from simple tasks to maintaining social connections. The caregiver, too, experiences exhaustion as they navigate the dual responsibilities of caregiving and managing other aspects of family life.

Other variables in the cancer equation include disruptions to routine, lifestyle adjustments, and the strain on relationships. The daily rhythms of family life are inevitably disrupted by medical appointments, treatment regimens, and the unpredictability of the disease. Adjusting to a 'new normal' becomes a collective effort for the family. Lifestyle changes, such as dietary modifications and restrictions, can add an additional layer of complexity to an already challenging situation.

The impact of cancer on a family is multi-faceted and pervasive. From the tangible financial burdens to the intangible emotional toll, every aspect of family life is touched by the presence of this formidable adversary. Navigating these challenges requires resilience, support, and a collective commitment to weathering the storm. Cancer not only tests the strength of an individual but also the bonds that tie a family together. The best weapon against cancer is prevention. Choosing to live a healthy lifestyle has proven to lower the risk of getting cancer. As you have read by now in this book diet is the biggest part of living a healthy lifestyle, the other big part is keeping toxins (bad chemistry) out of your body. Our clients on the P53 Diet website have had great success with their cancer & other ailments when choosing to eat a plant-based diet. Listed below are types of common cancers and ailments.

Breast Cancer

Breast cancer is a malignant condition characterized by the uncontrolled growth of abnormal cells within the breast tissue. It is one of the most prevalent forms of cancer, affecting both men and women, although it is far more common in women. The disease can originate in various parts of the breast, including the ducts that carry milk to the nipple or the glands that produce milk.

The development of breast cancer is a complex interplay of genetic, hormonal, and environmental factors. While certain genetic mutations, such as BRCA1 and BRCA2, are known to increase the risk of breast cancer, most cases occur in individuals with no family history of the disease. Hormonal influences, particularly estrogen, play a crucial role, and factors like early menstruation, late menopause, or hormone replacement therapy can contribute to an elevated risk.

There are several types of breast cancer, classified based on the specific cells in the breast that become cancerous. Ductal carcinoma in situ (DCIS) involves abnormal cells in the lining of a duct but has not spread beyond it. Invasive ductal carcinoma (IDC) is the most common type, where cancer cells invade nearby tissues. Lobular carcinoma in situ (LCIS) is abnormal cell growth within the lobules, while invasive lobular carcinoma (ILC) is characterized by cancer cells spreading beyond the lobules.

Detecting breast cancer at an early stage is crucial for successful treatment. Regular screening methods, such as mammograms and self-examinations, can aid in early identification. Symptoms may include a lump in the breast or underarms, changes in breast size or shape, nipple changes, or skin alterations.

Colon Cancer

Colon cancer, also known as colorectal cancer, is a type of cancer that originates in the colon or rectum, which are parts of the large intestine. It is one of the most common forms of cancer worldwide and develops when normal cells in the lining of the colon or rectum undergo a series of genetic mutations that lead to the uncontrolled growth of cells.

These abnormal cells can form a mass or tumor, which, if not detected and treated early, can invade nearby tissues and spread to other parts of the body through the bloodstream or lymphatic system.

The cells involved in colon cancer are primarily the epithelial cells that line the inner surface of the colon and rectum. The large intestine plays a crucial role in the final stages of digestion, absorbing water and electrolytes from undigested food and forming solid waste. The inner lining, or mucosa, of the colon and rectum, is composed of epithelial cells, which are responsible for the absorption of nutrients and the secretion of mucus. When these cells undergo genetic mutations, they can transform into cancerous cells, initiating the development of colon cancer.

The most common type of colon cancer is adenocarcinoma, which arises from the glandular cells in the lining of the colon. These glandular cells produce mucus to lubricate the passage of stool through the intestines. Other less common types of colon cancer include carcinoid tumors, gastrointestinal stromal tumors (GISTs), lymphomas, and sarcomas. However, adenocarcinoma accounts for the majority of cases.

The development of colon cancer is often a slow process that begins with the formation of small, noncancerous growths called polyps on the inner lining of the colon or rectum. Over time, some of these polyps can undergo genetic changes, becoming cancerous. Not all polyps develop into cancer, but detecting and removing them early can significantly reduce the risk of colon cancer.

Risk factors for colon cancer include age, family history of colorectal cancer, personal history of colorectal cancer or certain types of polyps, inflammatory bowel diseases such as Crohn's disease or ulcerative colitis, and certain genetic syndromes. Lifestyle factors, such as a diet high in red and processed meats, a low-fiber diet, lack of physical activity, obesity, smoking, and heavy alcohol use, also contribute to an increased risk of developing colon cancer.

Symptoms of colon cancer may include changes in bowel habits, persistent abdominal discomfort, unexplained weight loss, fatigue, blood in the stool, and a feeling that the bowel does not empty completely. However, in the early stages, colon cancer may not cause noticeable symptoms, underscoring the importance of regular screening.

Colon cancer is a type of cancer that originates in the colon or rectum, with the primary cells involved being the epithelial cells of the intestinal lining. Early detection through regular screening and awareness of risk factors is crucial.

Prostate Cancer

Prostate cancer is a type of cancer that develops in the prostate, a small walnut-shaped gland in men that produces seminal fluid, the fluid that nourishes and transports sperm. It is one of the most common types of cancer in men, particularly in older individuals. While many prostate cancers grow slowly and may not cause noticeable symptoms for years, some can be aggressive and spread quickly.

The prostate is located just below the bladder and in front of the rectum. It surrounds the urethra, the tube that carries urine from the bladder and semen from the reproductive system out through the penis. The cells in the prostate gland undergo a controlled process of cell growth and division to replace old cells and maintain the normal functioning of the gland. However, when this process goes awry, cancer can develop.

Prostate cancer begins when normal cells in the prostate undergo changes in their DNA. These changes cause the cells to grow and divide at an accelerated rate, forming a tumor. The exact cause of these DNA changes is not always clear, but age, family history, and ethnicity are known risk factors. Men over the age of 50, those with a family history of prostate cancer, and African-American men are at a higher risk of developing prostate cancer.

The cells involved in prostate cancer are primarily the epithelial cells that make up the glandular tissue of the prostate. These cells are responsible for producing the fluid that combines with sperm to create semen. When these epithelial cells undergo genetic mutations, they can transform into cancer cells and initiate the development of a malignant tumor. Over time, if left untreated, these cancerous cells can invade nearby tissues and spread to other parts of the body through the bloodstream or lymphatic system.

Prostate cancer is often categorized based on its aggressiveness and how quickly it is likely to grow and spread. The two main types are localized prostate cancer, which is confined to the prostate gland, and advanced prostate cancer, which has spread beyond the prostate to other parts of the body.

Early-stage prostate cancer may not exhibit noticeable symptoms, making regular screenings, such as the prostate-specific antigen (PSA) test and digital rectal exam (DRE), crucial for early detection. As cancer progresses, symptoms may include difficulty urinating, blood in the urine or semen, erectile dysfunction, and pain in the back, hips, or pelvis.

Prostate cancer is a significant health concern for men, particularly as they age. Understanding the cells involved in its development, and the risk factors, is crucial for early detection. Regular screenings and awareness can play a pivotal role in improving outcomes for individuals diagnosed with prostate cancer.

Lung Cancer

Lung cancer is a devastating and often fatal disease characterized by the uncontrolled growth of abnormal cells in the tissues of the lungs. It is one of the most common types of cancer worldwide and is a leading cause of cancer-related deaths. Understanding the cellular basis of lung cancer is crucial for developing effective treatments and prevention strategies.

The cells involved in lung cancer are primarily epithelial cells, which line the airways and make up the majority of lung tissue. Lung cancer is broadly classified into two main types based on the histological characteristics of the cancer cells: non-small cell lung cancer (NSCLC) and small cell lung cancer (SCLC).

Non-small cell lung cancer (NSCLC) comprises about 85% of all lung cancer cases. The three main subtypes of NSCLC are adenocarcinoma, squamous cell carcinoma, and large cell carcinoma. Adenocarcinoma is the most common subtype and often originates in the peripheral lung tissue. Squamous cell carcinoma typically arises in the central airways, while large cell carcinoma is a less common and more aggressive subtype.

Adenocarcinoma is associated with the cells that produce mucus and other fluids, whereas squamous cell carcinoma involves the flat cells lining the airways. Large cell carcinoma is characterized by large, abnormal cells that can occur in any part of the lung. Each of these subtypes has distinct features, prognosis, and response to treatment.

Small cell lung cancer (SCLC) accounts for about 15% of lung cancer cases and is often characterized by the rapid growth of small, round cells. SCLC is strongly associated with smoking, and it tends to be more aggressive than NSCLC. This type of lung cancer is notorious for its tendency to metastasize early in the course of the disease, making it challenging to treat effectively.

The development of lung cancer is a multistep process involving genetic mutations that accumulate over time. Exposure to carcinogens, such as those found in tobacco smoke, is a major risk factor for these mutations. Mutations in specific genes, such as TP53, EGFR, and KRAS, are commonly associated with lung cancer. These mutations disrupt the normal regulation of cell growth and division, leading to the formation of tumors.

In addition to genetic factors, environmental exposures, such as air pollution, radon gas, and occupational exposures to asbestos and other carcinogens, contribute to the development of lung cancer. Early detection of lung cancer is challenging, as symptoms often do not manifest until the disease has reached an advanced stage.

Lung cancer is a complex and heterogeneous disease involving the uncontrolled growth of abnormal cells in the lungs. The cellular basis of lung cancer is intricately linked to genetic mutations and environmental exposures, with different subtypes exhibiting distinct characteristics.

Bladder Cancer

Bladder cancer is a type of cancer that originates in the tissues of the bladder, a hollow organ in the pelvic region responsible for storing urine. The development of bladder cancer is often associated with the uncontrolled growth of abnormal cells within the bladder lining. This condition can be classified into various types, with the majority of cases being urothelial carcinoma, also known as transitional cell carcinoma.

The bladder is composed of several layers, and urothelial cells, also called transitional cells, form the innermost layer of the bladder lining. These cells have the unique ability to stretch as the bladder fills with urine and contract when it empties. Urothelial carcinoma arises when the normal growth and repair mechanisms of these cells are disrupted, leading to the formation of cancerous tumors.

Several risk factors contribute to the development of bladder cancer. Smoking is one of the most significant risk factors, as it introduces harmful chemicals into the body, which are then filtered through the kidneys and concentrated in the urine. Chronic exposure of the bladder lining to these carcinogens increases the likelihood of cellular abnormalities and cancerous transformations. Other risk factors include advanced age, male gender (as men are more prone to bladder cancer than women), exposure to certain industrial chemicals, a history of chronic bladder irritation or inflammation, and a family history of bladder cancer.

The symptoms of bladder cancer can vary, but common signs include blood in the urine (hematuria), frequent urination, pain or a burning sensation during urination, and back or pelvic pain. It is important to note that these symptoms can also be indicative of other urinary tract issues, and a comprehensive medical evaluation is necessary for an accurate diagnosis.

Diagnosis of bladder cancer often involves a combination of a medical history review, physical examination, and various diagnostic tests. Urinalysis may reveal the presence of blood in the urine, while imaging studies such as CT scans or ultrasounds can help visualize abnormalities in the bladder. The definitive diagnosis is typically made through cystoscopy, a procedure in which a thin, flexible tube with a camera is inserted into the bladder to directly visualize and biopsy suspicious areas.

Prevention of bladder cancer involves lifestyle modifications such as quitting smoking, maintaining a healthy diet, staying hydrated, and minimizing exposure to occupational carcinogens. Regular medical check-ups, especially for individuals with risk factors, are crucial for early detection.

Bladder cancer is a complex condition involving the uncontrolled growth of abnormal cells, primarily urothelial cells lining the bladder. Understanding the risk factors, symptoms, and diagnostic procedures is essential for timely intervention and effective management of this disease.

Liver Cancer

Liver cancer, also known as hepatic cancer, is a type of malignancy that originates in the cells of the liver. The liver, a vital organ in the human body, plays a crucial role in various physiological processes, including metabolism, detoxification, and the synthesis of proteins. Liver cancer is a formidable disease characterized by the uncontrolled growth of abnormal cells within the liver tissue, often leading to the formation of tumors.

The liver is composed of different types of cells, and liver cancer can arise from various cell types. The majority of liver cancers, approximately 75-85%, are hepatocellular carcinoma (HCC). Hepatocellular carcinoma develops from hepatocytes, which are the main functional cells of the liver responsible for performing its diverse functions. These cells are susceptible to mutations that can trigger uncontrolled growth, leading to the development of cancerous tumors.

Apart from hepatocellular carcinoma, there are other types of liver cancer, albeit less common. Cholangiocarcinoma, also known as bile duct cancer, originates in the cells lining the bile ducts within the liver. Hepatoblastoma is a rare form of liver cancer that typically occurs in children under the age of 3 and develops from immature liver cells. Angiosarcoma and hemangiosarcoma are cancers that originate in the blood vessels of the liver.

The causes of liver cancer are multifactorial, and several risk factors are associated with its development. Chronic infection with hepatitis B or C viruses, excessive alcohol consumption, non-alcoholic fatty liver disease (NAFLD), cirrhosis, and exposure to certain toxins or chemicals are among the risk factors that can increase the likelihood of developing liver cancer. Genetic factors and underlying liver conditions may also contribute to the development of this malignancy.

Liver cancer often presents with few symptoms in its early stages, making it challenging to detect. As the disease progresses, symptoms such as unexplained weight loss, abdominal pain or swelling, jaundice, and changes in bowel habits may manifest. Diagnosis typically involves imaging studies, blood tests, and sometimes a biopsy to confirm the presence of cancerous cells.

Liver cancer is a formidable disease that can arise from various types of liver cells. Hepatocellular carcinoma, originating in hepatocytes, is the most common form.

Ovarian Cancer

Ovarian cancer is a type of cancer that begins in the ovaries, the female reproductive organs responsible for producing eggs and hormones such as estrogen and progesterone. It is one of the most common gynecological cancers and a leading cause of cancer-related deaths among women.

The ovaries are small, almond-shaped organs located on either side of the uterus. Ovarian cancer typically develops in the epithelial cells, which form the outer surface of the ovaries. These cells play a crucial role in the normal functioning of the ovaries, including the release of eggs during the menstrual cycle.

There are several subtypes of ovarian cancer, and they are classified based on the specific cells involved. The main subtypes include epithelial ovarian cancer, germ cell ovarian cancer, and stromal ovarian cancer.

- **Epithelial Ovarian Cancer (EOC):**
    - *Serous carcinoma:* This is the most common subtype of epithelial ovarian cancer, accounting for approximately 70-80% of cases. It typically originates in the cells lining the fallopian tubes and the surface of the ovaries.
    - *Mucinous carcinoma:* This subtype arises from cells that produce mucus and is less common, representing around 3-4% of cases.
    - *Endometrioid carcinoma:* Similar to mucinous carcinoma, endometrioid carcinoma is less common and often associated with endometriosis.
- **Germ Cell Ovarian Cancer:**
    - Germ cells are the reproductive cells that develop into eggs. Germ cell ovarian cancer is relatively rare and tends to occur in younger women. Examples include dysgerminoma, yolk sac tumor, and immature teratoma.
- **Stromal Ovarian Cancer:**
    - Stromal cells provide structural support to the ovaries and produce hormones. Stromal ovarian cancer is rare and

often diagnosed at an early stage. The most common subtype is granulosa cell tumor.

Ovarian cancer is challenging to detect in its early stages because symptoms may be vague and nonspecific. Common symptoms include bloating, pelvic or abdominal pain, difficulty eating, and a frequent need to urinate. Due to the lack of early symptoms, ovarian cancer is often diagnosed at an advanced stage, making it more difficult to treat successfully.

Several risk factors are associated with an increased likelihood of developing ovarian cancer, including a family history of the disease, certain genetic mutations (such as BRCA1 and BRCA2), age, and a history of hormone replacement therapy.

Ovarian cancer is a complex disease involving different cell types within the ovaries. Its diverse subtypes pose challenges in terms of early detection and effective treatment.

Melanoma

Melanoma is a type of skin cancer that originates in the cells responsible for producing pigment, known as melanocytes. These cells are primarily found in the skin but can also be present in other parts of the body, such as the eyes and mucous membranes. Melanoma is considered the most serious form of skin cancer due to its potential to metastasize, spreading to other organs and tissues.

Melanocytes produce a pigment called melanin, which gives color to the skin, hair, and eyes. The primary function of melanin is to absorb ultraviolet (UV) radiation from the sun, protecting the skin from its harmful effects. However, when melanocytes undergo malignant transformation, they can form cancerous growths known as melanomas.

The exact causes of melanoma are complex and involve a combination of genetic and environmental factors. Exposure to UV radiation from the sun or artificial sources, such as tanning beds, is a significant risk factor. Individuals with fair skin, light hair, and a history of sunburns are more susceptible to developing melanoma. Additionally, a family history of the disease or a personal history of atypical moles can increase the risk.

Melanoma often begins as a new mole or a change in the appearance of an existing mole. The ABCDE rule is a helpful guide for recognizing potential signs of melanoma:

A – ***Asymmetry:*** One half of the mole does not match the other.

B – ***Border irregularity:*** The edges are irregular, notched, or blurred.

C – ***Color:*** The color is not uniform and may include shades of brown, black, red, white, or blue.

D – ***Diameter:*** The mole is larger than the size of a pencil eraser.

E – ***Evolution:*** The mole is changing in size, shape, or color.

The cancerous transformation in melanoma occurs when the DNA in melanocytes is damaged, leading to uncontrolled cell growth. Mutations in certain genes, such as BRAF and NRAS, are commonly associated with melanoma development. As these mutated cells multiply, they can invade nearby tissues and spread to distant organs through the lymphatic system or bloodstream.

There are different types of melanoma, including superficial spreading melanoma, nodular melanoma, lentigo maligna melanoma, and acral lentiginous melanoma. Each type has distinct characteristics and growth patterns, influencing the prognosis and treatment approach.

Melanoma is a potentially deadly form of skin cancer originating in melanocytes. Various risk factors contribute to its development, with UV radiation exposure being a primary concern. The ABCDE rule helps individuals recognize potential signs of melanoma, emphasizing the importance of early detection.

Brain Cancer

Brain cancer is a complex and challenging medical condition characterized by the abnormal growth of cells within the brain. This devastating disease poses significant threats to both the structure and function of the central nervous system, often leading to severe health implications. To comprehend the intricacies of brain cancer, it is crucial to explore the types of cells involved and the mechanisms that drive their uncontrolled proliferation.

The human brain is an incredibly intricate organ composed of diverse cell types, each with distinct functions and responsibilities. The primary cell types implicated in brain cancer are glial cells and neurons. Glial cells, which include astrocytes, oligodendrocytes, and ependymal cells, play essential roles in supporting and nourishing neurons. These cells maintain the structural integrity of the brain, provide nutrients, and insulate nerve fibers. However, when these glial cells undergo malignant transformation, they give rise to gliomas, the most common type of primary brain cancer.

Gliomas are further classified based on the specific glial cell from which they originate. Astrocytomas arise from astrocytes, oligodendrogliomas from oligodendrocytes, and ependymomas from ependymal cells. These tumors can occur in various regions of the brain, leading to diverse symptoms and challenges in diagnosis and treatment.

The second major category of brain tumors involves cancer that originates from neurons. While less common than gliomas, neuronal tumors can still cause significant morbidity. Medulloblastomas, for instance, are malignant tumors that develop in the cerebellum and primarily affect children. These tumors arise from primitive neuroectodermal cells, which have the potential to differentiate into both neuronal and glial cell types.

The underlying cause of brain cancer is often attributed to genetic mutations that disrupt the normal regulatory mechanisms controlling cell growth and division. Environmental factors, exposure to certain chemicals or radiation, and genetic predispositions can contribute to the development of these mutations. Once these alterations occur, the affected cells evade the body's natural control mechanisms, leading to uncontrolled proliferation and the formation of tumors.

The symptoms of brain cancer can vary widely depending on the location, size, and type of the tumor. Common symptoms include persistent headaches, seizures, changes in vision, coordination difficulties, and cognitive impairments.

Non-Hodgkin Lymphoma (NHL)

Non-Hodgkin lymphoma (NHL) is a type of cancer that originates in the lymphatic system, a vital component of the body's immune system. The lymphatic system includes lymph nodes, spleen, thymus, and bone marrow, and it plays a crucial role in maintaining fluid balance, filtering harmful substances, and producing immune cells. Non-Hodgkin lymphoma encompasses a diverse group of blood cancers that involve the uncontrolled proliferation of lymphocytes, a type of white blood cell.

Lymphocytes are a key part of the immune system, responsible for identifying and eliminating foreign invaders, such as bacteria, viruses, and abnormal cells. In NHL, these lymphocytes undergo malignant transformations, leading to the formation of cancerous cells. Unlike Hodgkin lymphoma, which is characterized by the presence of specific abnormal cells called Reed-Sternberg cells, non-Hodgkin lymphoma is a heterogeneous disease with various subtypes, each characterized by distinct features and behaviors.

The two main types of lymphocytes involved in NHL are B lymphocytes (B cells) and T lymphocytes (T cells). B-cell lymphomas are more prevalent, constituting the majority of non-Hodgkin lymphoma cases. These cancers originate from abnormal B cells that fail to undergo the normal process of maturation and instead multiply uncontrollably. Subtypes of B-cell lymphomas include diffuse large B-cell lymphoma (DLBCL), follicular lymphoma, mantle cell lymphoma, and Burkitt lymphoma, among others.

On the other hand, T-cell lymphomas arise from malignant transformations of T cells. T-cell lymphomas are less common than B-cell lymphomas, and they exhibit a diverse range of subtypes, including peripheral T-cell lymphoma, anaplastic large-cell lymphoma, and cutaneous T-cell lymphoma. The classification of non-Hodgkin lymphomas is continually evolving as researchers gain a deeper understanding of the molecular and genetic factors contributing to the disease.

The exact cause of non-Hodgkin lymphoma remains largely unknown, but certain risk factors have been identified. These include age, with the risk increasing as individuals get older, as well as a compromised immune system due to conditions such as immunosuppressive medications. Exposure to certain chemicals, infections, and a family history of lymphomas may also contribute to the development of NHL.

Symptoms of non-Hodgkin lymphoma can vary depending on the specific subtype and the organs involved. Common symptoms include swollen lymph nodes, fever, night sweats, unexplained weight loss, fatigue, and changes in appetite. Diagnosis typically involves a combination of imaging studies, blood tests, and the biopsy of affected lymph nodes or other tissues.

Non-Hodgkin lymphoma is a complex and diverse group of blood cancers that involve the abnormal proliferation of lymphocytes in the lymphatic system. B-cell and T-cell lymphomas are the two main types, each with numerous subtypes exhibiting distinct features.

Kidney Cancer

Kidney cancer, also known as renal cell carcinoma (RCC), is a type of cancer that originates in the kidneys, the bean-shaped organs responsible for filtering waste products from the blood and producing urine. These vital organs play a crucial role in maintaining the body's overall health by regulating electrolyte balance, blood pressure, and red blood cell production.

The majority of kidney cancers are renal cell carcinomas, accounting for about 90% of cases. These cancers develop in the lining of the small tubes (tubules) within the kidneys. Understanding the cellular basis of kidney cancer requires delving into the intricate world of renal cells.

The kidneys consist of various types of cells, each with specific functions. The primary cells involved in kidney cancer are the renal tubular epithelial cells. These cells line the tubules and are integral to the filtration process. Renal cell carcinoma arises when mutations occur in the DNA of these epithelial cells, leading to uncontrolled cell growth and the formation of tumors.

There are several subtypes of renal cell carcinoma, each associated with distinct cellular characteristics. Clear cell renal cell carcinoma is the most common subtype, representing around 75% of all cases. It is named for the clear appearance of the cancer cells when viewed under a microscope. Other subtypes include papillary renal cell carcinoma, chromophobe renal cell carcinoma, and collecting duct renal cell carcinoma, each with its unique cellular features.

The exact cause of kidney cancer remains elusive, but certain risk factors are known to increase the likelihood of its development. Smoking, obesity, hypertension, and a family history of kidney cancer are among the risk factors associated with this disease. Additionally, certain genetic conditions, such as von Hippel-Lindau (VHL) syndrome, predispose individuals to the development of renal cell carcinoma.

Symptoms of kidney cancer can vary, but they often include blood in the urine, persistent pain or pressure in the side or lower back, fatigue, unexplained weight loss, and a palpable mass or lump in the abdominal area.

Diagnosis typically involves imaging studies such as CT scans, MRIs, and ultrasounds, along with a biopsy to confirm the presence of cancerous cells.

Kidney cancer, or renal cell carcinoma, is a formidable disease originating in the renal tubular epithelial cells of the kidneys. Understanding the cellular basis of kidney cancer is vital for developing effective diagnostic and treatment strategies.

Thyroid Cancer

Thyroid cancer is a type of cancer that originates in the cells of the thyroid gland, a small butterfly-shaped gland located in the front of the neck, just below the Adam's apple. The thyroid gland plays a crucial role in regulating various metabolic processes in the body by producing hormones, primarily thyroxine (T4) and triiodothyronine (T3). These hormones are essential for maintaining the body's metabolism, energy levels, and overall growth and development.

The development of thyroid cancer occurs when normal cells in the thyroid gland undergo genetic mutations, leading to uncontrolled growth and the formation of a tumor. The thyroid gland consists of two main types of cells: follicular cells and parafollicular cells, also known as C cells. Both cell types can give rise to different types of thyroid cancer.

Follicular cells are responsible for producing the thyroid hormones T3 and T4. When these cells become cancerous, they can lead to the formation of differentiated thyroid cancers, such as papillary thyroid cancer and follicular thyroid cancer. Papillary thyroid cancer is the most common type, accounting for about 80% of all thyroid cancer cases. It tends to grow slowly and has a favorable prognosis. Follicular thyroid cancer is less common but still represents a significant proportion of thyroid cancer diagnoses.

Parafollicular cells, or C cells, produce calcitonin, a hormone that helps regulate calcium levels in the body. When C cells undergo cancerous changes, medullary thyroid cancer (MTC) can develop. Medullary thyroid cancer accounts for a smaller percentage of thyroid cancers, but it is often more aggressive than differentiated thyroid cancers. MTC can occur sporadically or be inherited as part of a genetic syndrome, such as multiple endocrine neoplasia type 2 (MEN2).

There is also a rare and highly aggressive form of thyroid cancer known as anaplastic thyroid cancer. This type of cancer often arises from pre-existing differentiated thyroid cancers that have undergone a transformation into a more undifferentiated and rapidly growing state.

Thyroid cancer is more common in women than men, and the risk increases with age. While the exact cause of thyroid cancer is often unknown, certain risk factors may contribute to its development, including a family history of thyroid cancer, exposure to high levels of radiation, and certain genetic conditions.

Early detection and treatment play a crucial role in managing thyroid cancer. Common diagnostic methods include thyroid ultrasound, fine-needle aspiration biopsy, and blood tests to assess thyroid hormone levels.

Thyroid cancer involves the abnormal growth of cells in the thyroid gland, impacting both follicular and parafollicular cells. Differentiated thyroid cancers, originating from follicular cells, include papillary and follicular thyroid cancer. Medullary thyroid cancer arises from C cells, while anaplastic thyroid cancer is a more aggressive and less common form. Early diagnosis is essential for managing thyroid cancer and improving patient outcomes.

Leukemia

Leukemia is a type of cancer that affects the blood and bone marrow, disrupting the normal production of blood cells. It is characterized by the uncontrolled growth of abnormal cells, typically white blood cells, which are an integral part of the body's immune system. The word "leukemia" is derived from the Greek words "leukos," meaning white, and "haima," meaning blood. This aptly reflects the disease's association with the abnormal proliferation of white blood cells.

In a healthy individual, blood cells are produced in the bone marrow, a spongy tissue found in the center of bones. There are three main types of blood cells: red blood cells (RBCs), white blood cells (WBCs), and platelets. Each type has a specific function in maintaining the body's health and functionality. Leukemia primarily affects the white blood cells, which play a crucial role in the immune system's defense against infections.

Leukemia can be broadly classified into four main types based on the rate of progression and the types of white blood cells involved: acute lymphoblastic leukemia (ALL), acute myeloid leukemia (AML), chronic lymphocytic leukemia (CLL), and chronic myeloid leukemia (CML). The classification is based on the specific type of white blood cell that undergoes malignant transformation.

In acute leukemias, the abnormal cells, often referred to as blasts, multiply rapidly and crowd out normal cells. Acute lymphoblastic leukemia primarily affects immature lymphoid cells, while acute myeloid leukemia affects immature myeloid cells. These rapidly progressing forms of leukemia require prompt and aggressive treatment.

Chronic leukemias, on the other hand, progress more slowly, allowing some mature cells to function relatively normally. Chronic lymphocytic leukemia involves abnormal lymphocytes, and chronic myeloid leukemia affects mature myeloid cells. While chronic leukemias may not require immediate intervention, they still necessitate ongoing monitoring and treatment.

The cells involved in leukemia originate from the bone marrow, where genetic mutations occur, leading to the abnormal proliferation of white blood cells. These mutations disrupt the normal processes of cell growth and division, causing the accumulation of immature and dysfunctional cells. The exact cause of these mutations is often unknown, although certain risk factors, such as exposure to radiation, certain chemicals, and genetic predisposition, may contribute to the development of leukemia.

The symptoms of leukemia can vary but often include fatigue, weakness, frequent infections, unexplained weight loss, and easy bruising or bleeding. Diagnosis typically involves blood tests, bone marrow biopsy, and imaging studies to determine the extent of the disease.

Leukemia is a type of cancer characterized by the uncontrolled growth of abnormal white blood cells, disrupting the normal production of blood cells in the bone marrow. The specific type of leukemia is determined by the affected white blood cells and the rate of disease progression.

Esophageal Cancer

Esophageal cancer is a malignancy that develops in the esophagus, the muscular tube connecting the throat to the stomach. This type of cancer occurs when cells in the lining of the esophagus undergo abnormal changes and start to divide and grow uncontrollably. The esophagus plays a crucial role in transporting food and liquids from the mouth to the stomach for digestion, and any disruption in its normal function can have significant consequences.

There are two primary types of esophageal cancer: squamous cell carcinoma and adenocarcinoma. Each type originates from different cells in the esophageal lining, and their incidence varies based on geographic and demographic factors.

- **Squamous Cell Carcinoma:**
- Squamous cell carcinoma typically arises in the squamous cells that line the upper part of the esophagus. These flat, scale-like cells are responsible for protecting the esophagus from the wear and tear associated with the passage of food. Squamous cell carcinoma used to be the more common type of esophageal cancer globally, but its prevalence has decreased in some regions.
- **Adenocarcinoma:**
- Adenocarcinoma, on the other hand, originates in the glandular cells of the lower part of the esophagus. These glandular cells produce mucus and are not normally present in the esophagus; however, due to a condition called Barrett's esophagus, which is often associated with chronic gastroesophageal reflux disease (GERD), the normal squamous cells may be replaced by glandular cells. Over time, these glandular cells can undergo malignant transformation, leading to adenocarcinoma.

Esophageal cancer often goes unnoticed in its early stages because symptoms may not manifest until the disease has progressed. Common symptoms include difficulty swallowing, chest pain, weight loss, and persistent coughing. As the cancer advances, it can invade nearby tissues and organs, making it more challenging to treat.

Several risk factors contribute to the development of esophageal cancer. These include chronic irritation of the esophagus (such as from smoking or heavy alcohol consumption), obesity, a history of certain precancerous conditions like Barrett's esophagus, and genetic factors. Additionally, individuals with a diet lacking in fruits and vegetables may be at an increased risk.

Diagnosis typically involves endoscopy, where a flexible tube with a camera is passed through the esophagus to examine the tissue and collect biopsy samples. Imaging tests such as CT scans may also be used to determine the extent of the cancer.

Esophageal cancer is a formidable disease that arises from the abnormal growth of cells in the esophageal lining. Squamous cell carcinoma and adenocarcinoma are the two primary types, each originating from different cells within the esophagus. Early detection and a multidisciplinary approach to treatment are crucial for improving outcomes and enhancing the quality of life for individuals diagnosed with esophageal cancer.

Other Ailments

Crohn's Disease

Crohn's disease is a chronic inflammatory bowel disease (IBD) characterized by inflammation of the digestive tract. Named after the physician Burrill B. Crohn, who first described the condition in 1932 along with colleagues Leon Ginzburg and Gordon D. Oppenheimer, Crohn's disease can affect any part of the gastrointestinal tract, from the mouth to the anus. It most commonly impacts the small intestine and the beginning of the colon.

The exact cause of Crohn's disease remains unclear, but it is believed to involve a combination of genetic, environmental, and immune system factors. Certain genetic mutations may make individuals more susceptible to the disease, and environmental factors such as diet, smoking, and infections may trigger its onset or exacerbate symptoms. Additionally, an overactive immune system may play a role in the inflammation seen in Crohn's disease, as the body's immune cells mistakenly attack the gastrointestinal tract.

One of the hallmarks of Crohn's disease is the chronic inflammation that occurs in the affected areas of the digestive tract. This inflammation can lead to a variety of symptoms, including abdominal pain, diarrhea, weight loss, fatigue, and malnutrition. The severity and course of the disease can vary widely among individuals, with some experiencing periods of remission and others facing continuous symptoms.

Living with Crohn's disease can be challenging, as the unpredictable nature of the condition can significantly impact an individual's quality of life. Support from healthcare professionals, family, and friends is crucial in managing the physical and emotional aspects of the disease. Additionally, support groups and patient advocacy organizations can provide valuable resources and a sense of community for individuals with Crohn's disease.

A plant-based diet has emerged as a promising approach to the management and potential reversal of Crohn's disease, a condition that affects millions worldwide. While conventional treatments often involve medication and, in severe cases, surgery, recent research suggests that adopting a plant-based diet may offer a holistic and natural solution to alleviate symptoms and promote healing.

The anti-inflammatory properties of plant-based foods play a crucial role in managing this condition. Fruits, vegetables, whole grains, legumes, and nuts are rich in antioxidants and fiber, which can help reduce inflammation and promote a healthier gut microbiome.

Studies have shown that individuals with Crohn's disease who adopt a plant-based diet often experience improvements in symptoms. The high fiber content aids in bowel regularity, reducing the frequency and severity of flare-ups. Additionally, plant-based diets are typically lower in saturated fats, which may contribute to inflammation, and higher in beneficial nutrients like vitamins, minerals, and phytochemicals that support overall health.

The role of plant-based diets in modulating the gut microbiota is particularly relevant to Crohn's disease. A diverse and balanced microbiome is associated with better gut health, and plant-based foods provide a variety of nutrients that support the growth of beneficial bacteria. This positive shift in the microbial composition can contribute to the reduction of inflammation and the restoration of intestinal integrity.

While more research is needed to fully understand the mechanisms and long-term effects of a plant-based diet on Crohn's disease, the existing evidence suggests that embracing a diet centered around whole, plant-based foods may hold promise as a complementary strategy for managing and potentially reversing the symptoms of this challenging condition.

Type 2 Diabetes

A plant-based diet has emerged as a promising and effective approach to addressing and even reversing Type 2 diabetes, a chronic condition characterized by insulin resistance and elevated blood sugar levels. Research and clinical studies have provided compelling evidence of the positive impact that a diet centered around plant-based foods can have on managing and, in some cases, reversing this metabolic disorder.

One key factor contributing to the effectiveness of a plant-based diet in combating Type 2 diabetes is its ability to improve insulin sensitivity. Plant-based foods are generally rich in fiber, antioxidants, and micronutrients, which play crucial roles in regulating blood sugar levels and reducing inflammation. Fiber, in particular, slows down the absorption of glucose, preventing rapid spikes in blood sugar after meals and promoting better insulin function.

Furthermore, plant-based diets are typically low in saturated fats and cholesterol, reducing the risk of obesity and cardiovascular complications associated with Type 2 diabetes. Weight loss, often a beneficial outcome of adopting a plant-based lifestyle, is directly linked to improved insulin sensitivity and glycemic control.

Several studies have demonstrated the positive outcomes of plant-based diets in clinical settings. For instance, research published in the American Journal of Clinical Nutrition has shown that individuals who follow a plant-based diet experience significant improvements in HbA1c levels, a key marker of long-term blood sugar control. Additionally, a study conducted by the Physicians Committee for Responsible Medicine found that participants following a low-fat, plant-based diet experienced better insulin sensitivity and lower cholesterol levels compared to those following conventional diabetes diets.

The evidence supporting the role of a plant-based diet in reversing Type 2 diabetes is substantial and continues to grow. By prioritizing whole, plant-based foods such as the P53 Diet, individuals may not only manage their condition more effectively but also witness improvements that could potentially lead to the reversal of Type 2 diabetes, offering hope for a healthier and more sustainable approach to diabetes management.

Heart Disease

In recent years, there has been a growing body of evidence supporting the idea that a plant-based diet can play a pivotal role in reversing heart disease. Prominent figures in the field of nutrition, such as Michael Greger M.D., have championed the benefits of embracing a diet rich in fruits, vegetables, whole grains, and legumes. This dietary approach not only addresses cardiovascular health but has also shown promising signs of actually reversing the progression of heart disease.

Heart disease remains a leading cause of morbidity and mortality worldwide. Traditional treatments often focus on medication and surgical interventions, but emerging research suggests that a plant-based diet can be a powerful tool in preventing and even reversing heart disease. Michael Greger, a renowned physician and author of *"How Not to Die,"* emphasizes the profound impact of diet on heart health. He states, "The vast majority of premature deaths can be prevented with simple changes in diet and lifestyle. Plant-based diets have been shown to reverse the progression of even severe coronary artery disease."

One of the key mechanisms through which a plant-based diet exerts its positive effects on heart health is by reducing cholesterol levels. Elevated levels of cholesterol, particularly low-density lipoprotein (LDL) cholesterol, are a major risk factor for heart disease. Greger points out, *"Plants don't have cholesterol. Animal products have cholesterol, and that's what clogs up arteries."* By eliminating or significantly reducing animal products from the diet, individuals can lower their cholesterol levels and, consequently, decrease their risk of heart disease.

Inflammation plays a crucial role in the development and progression of heart disease. A plant-based diet is inherently anti-inflammatory, as it is rich in antioxidants and phytochemicals that combat oxidative stress and inflammation. Greger notes, *"In every population studied, the more plant-based people were eating, the lower their levels of inflammation."* This anti-inflammatory effect contributes to the overall improvement of cardiovascular health and helps in reversing the damage caused by chronic inflammation.

The endothelium, the inner lining of blood vessels, plays a vital role in cardiovascular health. Dysfunction of the endothelium is a hallmark of heart disease. Research indicates that a plant-based diet can enhance endothelial function, promoting better blood flow and reducing the risk of arterial plaque formation. Greger explains, *"The endothelium likes it when you eat greens. It secretes a vasodilator, a blood vessel-relaxing chemical called nitric oxide."* This improvement in endothelial function is a key factor in the reversal of heart disease.

The impact of a plant-based diet on heart disease is not just theoretical; numerous real-life success stories attest to its effectiveness. Greger often shares anecdotes of patients who have experienced significant improvements in their cardiovascular health by adopting a plant-based lifestyle. These stories serve as inspirational examples of how dietary changes can lead to tangible and life-changing results.

The evidence supporting the ability of a plant-based diet to reverse heart disease is compelling and continues to grow. Michael Greger's advocacy for plant-based nutrition underscores the transformative potential of dietary choices in promoting cardiovascular health. Embracing a diet centered on plant foods not only addresses the root causes of heart disease but also provides a sustainable and holistic approach to improving overall well-being. As the scientific community and public awareness continue to align with the benefits of plant-based living, the potential for a widespread positive impact on heart health remains promising. Dr. Michael Greger's M.D. book *"How Not to Die"* is a great read on how a plant-based diet works.

Cirrhosis

In recent years, there has been a growing body of evidence suggesting that adopting a plant-based diet may hold the key to reversing cirrhosis, a condition characterized by scarring of the liver tissue. Cirrhosis is often the result of chronic liver diseases, such as hepatitis or alcohol-related liver disease, and its progression can lead to liver failure. Traditional treatments have focused on managing symptoms and preventing further damage, but emerging research indicates that a plant-based diet might offer a promising avenue for actual recovery.

A plant-based diet emphasizes the consumption of whole, unprocessed plant foods such as fruits, vegetables, legumes, nuts, and whole grains while excluding or minimizing animal products. This dietary approach is rich in antioxidants, fiber, and various phytochemicals, which have been associated with anti-inflammatory and liver-protective properties.

Chronic inflammation is a common denominator in the progression of liver diseases, including cirrhosis. Plant-based diets, abundant in antioxidants and anti-inflammatory compounds, may help modulate the inflammatory response. Fruits and vegetables, in particular, are rich in vitamins, minerals, and phytonutrients that have been shown to quell inflammation and promote healing.

The liver plays a central role in detoxifying the body by breaking down and eliminating toxins. Plant-based diets may facilitate this process by providing the necessary nutrients for optimal liver function. Cruciferous vegetables like broccoli and Brussels sprouts contain sulfur compounds that support the liver's detoxification pathways, potentially aiding in the removal of harmful substances contributing to cirrhosis.

Obesity and metabolic syndrome are risk factors for liver diseases, including cirrhosis. Plant-based diets have been linked to weight loss and improved metabolic markers, such as insulin sensitivity and lipid profiles. By promoting a healthy weight and metabolic balance, a plant-based diet may indirectly contribute to the reversal of cirrhosis by addressing underlying risk factors.

The gut-liver axis is a crucial connection in liver health. Plant-based diets, high in fiber and prebiotics, promote a diverse and healthy gut microbiota. A balanced gut microbiome is associated with reduced inflammation and improved liver function. Fermented foods like sauerkraut and kimchi, common in plant-based diets, further contribute to gut health and may positively impact cirrhosis reversal.

While research on the direct impact of plant-based diets on cirrhosis reversal is still in its early stages, some studies and anecdotal evidence suggest promising results. Cases have been documented where individuals with cirrhosis experienced improvements in liver function, reduction in fibrosis, and even regression of cirrhotic changes after adopting a plant-based lifestyle.

The potential for a plant-based diet to reverse cirrhosis represents a promising area of exploration in the field of liver health. By addressing inflammation, supporting detoxification, promoting weight management, and restoring gut health, a plant-based approach may offer a holistic strategy for mitigating the effects of cirrhosis. However, it is essential to note that individual responses may vary, and further rigorous research is needed to establish the efficacy and mechanisms behind the observed benefits. As our understanding of the intricate relationship between diet and liver health evolves, embracing a plant-based lifestyle holds the promise of not only preventing but potentially reversing the debilitating effects of cirrhosis.

Arthritis

Arthritis, a common and debilitating condition affecting millions worldwide, is characterized by inflammation in the joints leading to pain, stiffness, and decreased mobility. While traditional treatments often involve medications and lifestyle modifications, emerging research suggests that adopting a plant-based diet may offer significant relief for arthritis sufferers. The link between dietary choices and arthritis has gained attention as more evidence supports the potential benefits of plant-based eating patterns in managing inflammation and improving overall joint health.

Arthritis encompasses a variety of conditions, with osteoarthritis and rheumatoid arthritis being the most prevalent forms. Both conditions involve inflammation in the joints, which can contribute to pain and damage over time. Inflammation is the body's natural response to injury or infection, but in chronic conditions like arthritis, it becomes persistent and contributes to tissue damage.

Plant-based diets, rich in fruits, vegetables, whole grains, nuts, and seeds, are known for their anti-inflammatory properties. These foods are packed with antioxidants, vitamins, and phytochemicals that can help counteract inflammation. Research suggests that the compounds found in plant-based foods may play a crucial role in reducing inflammation markers in the body, offering potential relief for arthritis sufferers.

One key component of a plant-based diet that has shown promise in managing arthritis is the inclusion of omega-3 fatty acids. Found abundantly in flaxseeds, chia seeds, walnuts, and algae-based supplements, omega-3 fatty acids have been associated with reduced inflammation and improved joint function. Some studies indicate that these essential fatty acids may help alleviate symptoms in rheumatoid arthritis patients.

The link between gut health and arthritis is an emerging area of research, and plant-based diets are known to promote a healthy gut microbiome. High-fiber foods, such as fruits, vegetables, and whole grains, support the growth of beneficial gut bacteria. A balanced and diverse gut microbiome has been associated with a reduced risk of inflammatory conditions, including arthritis. By fostering a healthy gut environment, a plant-based diet may indirectly contribute to the management of arthritis symptoms.

Maintaining a healthy weight is crucial for arthritis management, especially in osteoarthritis cases where excess weight can exacerbate joint pain. Plant-based diets are often associated with weight loss and weight maintenance due to their emphasis on nutrient-dense, low-calorie foods. By helping individuals achieve and maintain a healthy weight, a plant-based diet may alleviate the burden on joints and reduce arthritis symptoms.

While more research is needed to fully understand the intricate relationship between diet and arthritis, the evidence supporting the benefits of a plant-based diet in managing arthritis symptoms is growing. By embracing a diet rich in anti-inflammatory foods, individuals with arthritis may find relief from pain and improved joint function. As always, consulting with healthcare professionals and nutritionists is crucial when considering significant dietary changes, but the promising findings suggest that plant-based eating patterns could play a role in enhancing the quality of life for those living with arthritis.

Gout

A plant-based diet has emerged as a promising approach to managing and even reversing the symptoms of gout, a form of inflammatory arthritis caused by the accumulation of urate crystals in the joints. Gout is often associated with high levels of uric acid in the blood, and dietary choices play a crucial role in either exacerbating or alleviating this condition. Research and clinical studies have increasingly highlighted the benefits of adopting a plant-based diet in mitigating gout symptoms and promoting overall joint health.

One of the key reasons why a plant-based diet is beneficial for individuals with gout is its impact on reducing uric acid levels. Plant-based foods are generally lower in purines, compounds that contribute to the production of uric acid in the body. Purines are found in higher concentrations in animal products such as red meat, organ meats, and seafood. By shifting to a plant-based diet, individuals can lower their purine intake, subsequently decreasing the production of uric acid and reducing the likelihood of gout attacks.

Moreover, plant-based diets are rich in fiber, which plays a crucial role in promoting gut health and regulating the body's metabolism. High-fiber foods help in the excretion of uric acid through the urine, preventing its accumulation in the joints. Fruits, vegetables, whole grains, and legumes are excellent sources of dietary fiber that not only aid in digestion but also contribute to the overall well-being of individuals with gout.

Studies have shown that certain plant-based foods possess anti-inflammatory properties, which can be particularly beneficial for individuals with gout experiencing joint inflammation and pain. Foods like berries, cherries, and leafy greens contain compounds that can help reduce inflammation and alleviate symptoms associated with gout. Cherries, in particular, have been linked to lower levels of uric acid and a decreased risk of gout attacks.

The emphasis on plant-based protein sources is another notable aspect of a plant-based diet that can positively impact individuals with gout. While animal proteins may contribute to higher levels of uric acid, plant-based protein sources like legumes, tofu, and quinoa provide a healthier alternative. These plant-based protein sources not only offer essential nutrients but also contribute to the overall balance of a gout-friendly diet.

Adopting a plant-based diet also encourages a higher intake of water-rich foods, promoting hydration. Increased hydration is essential for individuals with gout as it helps in flushing out excess uric acid from the body. Hydration is crucial in preventing the crystallization of urate in the joints, reducing the frequency and severity of gout attacks.

It is important to note that while a plant-based diet has shown promise in managing gout, individual responses may vary. Consulting with healthcare professionals, including dietitians or rheumatologists, is crucial for personalized dietary recommendations based on the specific needs and health status of each individual. Additionally, lifestyle factors such as regular physical activity and weight management complement the benefits of a plant-based diet in managing gout effectively.

The evidence supporting the potential of a plant-based diet in reversing the symptoms of gout is compelling. By focusing on nutrient-dense, plant-based foods, individuals with gout can address the root causes of the condition, including high uric acid levels and inflammation. As part of a comprehensive approach to managing gout, adopting a plant-based diet offers a holistic and sustainable solution that aligns with overall health and well-being.

Lupus

While there is currently no cure for lupus, emerging research suggests that adopting a plant-based diet may offer potential benefits in managing and even reversing symptoms of this autoimmune disease. Lupus is a chronic condition where the immune system mistakenly attacks healthy tissues, leading to inflammation and damage in various organs of the body. The impact of diet on autoimmune diseases is an area of growing interest, and several studies have explored the relationship between a plant-based diet and lupus.

A plant-based diet is centered around whole, unprocessed plant foods such as fruits, vegetables, whole grains, legumes, nuts, and seeds while avoiding animal products. This dietary approach is rich in antioxidants, phytochemicals, and anti-inflammatory compounds, which may help modulate the immune system and reduce inflammation, key factors in the progression of lupus.

One of the potential benefits of a plant-based diet for lupus patients lies in its ability to reduce inflammation. Chronic inflammation is a hallmark of lupus and is responsible for much of the damage to organs and tissues. Plant-based diets are known to have anti-inflammatory effects, primarily due to the abundance of antioxidants and polyphenols found in plant foods. These compounds help neutralize free radicals and reduce oxidative stress, which is often elevated in individuals with lupus.

Moreover, plant-based diets may positively influence the gut microbiota, the trillions of microorganisms residing in the digestive tract. Research has suggested a link between the gut microbiome and autoimmune diseases, including lupus. A plant-based diet, rich in fiber and diverse plant compounds, promotes the growth of beneficial bacteria in the gut, which can have anti-inflammatory effects and contribute to overall immune system balance.

Several studies have provided evidence supporting the potential benefits of a plant-based diet in lupus management. A study published in the journal *"Arthritis Research & Therapy"* found that lupus patients following a plant-based diet experienced improvements in disease activity, inflammatory markers, and overall well-being compared to those following a standard diet.

Another study published in *"Nutrition & Diabetes"* reported that a plant-based diet reduced levels of certain antibodies associated with lupus, suggesting a positive impact on the autoimmune response.

It is important to note that while these studies show promising results, more research is needed to establish a definitive link between a plant-based diet and the reversal of lupus.

A holistic approach to lupus management, which may include, lifestyle modifications, and dietary changes, can contribute to a comprehensive and personalized treatment plan for individuals living with this autoimmune condition.

Erectile Dysfunction

A plant-based diet, rich in fruits, vegetables, whole grains, and legumes, has gained recognition for its potential health benefits, including its positive impact on cardiovascular health. In recent years, there has been growing evidence suggesting that adopting a plant-based lifestyle may also play a role in improving erectile dysfunction (ED), a condition that affects a significant number of men worldwide.

Erectile dysfunction is often associated with underlying cardiovascular issues, as the health of the blood vessels is crucial for proper erectile function. The arteries that supply blood to the penis can become narrowed or blocked due to atherosclerosis, a condition characterized by the accumulation of plaque in the arteries. A plant-based diet has been shown to address many of the risk factors associated with cardiovascular disease, potentially leading to improvements in erectile function.

One key benefit of a plant-based diet is its ability to lower cholesterol levels. Plant-based foods are typically low in saturated fats and devoid of cholesterol, contributing to a reduction in overall cholesterol levels. High cholesterol is a major risk factor for atherosclerosis, and by adopting a plant-based diet, individuals may experience improvements in blood flow, which is essential for achieving and maintaining an erection.

Arginine, a conditional amino acid, is indeed believed to play a role in improving erectile dysfunction (ED). Arginine is a precursor to nitric oxide, a molecule that helps relax blood vessels and improve blood flow. This is significant in the context of ED because proper blood flow to the penis is crucial for achieving and maintaining an erection. See the chapter *"Amino Acids"* for data on all the amino acids.

When arginine is consumed, it can be converted into nitric oxide in the body. Nitric oxide helps dilate blood vessels, including those in the penis, leading to increased blood flow. This mechanism is similar to how some medications for ED work, as they also enhance the effects of nitric oxide.

Foods rich in arginine include nuts, seeds, and legumes. However, it's essential to note that while arginine supplementation or dietary adjustments may be beneficial for some individuals with ED, results can vary. In conclusion, arginine, through its role in nitric oxide production, is considered by some as a potential natural approach to improving erectile function. As with any health-related strategy, individual responses can differ, and professional guidance is crucial for a comprehensive and personalized approach to addressing erectile dysfunction.

Plant-based diets are rich in antioxidants, which play a crucial role in protecting the body's cells, including those in the blood vessels. Oxidative stress and inflammation are factors that contribute to the development and progression of atherosclerosis. The abundance of antioxidants in plant-based foods helps combat oxidative stress and inflammation, potentially promoting a healthier vascular system.

Additionally, a plant-based diet may positively influence other lifestyle factors that contribute to erectile dysfunction, such as obesity and diabetes. Plant-based diets tend to be lower in calorie density and can be effective in weight management. Obesity is a known risk factor for ED, and losing excess weight through a plant-based approach may lead to improvements in both cardiovascular health and erectile function.

While research on the specific effects of a plant-based diet on erectile dysfunction is still evolving, the existing evidence suggests a promising connection between plant-based eating and improved sexual health.

11

Vegetables & Spices

In the tapestry of a well-balanced and healthy diet, vegetables emerge as the vibrant threads that weave together the essential nutrients vital for the human body. Packed with vitamins, minerals, fiber, and an array of phytochemicals, vegetables play a pivotal role in promoting overall well-being. This book delves into the intricacies of why vegetables are not only good but indispensable for the human body, exploring the diverse ways in which they contribute to our health.

Vegetables are a nutritional powerhouse, providing an extensive array of essential vitamins and minerals crucial for various bodily functions. Leafy greens like spinach and kale are abundant sources of vitamin K, vital for blood clotting and bone health. Carrots and sweet potatoes boast high levels of beta-carotene, a precursor to vitamin A, essential for vision, immune function, and skin health. Cruciferous vegetables such as broccoli and Brussels sprouts are rich in vitamin C, an antioxidant that supports the immune system and aids in collagen formation.

Minerals such as potassium, found in abundance in vegetables like potatoes, play a crucial role in maintaining proper fluid balance, nerve transmission, and muscle contractions. Magnesium, present in leafy greens, nuts, and seeds, contributes to energy production, muscle function, and bone health. The diverse nutrient profile of vegetables ensures that the body receives a spectrum of essential elements, promoting optimal physiological functioning.

One of the standout features of vegetables is their high fiber content. Fiber, a non-digestible carbohydrate, comes in two forms – soluble and insoluble – each offering unique benefits for digestive health. Soluble fiber, found in foods like oats, beans, and fruits, forms a gel-like substance in the digestive tract, slowing down the absorption of nutrients and helping regulate blood sugar levels. Insoluble fiber, prevalent in vegetables like celery and cauliflower, adds bulk to the stool, promoting regular bowel movements and preventing constipation.

A diet rich in fiber has been linked to a reduced risk of various digestive disorders, including diverticulitis and irritable bowel syndrome. It also contributes to a feeling of fullness, aiding in weight management by curbing excessive calorie intake. The digestive benefits of vegetables extend beyond mere nutrient provision, emphasizing their integral role in maintaining a healthy gut.

Vegetables are replete with antioxidants, compounds that neutralize harmful free radicals in the body. Free radicals, generated through natural processes and environmental exposures, can damage cells and contribute to aging and chronic diseases. Antioxidants, such as vitamin C, vitamin E, and beta-carotene, help counteract this oxidative stress, mitigating the risk of various health conditions, including heart disease and certain cancers.

The diverse spectrum of phytochemicals in vegetables adds another layer to their antioxidant prowess. For instance, the flavonoids in berries and citrus fruits have been associated with cardiovascular health, while the sulforaphane in cruciferous vegetables exhibits potent anti-cancer properties. By incorporating a rainbow of vegetables into one's diet, individuals can harness the synergistic effects of these antioxidants, building a robust defense against oxidative damage.

Vegetable consumption has been linked to a lower risk of chronic diseases, making them an essential component of preventive healthcare. A diet rich in vegetables is associated with a reduced risk of heart disease, stroke, and hypertension. The fiber, potassium, and antioxidants in vegetables contribute to cardiovascular health by promoting healthy blood pressure, cholesterol levels, and overall vascular function.

The anti-inflammatory properties of many vegetables play a crucial role in preventing and managing chronic inflammatory conditions such as arthritis and inflammatory bowel diseases. The abundance of nutrients like vitamin K and calcium in leafy greens supports bone health, reducing the risk of osteoporosis and fractures.

In the era of sedentary lifestyles and processed foods, the prevalence of obesity and metabolic disorders has surged. Vegetables, with their low-calorie density and high nutrient content, present a valuable tool for weight management. The fiber in vegetables promotes satiety, reducing overall calorie intake and contributing to weight loss or weight maintenance.

Complex carbohydrates in vegetables, such as those found in sweet potatoes and quinoa, provide a sustained release of energy, helping regulate blood sugar levels. This characteristic is particularly beneficial for individuals with diabetes or those at risk of developing the condition. The combination of fiber, vitamins, and minerals in vegetables supports metabolic health, offering a holistic approach to combating the obesity epidemic and related metabolic disorders.

Emerging research suggests a link between vegetable consumption and cognitive health. Vegetables rich in antioxidants, such as leafy greens and cruciferous vegetables, may help protect the brain from oxidative stress and inflammation, factors implicated in age-related cognitive decline and neurodegenerative diseases like Alzheimer's.

Additionally, certain nutrients in vegetables, such as folate and vitamin K, play a role in cognitive function. Folate, found in abundance in leafy greens and legumes, is essential for the synthesis of neurotransmitters and has been associated with a lower risk of cognitive impairment. Vitamin K, prevalent in kale and broccoli, is involved in processes that support brain health, including myelin formation and the synthesis of sphingolipids, crucial components of brain cell membranes.

The profound impact of vegetables on human health is undeniable. From their rich nutrient profile to their role in preventing chronic diseases, promoting digestive health, and supporting cognitive function, vegetables stand as nutritional powerhouses that deserve a prominent place on every plate. Embracing a diverse and colorful array of vegetables ensures a comprehensive intake of essential vitamins, minerals, fiber, and phytochemicals, contributing to the vitality and longevity of the human body. As we navigate the complexities of modern lifestyles, prioritizing the inclusion of vegetables in our diets becomes not only a culinary choice but a cornerstone of holistic well-being.

Phytochemicals

In the next few chapters, I will talk about the phytochemicals found in vegetables, fruit, nuts, seeds, and whole grains, and the power of healing these foods have on our bodies. When you are at the store shopping for your family organic has been proven to carry fewer pesticides than the non-organic fruit and vegetables. Please make wise choices for your family. The phytochemicals found in whole plant foods are what give us the power to keep us healthy.

What are phytochemicals? The word "phyto" comes from the Greek word meaning "plant" and the chemicals means naturally produced by plants. A lot of the chemicals found in plants are bio-active which helps our bodies to protect themselves from harm like cancer and pathogens, they can also help to regulate the secretion of enzymes and hormones. Phytochemicals give fruits and vegetables their color and their aromas. When you hear the phrase "Eat the Rainbow" it means to eat an array of colors in your plant-based food diet. Those different colors will give your body different phytochemicals that do different things for your body. Always choose plant-based foods. Try not to give supplements to replace whole plant foods. Research has shown us that a lot of the supplements do not give us the same phytochemicals as eating plant-based foods.

Phytochemicals are broken up into groups based on the chemistry contained in that food. Listed below is a brief list of food phytochemicals and the health benefits of them:

- **Alkaloids** - Organic compounds that contain basic nitrogen atoms. Alkaloids act as a depressant on the central nervous system or as a stimulant such as coffee. Alkaloids are used widely in the drug industry. Some alkaloids can be very harmful in large doses.
- **Anthocyanins** - Belong to the Flavonoids group. They give the dark blue pigments of fruit or vegetables like blueberry, raspberry, purple cauliflower, black rice, red cabbage, and more. Research has shown that Anthocyanins help reduce the risk of heart disease in women by decreasing blood pressure and preventing arterial stiffness. Anthocyanins have also been shown to lower LDL cholesterol. Studies have shown that Anthocyanins play a role in inhibiting tumor growth in the esophagus. They also show promise in preventing the spread of certain cancers.

- **Carotenoids** - Carotenoids have been shown to decrease the risk of certain cancers and diseases of the eyes. The β-Carotene can be converted to vitamin A. Lutein and Zeaxanthin play a protective role by absorbing the damaging blue light that hits the eyes. Eating foods rich in β-Carotene has been shown to help fight against lung cancer. Lycopene has been found to help protect the skin and tissues. Carotenoids are found in orange, yellow, and red fruits and vegetables.
- **Coumestans** - Known as phytoestrogens, it is a derivative of coumarin. These phytochemicals are found in lima beans, split peas, pinto beans, and more. Research has shown that phytoestrogens can lower the risk of breast cancer, colon cancer, as well as endometrial cancer.
- **ECGC (catechins)** - Found in green tea and grapes has proven to be a strong antioxidant that can modulate different components of the NF-ƙB pathway
- **Flavan-3-Ols** - The Flavan-3-Ols are potent antioxidants that help protect cells from the damage that is caused by free radicals. Substances found in the flavanols-3-ols like Catechin have been shown to help fight hepatitis as well as inflammation of cells in the brain. These antioxidants also help with the ruction of blood glucose levels. Epigallocatechin Gallate has been shown to reduce LDL cholesterol as well as lowering high blood pressure. Epigallocatechin Gallate has also been shown to help treat certain cancers such as breast, cervical, prostate, and skin cancers. Some research indicates that Epigallocatechin Gallate has helped prevent Huntington's disease.
- **Flavonols** - Flavonols such as Kaempferol found in foods such as apples, grapes, leeks, onions, and more, play a role as a chemopreventive agent meaning that it inhibits the formation of cancer cells. Myricetin has been shown to have anticancer properties, as well as anti-inflammatory effects. Myricetin and Quercetin have also been shown to help prevent LDL oxidation. Quercetin has

been found to reduce the risk of cancers such as breast, colon, gastric, ovarian, and prostate. Quercetin has also been shown to reduce the levels of Notch 2 protein, which leads to the reduction proliferation rate of cancer cells.

- **Flavanones** - Flavanones help reduce the risk of diabetes. They have also been shown to fight against the damage caused by free radicals. Flavanones help protect the retina in the eyes. Hesperidin also helps build up collagen with the support of vitamin C. This helps the skin and the joints. It also helps with the lowering of LDL cholesterol.
- **Flavones** - Flavones play a crucial role in plant signaling and defense. Flavones also have great antioxidant powers. They also have been shown to lower the risk of certain cancers. Flavones can reduce hypertension and obesity. Flavones have been shown to limit the ability of the cell migration which can lessen the metastasis.
- **Isoflavones** - Isoflavones are phytoestrogens and have been shown to provide a variety of benefits. Isoflavones help to fight the oxidation of LDL cholesterol. Isoflavones which is found in soya (soybeans) has been studied, and the finding stated that the consumption of soy isoflavones helps reduce the risk of breast cancer. The soy isoflavones which some women avoid because of the estrogen binding don't realize that there is an alpha estrogen receptor and a beta estrogen receptor. The soy isoflavones always are known as weak estrogen binds to the beta receptor. The alpha receptor binding triggers cell proliferation, and the beta receptor binding decreases it.
- **Hydrocinnamic Acids** - Research has found that caffein acid and ferulic acid have great anticancer properties. Hydrocinnamic acids also help to protect against UV damage to the skin. Hydrocinnamic acids have also been shown to help reduce body fat by forcing the cell to use body fat as the cell fuel source. Hydro-

cinnamic Acids can be found in foods such as apples, artichokes, blueberries, carrots, cherries, coffee, lettuce, pears, and wheat.

- **Lignans** - Studies have shown that a higher intake of lignans has a reduced risk of breast, endometrial, ovarian, and prostate cancers. A study done in 2009 suggests that postmenopausal that had high intakes of lignans had less body fat and lower blood sugars. Lignans are found in nuts and seeds as well as vegetables, fruit, and whole grains, flaxseed having the highest levels. Lignans have also been shown to lower the risk of cardiovascular disease.
- **Monophenols** - There is not a lot of research information on monophenols. They have been shown to have antioxidants that have been shown to fight free radicals in the body.
- **Monoterpenes** - Monoterpenes are found in foods such as broccoli, cabbage, carrots, and parsley. The limonene has been shown to help prevent breast and liver cancers.
- **Organosulfides** - The sulfur compounds of organosulfides have been shown to help fight gastric cancer and other cancers. The anticancer properties of garlic are widely known. Garlic has also been shown to promote anti-inflammatory activities by cytokine modulation in the blood. Sulfur-containing phytochemicals have also been shown to reduce blood pressure as well and help boost the immune system.
- **Phenolic Acids** - Ellagic acid has been shown to help boost the immune system. Capsaicin has been shown to help with inflammatory bowel disease (IBD) and stomach ulcers. Capsaicin has also been shown to help prevent headaches, migraines, and joint and muscle pain. The phytochemicals found in phenolic acids such as capsaicin and ellagic acid have been shown to help prevent the growth of tumors. Salicylic acid has also been shown to help prevent psoriasis and shingles. Salicylic acid also helps reduce the signs of aging.
- **Phytosterols** - Have long been known to help lower cholesterol. Research reports have stated that phytosterols help prevent

breast, lung, ovarian, and stomach cancers. The phytosterols also contain antioxidants that help fight against free radicals. The high levels of phytosterols are found in beans and nuts.

- **Proanthocyanidins** - Proanthocyanidins are a class of polyphenols found in plants. Proanthocyanidins are the main polyphenols found in red wine.
- **Saponins** - Saponins bind with bile salt and cholesterol which reduces blood cholesterol. Saponins also boost the immune system. They also help lower the risk of cancer by slowing the growth of the cancer cells.
- **Stilbenes** - Stilbene has been shown to help fight Hodgkin's Lymphoma by the phytochemical resveratrol which causes apoptosis on cell line L428. They support the protection against free radicals that can damage cells. Stilbene has also been found to help to lower the blood sugar. In other studies, resveratrol has been shown to help fight against Parkinson's disease and Alzheimer's disease.
- **Tannins** - Tannins are found in blueberries, chocolate, coffee, cranberries, grapes, persimmons, pomegranates, strawberries, red wine, and tea. Tannins have been shown to help boost the immune. Tannins have also been shown to help people with too much iron in the blood. Tannins are a great source of antioxidants. Tannins are also said to create headaches. The tannins in the plant act as a defense for the plant to prevent it from being consumed. Tannins have been found to help lower total cholesterol. Tannins have also been shown to lower the risk of cancer as well as reducing blood pressure.
- **Triterpenoids** - Triterpenoids are a class of terpenes that are found in apples, basil, cranberries, peppermint, and lavender. Triterpenoids have been shown to fight against breast and colon cancers. Triterpenoids have also been found to induce apoptosis in T-cell leukemia. Triterpenoids have also been shown to have antioxidant properties.

- **Ursolic Acid** - Ursolic acid is a natural compound found in various plants, particularly in the skin of fruits. It belongs to a class of compounds known as triterpenoids, which are organic chemicals with a specific molecular structure. Some common natural sources of ursolic acid include apples, rosemary, basil, oregano, thyme, and certain berries. It is often present in the waxy coating or peel of these fruits. Research has suggested that ursolic acid may have potential health benefits, including anti-inflammatory, antioxidant, and anti-cancer properties. Additionally, it has been investigated for its potential role in promoting muscle growth and fat loss.
- **Xanthophylls** - Xanthophylls are a class of carotenoids. Xanthophylls have been shown to help in the soothing of the stomach as well as reducing inflammation. These phytochemicals also help to protect the kidney from damage. Canthaxanthin and astaxanthin have been shown to help protect the skin from UV damage. Some studies have shown that Xanthophylls can help in the lowering of your blood pressure. Xanthophylls have also been shown to aid in the prevention of gum disease.

Spices

Many spices contain bioactive compounds that are believed to contribute to potential health benefits, including anti-cancer properties and other ailment-fighting attributes. Here's a brief overview:

- **Turmeric:** The cancer-fighting phytochemical in turmeric is curcumin. Curcumin is a polyphenol and a natural compound that gives turmeric its vibrant yellow color. It is known for its anti-inflammatory, antioxidant, and anti-cancer properties. Numerous studies have suggested that curcumin may have potential benefits in preventing and treating various types of cancer by interfering with cancer cell growth, proliferation, and survival.

- **Ginger:** The cancer-fighting phytochemical in ginger is gingerol. Gingerol is a bioactive compound and a member of the ginger family. It is well-known for its anti-inflammatory and antioxidant properties, and there is growing evidence suggesting that it may have potential anti-cancer effects.
  Studies have indicated that gingerol may interfere with various signaling pathways involved in cancer cell growth, proliferation, and apoptosis (programmed cell death). Additionally, gingerol has been investigated for its ability to inhibit angiogenesis, the process through which new blood vessels develop, which is crucial for tumor growth.
- **Cinnamon:** Cinnamon contains several phytochemicals, and one of them is cinnamaldehyde, which is often associated with potential health benefits, including anti-cancer properties. Cinnamaldehyde is responsible for the characteristic flavor and scent of cinnamon. While research is ongoing, some studies suggest that cinnamaldehyde may have anti-tumor effects.
- In addition to cinnamaldehyde, cinnamon also contains other compounds like cinnamic acid, coumarin, and various polyphenols, each of which may contribute to its potential health-promoting properties.
- **Garlic:** Garlic contains several bioactive compounds, and one of the key cancer-fighting phytochemicals in garlic is allicin. Allicin is produced when garlic is crushed or chopped, leading to the release of an enzyme called alliinase that converts the precursor compound alliin into allicin. Allicin is responsible for the distinctive smell of garlic and is associated with various health benefits, including potential anti-cancer properties. Studies have suggested that allicin may have anti-cancer effects by influencing different stages of cancer development. It has been investigated for its potential to inhibit the growth of cancer cells, induce apoptosis (programmed cell death), and interfere with processes involved in cancer progression.

- **Rosemary:** Rosemary contains several phytochemicals, and one of the key compounds believed to have potential cancer-fighting properties is rosmarinic acid. Rosmarinic acid is a polyphenolic compound that exhibits antioxidant and anti-inflammatory properties. Studies have explored the potential anti-cancer effects of rosmarinic acid, indicating its ability to inhibit the growth of cancer cells and influence various signaling pathways involved in cancer development. Additionally, rosemary as a whole contains other bioactive compounds, such as carnosol and ursolic acid, which have also been investigated for their potential health benefits, including anti-cancer properties.
- **Thyme:** Thyme contains several phytochemicals, and one of the compounds believed to contribute to its potential cancer-fighting properties is thymol. Thymol is a natural monoterpene phenol that exhibits antioxidant and anti-inflammatory properties.
- Research has explored the potential health benefits of thymol, including its anti-cancer effects. Thymol has been studied for its ability to inhibit the growth of cancer cells and interfere with various processes involved in cancer development. Additionally, thyme contains other bioactive compounds, such as carvacrol, luteolin, and rosmarinic acid, which may also contribute to its potential health-promoting properties.
- **Oregano:** Oregano contains several bioactive compounds, and one of the key compounds believed to have potential cancer-fighting properties is carvacrol. Carvacrol is a natural monoterpenoid phenol with antimicrobial, antioxidant, and anti-inflammatory properties. Research has explored the potential health benefits of carvacrol, including its anti-cancer effects. Studies have suggested that carvacrol may inhibit the growth of cancer cells and influence various signaling pathways involved in cancer development. In addition to carvacrol, oregano contains other bioactive compounds such as thymol, rosmarinic acid, and quercetin, which

also may contribute to its potential health-promoting properties, including possible anti-cancer effects.

- **Basil:** Basil contains various phytochemicals, and one of the compounds believed to have potential cancer-fighting properties is eugenol. Eugenol is a natural compound that belongs to the phenylpropanoids class and is known for its antioxidant and anti-inflammatory properties. Research has explored the potential health benefits of eugenol, including its anti-cancer effects. Studies suggest that eugenol may inhibit the growth of cancer cells and affect various pathways involved in cancer development. In addition to eugenol, basil also contains other bioactive compounds such as flavonoids, polyphenols, and essential oils, which may contribute to its potential health-promoting properties.
- **Sage:** Sage contains various phytochemicals, and one of the compounds believed to contribute to its potential cancer-fighting properties is rosmarinic acid. Rosmarinic acid is a polyphenolic compound with antioxidant and anti-inflammatory properties. Research has explored the potential health benefits of rosmarinic acid, including its anti-cancer effects. Studies suggest that rosmarinic acid may inhibit the growth of cancer cells and influence various signaling pathways involved in cancer development. In addition to rosmarinic acid, sage also contains other bioactive compounds such as flavonoids and essential oils, which may contribute to its potential health-promoting properties.
- **Fennel:** Fennel contains various phytochemicals, and one of the compounds believed to have potential cancer-fighting properties is anethole. Anethole is a natural compound with antioxidant and anti-inflammatory properties. Research has explored the potential health benefits of anethole, including its anti-cancer effects. Some studies have suggested that anethole may exhibit anti-tumor activities, potentially inhibiting the growth of cancer cells. In addition to anethole, fennel also contains other bioactive

compounds such as flavonoids and polyphenols, which may contribute to its potential health-promoting properties.

- **Cloves:** Cloves contain several bioactive compounds, and one of the compounds believed to contribute to their potential cancer-fighting properties is eugenol. Eugenol is a natural compound that has been studied for its antioxidant, anti-inflammatory, and potential anti-cancer effects. Research has explored the impact of eugenol on various cancer cell lines, suggesting that it may inhibit the growth of cancer cells and influence signaling pathways involved in cancer development. Additionally, cloves contain other bioactive compounds such as flavonoids and phenolic acids, which may also contribute to their potential health-promoting properties.
- **Coriander:** Coriander contains various phytochemicals, and one of the compounds believed to have potential cancer-fighting properties is linalool. Linalool is a terpenoid alcohol that exhibits antioxidant and anti-inflammatory properties.
- Research has explored the potential health benefits of linalool, including its anti-cancer effects. Some studies suggest that linalool may have inhibitory effects on the growth of cancer cells and could influence various signaling pathways involved in cancer development. In addition to linalool, coriander also contains other bioactive compounds, such as flavonoids, polyphenols, and essential oils, which may contribute to its potential health-promoting properties.
- **Cumin:** Cumin contains various phytochemicals, and one of the compounds believed to have potential cancer-fighting properties is cuminaldehyde. Cuminaldehyde is a natural compound that exhibits antioxidant and anti-inflammatory properties. Research has explored the potential health benefits of cuminaldehyde, including its anti-cancer effects. Studies suggest that cuminaldehyde may have inhibitory effects on the growth of cancer cells and could influence various signaling pathways involved in cancer

development. In addition to cuminaldehyde, cumin also contains other bioactive compounds, such as flavonoids, polyphenols, and essential oils, which may contribute to its potential health-promoting properties.

- **Cardamom:** Cardamom contains various bioactive compounds, and while it has been associated with potential health benefits, specific phytochemicals responsible for cancer-fighting properties in cardamom are not as extensively studied or well-established as in some other spices. However, cardamom does contain compounds that have shown antioxidant and anti-inflammatory properties, which are generally associated with potential health benefits, including potential anti-cancer effects. Some of the compounds in cardamom that may contribute to its health-promoting properties include **1,8-cineole:** Also known as eucalyptol, this compound has shown anti-inflammatory and antioxidant properties. **Limonene:** Known for its potential antioxidant and anti-cancer effects. **Terpinene:** Exhibits antioxidant properties.
- **Black pepper:** Black pepper contains piperine, a compound that is not traditionally considered a cancer-fighting phytochemical but has shown potential health benefits. Piperine is known for its bioavailability-enhancing properties, which means it can enhance the absorption of certain nutrients and other compounds in the body. While piperine itself may not be directly involved in cancer-fighting mechanisms, its ability to improve the absorption of other bioactive compounds, such as curcumin from turmeric, has led to investigations into potential synergistic effects for cancer prevention and treatment. Piperine has been studied for its role in enhancing the bioavailability of curcumin, which is known for its anti-inflammatory and potential anti-cancer properties.
- **Cayenne pepper:** Cayenne pepper contains capsaicin, a compound responsible for its spicy flavor. While capsaicin is not traditionally classified as a cancer-fighting phytochemical, it has been studied for various potential health benefits, including

anti-cancer effects. Research on capsaicin suggests that it may have several mechanisms that could contribute to its anti-cancer properties. Some studies have indicated that capsaicin may induce apoptosis (programmed cell death) in cancer cells, inhibit the growth of tumors, and interfere with angiogenesis (the formation of new blood vessels that supply tumors).

- **Paprika:** Paprika is a spice made from dried and ground peppers, and it contains various phytochemicals, including capsaicin, which is responsible for the spiciness in certain varieties of paprika. Capsaicin has been studied for potential health benefits, including its anti-cancer effects. Research on capsaicin suggests that it may have several mechanisms that could contribute to its anti-cancer properties. Some studies have indicated that capsaicin may induce apoptosis (programmed cell death) in cancer cells, inhibit the growth of tumors, and interfere with angiogenesis (the formation of new blood vessels that supply tumors). However, it's essential to note that the specific effects of capsaicin in paprika can vary depending on the type and concentration of the spice.
- **Nutmeg:** Nutmeg contains various phytochemicals, but it's not traditionally recognized as a spice with well-established cancer-fighting properties. However, nutmeg does contain certain compounds that have demonstrated antioxidant and anti-inflammatory properties. One of the key bioactive compounds in nutmeg is myristicin. Myristicin is a natural organic compound that contributes to the characteristic flavor and aroma of nutmeg. While myristicin has been studied for various potential health benefits, including antioxidant effects, its direct role in cancer prevention or treatment is not as extensively researched or established as in some other spices.
- **Mustard seeds:** Mustard seeds contain several bioactive compounds, and one of the compounds believed to contribute to their potential health benefits, including potential cancer-fighting properties, is allyl isothiocyanate (AITC). AITC is a type of

isothiocyanate, a class of compounds known for their potential anti-cancer effects. Research has suggested that AITC may have several mechanisms that could contribute to its anti-cancer properties. Studies have indicated that AITC can induce apoptosis (programmed cell death) in cancer cells, inhibit the growth of tumors, and interfere with various signaling pathways involved in cancer development.

- **Fenugreek:** Fenugreek contains various bioactive compounds, and one of the compounds believed to contribute to its potential health benefits, including potential cancer-fighting properties, is diosgenin. Diosgenin is a steroidal saponin, a type of natural steroid found in certain plants. Research has explored the potential health benefits of diosgenin, including its anti-cancer effects. Some studies have suggested that diosgenin may have inhibitory effects on the growth of cancer cells and could influence various signaling pathways involved in cancer development. In addition to diosgenin, fenugreek also contains other bioactive compounds such as flavonoids, alkaloids, and fiber, which may contribute to its potential health-promoting properties.
- **Dill:** Dill contains various bioactive compounds, but it is not traditionally recognized as a spice with well-established cancer-fighting properties. However, like many herbs and spices, dill does contain certain compounds that have demonstrated antioxidant and anti-inflammatory properties. One of the key components in dill is monoterpenes, including carvone and limonene. While these compounds have shown antioxidant effects and may contribute to the overall health-promoting properties of dill, their direct role in cancer prevention or treatment is not as extensively researched or established.
- **Mint:** Mint contains several phytochemicals that have been studied for potential health benefits, including antioxidant and anti-inflammatory properties. One of the compounds in mint, especially peppermint, is menthol. While menthol is not

traditionally classified as a cancer-fighting phytochemical, it has shown some interesting properties in research. Studies have suggested that menthol may have anti-inflammatory and antioxidant effects, and some research has explored its potential impact on cancer. For example, in certain studies, menthol has been investigated for its ability to inhibit the growth of cancer cells, particularly in relation to certain types of cancer.

- **Parsley:** Parsley contains various bioactive compounds, and while it's not traditionally classified as a spice, it is an herb that has been associated with potential health benefits, including antioxidant and anti-inflammatory properties. One of the key phytochemicals in parsley is myristicin. Myristicin is a natural organic compound that belongs to the class of compounds known as phenylpropanoids. Some studies have suggested that myristicin may have potential anti-cancer effects. Research has explored its ability to induce apoptosis (programmed cell death) in cancer cells and interfere with various pathways involved in cancer development.
- **Tarragon:** Tarragon contains various bioactive compounds, and one of the compounds believed to contribute to its potential health benefits, including potential cancer-fighting properties, is estragole (methyl chavicol). However, it's important to note that the presence of estragole has raised some concerns, as high doses of estragole have been associated with potential carcinogenic effects in animal studies. Research on estragole and tarragon is somewhat complex. While it has been studied for potential antioxidant and anti-inflammatory effects, its safety, especially in higher doses, has been a topic of investigation.
- **Bay leaves:** Bay leaves contain various phytochemicals, and one of the compounds believed to contribute to potential health benefits, including possible cancer-fighting properties, is parthenolide. Parthenolide is a sesquiterpene lactone with anti-inflammatory and antioxidant properties. Research has explored the potential

health benefits of parthenolide, including its anti-cancer effects. Some studies have suggested that parthenolide may inhibit the growth of cancer cells and induce apoptosis (programmed cell death) in certain types of cancer.

- **Chili powder:** Chili powder typically contains capsaicin, which is the compound responsible for the spiciness in chili peppers. Capsaicin is a type of phytochemical known as a capsaicinoid. While capsaicin is not traditionally classified as a cancer-fighting compound, it has been studied for various potential health benefits, including its potential effects on cancer. Research on capsaicin suggests that it may have several mechanisms that could contribute to its potential anti-cancer properties. Some studies have indicated that capsaicin may induce apoptosis (programmed cell death) in cancer cells, inhibit the growth of tumors, and interfere with angiogenesis (the formation of new blood vessels that supply tumors).
- **Allspice:** Allspice contains various phytochemicals, and one of the compounds believed to contribute to its potential health benefits, including possible cancer-fighting properties, is eugenol. Eugenol is a natural compound with antioxidant and anti-inflammatory properties. Research has explored the potential health benefits of eugenol, including its anti-cancer effects. Some studies have suggested that eugenol may inhibit the growth of cancer cells and influence various signaling pathways involved in cancer development.
- **Celery seeds:** Celery seeds contain various bioactive compounds, and one of the compounds believed to contribute to potential health benefits, including possible cancer-fighting properties, is apigenin. Apigenin is a flavonoid with antioxidant and anti-inflammatory properties. Research has explored the potential health benefits of apigenin, including its anti-cancer effects. Some studies have suggested that apigenin may inhibit the growth of

cancer cells and influence various signaling pathways involved in cancer development.

- **Caraway seeds:** Caraway seeds contain various bioactive compounds, and one of the compounds believed to contribute to potential health benefits, including possible cancer-fighting properties, is limonene. Limonene is a monoterpene compound found in certain plants, including citrus fruits and some spices. Research on limonene has explored its potential anti-cancer effects. Studies have suggested that limonene may inhibit the growth of cancer cells and interfere with various signaling pathways involved in cancer development. It's important to note that while limonene is found in caraway seeds, it may not be the sole contributor to any potential health benefits associated with caraway consumption.
- **Anise:** Anise contains various phytochemicals, and one of the compounds believed to contribute to potential health benefits, including possible cancer-fighting properties, is anethole. Anethole is a natural compound with antioxidant and anti-inflammatory properties. Research has explored the potential health benefits of anethole, including its anti-cancer effects. Some studies have suggested that anethole may exhibit inhibitory effects on the growth of cancer cells and influence various signaling pathways involved in cancer development.

It's essential to incorporate a variety of spices into a balanced diet for potential health benefits, and more research is needed to fully understand their impact on specific health conditions.

List of Commonly Used Vegetables

Artichoke

About: Belongs to the Asteraceae family. The artichoke roots are mainly from the Mediterranean and also in the state of Virginia in the U.S. as well as Southern Europe. The leaves on the outside and the heart are the parts that are eaten. Artichokes are a great source of dietary fiber. Artichokes are very low in calories. The active ingredients of artichokes are caffeoylquinic acids like Cynarin. The leaves from the artichoke have been shown to protect the liver. Fiber also plays a role in decreasing the amount of LDL cholesterol. Artichokes are a good source of antioxidants that fight the free radicals in the body. Artichokes also help with the flow of bile and fat to and from the liver thanks to the choleretic effect.

Cancer-Fighting: Helps with lowering the risk of colon cancer.

Phytochemicals: Flavonoid, α-Carotene, Cryptoxanthin, Lutein, Zeaxanthin.

Minerals: Calcium, Copper, Iron, Magnesium, Manganese, Phosphorus, Selenium, Zinc.

Vitamins: Vitamin A, Vitamin B1 (Thiamin), Vitamin B2 (Riboflavin), Vitamin B3 (Niacin), Vitamin B5 (Pantothenic Acid), Vitamin B6 (Pyridoxine), Vitamin C (ASCORBIC Acid), Choline, Vitamin E (Alpha-Tocopherol), Vitamin B9 (Folic Acid), Vitamin K (Phylloquinone).

Arugula

About: Belongs to the Brassicaceae family. Also known as salad rocket. A native plant in Central Asia, Morocco area Portugal, and Southern Europe. Arugula is an excellent source of vitamin A as well as vitamin K. Pregnant women with a high percentage of folic acid which helps prevent neural tube defects in the born baby. Arugula is also a great source of B vitamins. Arugula is high in antioxidants.

Cancer & Disease Fighting: Because of the Phytochemicals in arugula, can help lower the risk of getting breast cancer, cervical cancer, colon cancer, ovarian cancer, prostate cancer, and skin cancer because of the glucosinolates.

Phytochemicals: Glucosinolates, Indoles, Isothiocyanates, Sulforaphane, Thiocyanates.

Minerals: calcium, Copper, Iron, Magnesium, Manganese, Phosphorus, Selenium, Zinc.

Vitamins: Vitamin A, Vitamin C, Vitamin E, Vitamin K, Folic acid, Niacin, Pantothenic acid, Pyridoxine, Riboflavin, and Thiamin.

Asparagus

About: Belongs to the Asparagaceae family. Native in the Himalayas and Spain. Asparagus is very low in calories, but rich in proteins compared to other vegetables. It also has medium levels of dietary fiber. It has also been found to aid in hair growth. Asparagus has been found to help with irritable bowel syndrome. Vitamin K helps in promoting bone formation as well as preventing damage to the neurons. It is an excellent source of vitamins A, C, and K. Asparagus is an excellent source of iron and copper. Asparagus has also aided in the treatment of arthritis.

Cancer & Disease Fighting: It has been shown that asparagus helps fight against breast cancer, colon cancer, liver cancer, and skin cancer.

Phytochemicals: Flavonoids, Carotenes, Cryptoxanthins, Lutein, Zeaxanthin, Kaempferol, Quercetin, and Rutin.

Minerals: Calcium, Copper, Iron, Magnesium, Manganese, Phosphorus, Selenium, Zinc.

Vitamins: Vitamin A, Vitamin C, Vitamin E, Vitamin K, Folic Acid, Niacin, Pantothenic Acid, Pyridoxine, Riboflavin, Thiamin.

Acorn Squash

About: Acorn squash belongs to the Cucurbitaceae family. It carries a modest amount of nutrients. Helps with vision, and vitamin A content.

Cancer & Disease Fighting: Not enough research on Acorn Squash in the anti-cancer role.

Phytochemicals: Flavonoids, Carotenes, Lutein, Zeaxanthin.

Minerals: Calcium, Iron, Magnesium, Manganese, Phosphorus, Selenium, Zinc.

Vitamins: Vitamin A, Vitamin C, Folic Acid, Niacin, Pantothenic Acid, Pyridoxine, Riboflavin, Thiamin.

Bamboo Shoots

About: Bamboo plants are found native in East Asia. Bamboo shoots while modest in most nutrients carry a high amount of copper. Copper is needed in the production of red blood cells. Bamboo shoots are also a good source of potassium. Bamboo shoots are also high in fiber.

Cancer & Disease Fighting: Not enough research on bamboo shoots in the anti-cancer role.

Phytochemicals: Carotenoids, β-Carotene, Lignans, Phenolic Acids.

Minerals: Calcium, Copper, Iron, Magnesium, Manganese, Phosphorus, Selenium, Zinc.

Vitamins: Vitamin C, Vitamin E, Folic Acid, Niacin, Pantothenic Acid, Pyridoxine, Riboflavin, Thiamin.

Beets

About: Belongs to the Amaranthaceae family. Beets are a great source of folates. The beetroot helps boost the immune system by increasing the production of white blood cells. The beetroot also helps raise oxygen levels in the blood.

Cancer & Disease Fighting: Beets have been shown to have antiproliferative effects against colon cancer. The betacyanins are an anticancer agent for colon cancer when combined with the fiber.

Phytochemicals: Tocopherol-α, β-Carotene, Betanin, Polyphenols, Glycine betaine, Betacyanins.

Minerals: Calcium, Copper, Iron, Magnesium, Manganese, Zinc.

Vitamins: Vitamin A, Vitamin C, Vitamin E, Folic Acid, Niacin, Pantothenic Acid, Pyridoxine, Riboflavin, and Thiamin.

Bok Choy

About: Belongs to the Brassicaceae family. Once bok choy is digested, it is broken down into oxazolidines, thiocyanates, and nitriles. Bok choy is an excellent source of vitamin A, vitamin C, and vitamin K. Vitamin K is needed for stronger bones. Vitamin K has also played a role in Alzheimer's disease by decreasing neuronal damage in the brain. Bok choy is very low in calories and has no cholesterol.

Cancer & Disease Fighting: Bok choy has been found to help in the fight against colon cancer by glucosinolates.

Phytochemicals: Flavonoids, β-Carotene, Myrosinase.

Minerals: Calcium, Iron, Magnesium, Manganese, Phosphorus, Zinc.

Vitamins: Vitamin A, Vitamin C, Vitamin K, Folic Acid, Niacin, Pantothenic Acid, Pyridoxine, Riboflavin, and Thiamin.

Broccoli

About: Belongs to the Brassicaceae family. Broccoli is a part of the cruciferous group of vegetables. Broccoli is an excellent source of vitamin C. Researchers have stated that eating broccoli has helped with digestion issues such as colitis and leaky gut as compared to those in the study who did not eat broccoli. The fiber in the broccoli and the kaempferol also helps maintain a healthy stomach lining and helps keep healthy bacteria levels. In specific studies, broccoli has been shown to help protect the liver and its functions. It has also been known to lower cholesterol levels. Broccoli helps boost the immune system. The compound sulforaphane has been stated by researchers to aid in the prevention of Alzheimer's and other neurodegenerative diseases. The high levels of vitamin A and vitamin C have been shown to reduce hair loss. Broccoli should be part of your daily diet.

Cancer & Disease Fighting: Researchers have found broccoli to help protect against breast cancer, colon cancer, urinary bladder cancer, pancreatic and prostate cancer.

Phytochemicals: Glucosinolates, Isothiocyanates, Indoles, Sulforaphane, Carotenoids, Flavonoids, β-Carotene, Cryptoxanthin, Lutein, Zeaxanthin.

Minerals: Calcium, Copper, Iron, Magnesium, Manganese, Selenium, Zinc.

Vitamins: Vitamin A, Vitamin C, Vitamin E, Vitamin K, Folic Acid, Niacin, Pantothenic Acid, Pyridoxine, Riboflavin, and Thiamin.

Brussels Sprouts

About: Belongs to the Brassica family. Brussels sprouts are native to Belgium and Brazil. Brussels sprouts are a great source of vitamins A, C, and K.

Cancer & Disease Fighting: Because of the high antioxidant levels in Brussels sprouts have been shown to offer protection from colon and prostate cancer. The glucoside sinigrin has been shown in studies to fight colon cancer by causing apoptosis in pre-cancerous cells. The high vitamin K levels have been shown to play an essential role in bone health. Brussels sprouts have also been known to balance hormones in the body. Researchers have found that Brussels sprouts help with metabolism by helping burn calories faster. Brussels sprouts help boost the immune system.

Phytochemicals: Flavonoids, Polyphenols, Indoles, Isothiocyanates, Sulforaphane, Glucoside, Sinigrin.

Minerals: Calcium, Copper, Iron, Magnesium, Manganese, Phosphorus, Selenium, Zinc.

Vitamins: Vitamin A, Vitamin C, Vitamin K, Folic Acid, Niacin, Pantothenic Acid, Pyridoxine, Riboflavin, and Thiamin.

Butternut Squash

About: Belongs to the Cucurbitaceae family. It is in the same family as pumpkins. The high vitamin A content of this squash helps the body by protecting it against lung and oral cavity cancer (mouth). The seeds from this squash are a great source of the amino acid tryptophan.

Cancer & Disease Fighting: More research is needed.

Phytochemicals: Flavonoids, β-Carotene, Cryptoxanthin-b, Lutein.

Minerals: Calcium, Copper, Iron, Magnesium, Manganese, Phosphorus, Selenium, Zinc.

Vitamins: Vitamin A, Vitamin C, Vitamin E, Vitamin K, Folic Acid, Niacin, Pantothenic Acid, Pyridoxine, Riboflavin, and Thiamin.

Cabbage

About: Belongs to the Brassicaceae family. Cabbage found in Europe before 1,000 B.C. Cabbage contains sulfur chemicals thanks to the glucosinolates which are responsible for the pungent aroma and the bitter taste. Cabbage gas has also been shown to help protect cells from DNA damage. Scientists have also stated that cabbage has both antiviral and antibacterial effects.

Cancer & Disease Fighting: Researchers have found links between cruciferous vegetables, which cabbage is one of them, and lowering the risks of certain cancers such as breast cancer, colon cancer, lung cancer, and prostate cancer.

Phytochemicals: Carotenoids, β-Carotene, Lutein, Zeaxanthin, Glucosinolates, Indoles, Isothiocyanates, Nitriles, Thiocyanates, Indole-3-carcarbinol.

Minerals: Calcium, Iron, Magnesium, Manganese, Phosphorus, Zinc.

Vitamins: Vitamin A, Vitamin C, Vitamin K, Folic Acid, Niacin, Pantothenic Acid, Pyridoxine, Riboflavin, and Thiamin.

Carrots

About: Belongs to the Apiaceae family. Carrots are known to lower the risk of heart attacks, improve vision, and reduce cholesterol. Carrots have also been known to help with night vision. A study done on rats that were fed with carrots showed a delay in the growth of colon tumors. Carrots have also been known to help the immune system because of the β-Carotene that helps maintain healthy mucus membranes in the body that line the intestinal and respiratory tracts.

Cancer & Disease Fighting: The high carotene levels in carrots have been shown to have a 20% decrease in postmenopausal breast cancer. Carrots have been shown in human studies to cut lung cancer rates by 50% just by consuming just one carrot a day. Scientists have also stated the same high carotene in carrots also decreased the incidence rates of bladder, cervix, colon, esophagus, larynx, and prostate cancers in half.

Phytochemicals: Falcarinol, β-Carotene, Pectin, Myristicin, Alpha-Terpineol.

Minerals: Calcium, Iron, Magnesium, Manganese, Phosphorus, Potassium, Sodium Zinc.

Vitamins: Vitamin A, Vitamin C, Vitamin E, Vitamin K, Folic Acid, Niacin, Pantothenic Acid, Pyridoxine, Riboflavin, and Thiamin.

Cantaloupe

About: Belongs to the Cucurbitaceae family. Cantaloupe is a vegetable, but some people consider it a fruit. Cantaloupe is part of the squash family. Because of the strong levels of vitamin C, cantaloupes are great for lowering the risk of asthma. Research has shown us that cantaloupe can help reduce the risk of cancer by fighting free radicals. The high levels of vitamin A help boost the immune system by helping increase the production of white blood cells. Cantaloupe also helps the skin membrane by fighting off toxins. Researchers have found that cantaloupe can help prevent arthritis. Cantaloupe also helps control spikes in blood sugar.

Cancer & Disease Fighting: Cantaloupe helps fight cancer by the potent antioxidants that help fight tumors.

Phytochemicals: Serine, Carotenoids, Zeaxanthin.

Minerals: Calcium, Iron, Magnesium, Manganese, Potassium.

Vitamins: Vitamin A (beta-carotene), Vitamin C, Vitamin E, Vitamin K, Folic Acid, Niacin, Pantothenic Acid, Pyridoxine, Riboflavin, and Thiamin.

Cauliflower

About: Belongs to the Brassicaceae family. Cauliflower is a cruciferous vegetable along with broccoli, brussels sprouts, cabbage, and kale. Eating vegetables from the allium (garlic, leeks, onions) and the cruciferous group multiple times each week has been shown to reduce the risk of most cancers significantly. Cauliflower has a high level of vitamin C which helps fight the adverse effects caused by free radicals. Vitamin C also helps boost the immune system thanks to the glutathione. Cauliflower has been shown to help reduce the risk of brain disorders, help with weight loss, and help keep a hormonal balance.

Cancer & Disease Fighting: The phytonutrients found in cauliflower have been proven to help fight certain cancers such as breast, cervical, colon, ovarian, and prostate. One study showed that a high intake of cauliflower can reduce the advancement of prostate cancer.

Phytochemicals: Sulforaphane, Indole-3-Carbinol, Di-indolmethane, Isothiocyanates, Glucosinolates, Peroxidases, Isalexin, Glutathione.

Minerals: Calcium, Copper, Iron, Magnesium, Manganese, Potassium, Sodium, Zinc.

Vitamins: Vitamin C, Vitamin K, Folic Acid, Niacin, Pantothenic Acid, Pyridoxine, Riboflavin, and Thiamin.

Celery

About: Belongs to the Apiaceae family. Celery has been known to help the body in so many ways such as reducing blood pressure and lowering cholesterol. It also helps prevent urinary tract infections in women. Scientists have shown us that celery can lessen the pain and swelling in and around the joints. Pregnant women should talk to their doctor about celery and pregnancy. Celery has also been shown to give relief from both asthma and migraines. Research has stated that celery plays a crucial role in eye health. Vitamin C levels also help prevent the damage caused by free radicals. A study that was conducted in China showed a link to lower UTI symptoms in men. Celery has also been shown to boost the immune system. Celery has also been shown to help with weight loss due to its high fiber content.

Cancer & Disease Fighting: Scientists have found that celery has been known to inhibit stomach cancer as well as liver cancer in certain animals.

Phytochemicals: Flavonoids, Phthalides, Luteolin, Polyacetylenes.

Minerals: Calcium, Iron, Magnesium, Manganese, Phosphorus, Potassium, Sodium, Zinc.

Vitamins: Vitamin A, Vitamin C, Vitamin E, Vitamin K, Folic Acid, Niacin, Pantothenic Acid, Pyridoxine, Riboflavin, and Thiamin.

Corn

About: Belongs to the Poaceae family. Corn is also called maize. The calories from corn are mainly because of the simple carbohydrates like glucose and sucrose. Corn is used to produce food sweeteners. Corn has a high glycemic index. Corn oils are rich in vitamin E.

Cancer & Disease Fighting: Because of the high ferulic acid levels corn helps play a vital role in the prevention of certain cancers. The flavonoids play a role in fighting lung and oral cavity cancers. The lutein in corn helps prevent the oxidation of vitamin A and could help in the prevention of colon cancer.

Phytochemicals: Flavonoids, Lutein, β-Carotene, Cryptoxanthins, Xanthins.

Minerals: Calcium, Iron, Magnesium, Manganese, Phosphorus, Potassium, Selenium, Sodium, Zinc.

Vitamins: Vitamin A, Vitamin C, Vitamin K, Folic Acid, Niacin, Pantothenic Acid, Pyridoxine, Riboflavin, and Thiamin.

Cucumber

About: Belongs to the Cucurbitaceae. Cucumbers have a low-calorie intake. Cucumbers are a great source of silica which helps strengthen the connective tissues. Cucumbers contain ascorbic acid and caffein acids that help prevent water retention. This is why you see people using cucumbers on their eyes and burns to the skin. Cucumbers also help prevent the formation of kidney stones. Cucumbers are high in alkaline levels which help the pH levels in the body. Research has also shown us that cucumbers have the ability to counter the effects of uric acid.

Cancer & Disease Fighting: In a recent study, cucumbers were shown to slow skin cancer in animals.

Phytochemicals: ß-Carotene, Cucurbitacins, Cucumerin A and B, Lutein, Vitexins, Zeaxanthin.

Minerals: Calcium, Iron, Magnesium, Manganese, Phosphorus, Potassium, Zinc.

Vitamins: Vitamin A, Vitamin C, Vitamin K, Folic Acid, Pantothenic Acid, Pyridoxine, Riboflavin, Thiamin.

Edamame (soybeans)

About: Belongs to the Fabaceae family. Edamame is also known as soybeans. According to research edamame has been shown to help improve lung function in people with asthma. Edamame is also a great source of protein. Edamame has been shown to help with reducing the risk of cardiovascular disease. Soybeans have been shown in many studies to improve the human body in many ways. Edamame also helps strengthen the immune system and helps manage weight. Edamame contains high levels of manganese which is a co-factor for the antioxidant superoxide dismutase. Superoxide dismutase is an enzyme that allows the breakdown of free radicals.

Cancer & Disease Fighting: Research has shown that the compounds found in the soybeans isoflavones have caused apoptosis in HN4 squamous cell carcinoma of the head and neck cell lines.

Phytochemicals: Phytosterols, Campesterol, Sitosterol, Stigmasterol-Lecithins, Isoflavones.

Minerals: Calcium, Copper, Iron, Magnesium, Manganese, Phosphorus, Potassium, Zinc.

Vitamins: Vitamin C, Vitamin E, Vitamin K, Folic Acid, Pantothenic Acid, Pyridoxine, Riboflavin, and Thiamin.

Eggplant

About: Belongs to the Solanaceae family. Eggplant is low in fats, carbohydrates, and proteins. Research has shown that eggplants help control high blood cholesterol levels. Eggplant has also been shown to reduce the symptoms of anemia and also improve the digestive system.

Cancer & Disease Fighting: The antioxidant powers of eggplants have been shown to lower the risk of certain cancers such as skin cancer.

Phytochemicals: Anthocyanins.

Minerals: Calcium, Copper, Iron, Magnesium, Manganese, Potassium, Zinc.

Vitamins: Vitamin A, Vitamin C, Vitamin E, Vitamin K, Folic Acid, Pantothenic Acid, Pyridoxine, Riboflavin, and Thiamin.

Endive

About: Belongs to the Asteraceae family. Endive is also known as escarole and chicory. Endives carry high levels of vitamin A which are essential to maintaining healthy skin.

Cancer & Disease Fighting: The compounds found in endives have been shown to fight against certain cancers such as breast, cervix, and skin epidermoid carcinoma in vitro. A large study done in the Netherlands of 62,000 women showed that women eating endive can reduce the risk of ovarian cancer by 75% because of the compound kaempferol that causes apoptosis on the cell line.

Phytochemicals: Scyllo-inositol, Carotenoids, β-Carotene, Phenols, Kaempferol.

Minerals: Calcium, Copper, Iron, Magnesium, Manganese, Phosphorus, Selenium, Potassium, Zinc.

Vitamins: Vitamin A, Vitamin C, Vitamin E, Vitamin K, Folic Acid, Pantothenic Acid, Pyridoxine, Riboflavin, and Thiamin.

Fennel

About: Belongs to the Umbelliferae family. Fennel has been known to provide relief of intestinal cramps and spasms. Fennel has also been found to suppress the appetite. Fennel will also reduce water weight.

Cancer & Disease Fighting: The compound anethole found in fennel has been shown in multiple studies to reduce inflammation and reduce the risks of certain cancers.

Phytochemicals: Flavonoids, Phytoestrogens.

Minerals: Calcium, Copper, Iron, Magnesium, Manganese, Phosphorus, Selenium, Potassium, Sodium, Zinc.

Vitamins: Vitamin A, Vitamin C, Folic Acid, Pantothenic Acid, Pyridoxine, Riboflavin, and Thiamin.

Garlic

About: Belongs to the Liliaceae family. Garlic has very high levels of pyridoxine (vitamin B6). The allicin in garlic has been shown to decrease blood vessel stiffness by the release of nitric oxide (NO); this will cause a reduction in blood pressure. Garlic is excellent for helping boost the immune system by the compound found in garlic called allicin. When garlic is chewed or crushed it turns into allicin.

Cancer & Disease Fighting: Garlic has been found in many studies to be the top vegetable in the fight against cancer. Studies show that garlic also protects against cancers caused by nitrosamines. Nitrosamines are found in preserved meats. Eating garlic is one of the best defenses in the apoptosis of cancer cells. The risk of prostate cancer significantly decreased with the daily consumption of garlic. Researchers found garlic is also associated with a decrease in stomach cancer. Garlic is the number one vegetable to stop cell proliferation in seven different cancer cell lines.

Phytochemicals: Flavonoids, Alliin, Allicin, Alliinase, S-allyl cysteine, Diallyl disulfide.

Minerals: Calcium, Copper, Iron, Magnesium, Manganese, Selenium, Potassium, Zinc.

Vitamins: Vitamin C, Vitamin E, Vitamin K, Folic Acid, Pantothenic Acid, Pyridoxine, Riboflavin, and Thiamin.

Green Beans

About: Belongs to the Fabaceae family. Green beans are a good source of vitamin A and vitamin C. Green beans are low in calories

Cancer & Disease Fighting: More research is needed on the role of green beans and cancer.

Phytochemicals: Flavonoids, Carotenoids, β-Carotene, Lutein, Zeaxanthin.

Minerals: Calcium, Iron, Magnesium, Manganese, Phosphorus, Potassium, Zinc.

Vitamins: Vitamin A, Vitamin C, Vitamin K, Folic Acid, Pantothenic Acid, Pyridoxine, Riboflavin, and Thiamin.

Green Peas

About: Belongs to the Fabaceae family. Green peas are also known as garden peas or English peas. Green peas are a great source of protein. Peas have also been shown to fight several allergic reactions in vitro. Peas are also low in calories. The high vitamin K levels in foods have been shown to help fight neuronal damage in the brain.

Cancer & Disease Fighting: Research has shown that peas inhibit the proliferation of colon cancer cells.

Phytochemicals: Flavonoids, Polyphenols, Phytosterols.

Minerals: Calcium, Copper, Iron, Magnesium, Manganese, Selenium, Potassium, Zinc.

Vitamins: Vitamin A, Vitamin C, Vitamin E, Vitamin K, Folic Acid, Pantothenic Acid, Pyridoxine, Riboflavin, and Thiamin.

Kale

About: Belongs to the Brassicaceae family. Kale is loaded with vitamins A, C, and K. Vitamin K has been shown to promote bone health as well as limit neuronal damage in the brain. Kale has been known to boost the immune system due to the high levels of vitamin C.

Cancer & Disease Fighting: Foods that are rich in vitamin A have been shown to protect against lung cancer. Multiple studies have been conducted in vitro on skin cancer with very positive results.

Phytochemicals: Flavonoids, Glucosinolates, Carotenoids, Indole-3-carbinol, Sulforaphane, β-Carotene, Lutein, Zeaxanthin, Kaempferol, Quercetin, Isorhamnetin.

Minerals: Calcium, Copper, Iron, Magnesium, Manganese, Potassium, Phosphorus, Selenium, Sodium, Zinc.

Vitamins: Vitamin A, Vitamin C, Vitamin K, Folic Acid, Pantothenic Acid, Pyridoxine, Riboflavin, and Thiamin.

Leeks

About: Belongs to the Alliaceae family. Leeks are found in parts of Europe and Asia.

Cancer & Disease Fighting: Leeks in the allium group like garlic have been shown to be a powerful food against the growth of cancer by causing apoptosis of certain cancer cell lines.

Phytochemicals: Flavonoids, Allicin, Diallyl Disulfide, Diallyl Trisulfide, Allyl Propyl Disulfide, Carotenoids, Lutein, Xanthin.

Minerals: Calcium, Copper, Iron, Magnesium, Manganese, Potassium, Phosphorus, Selenium, Sodium, Zinc.

Vitamins: Vitamin A, Vitamin C, Vitamin E, Vitamin K, Folic Acid, Pantothenic Acid, Pyridoxine, Riboflavin, and Thiamin.

Lettuce

About: Belongs to the Asteraceae family. Lettuce is very low in calories. Lettuce is loaded with vitamin A.

Cancer & Disease Fighting: Researchers have shown lettuce to inhibit the growth of leukemia and breast cancer.

Phytochemicals: Carotenoids, β-Carotene, Lutein, Zeaxanthin.

Minerals: Calcium, Copper, Iron, Magnesium, Manganese, Potassium, Phosphorus, Sodium, Zinc.

Vitamins: Vitamin A, Vitamin C, Vitamin E, Vitamin K, Folic Acid, Pantothenic Acid, Pyridoxine, Riboflavin, and Thiamin.

Okra

About: Belongs to the Malvaceae family. Researchers have found okra to help improve digestion and help prevent constipation. Okra was also found in a study conducted in China to help reduce fatigue in mice. More research is needed on human trials to confirm these results.

Cancer & Disease Fighting: Okra has been found to inhibit cell proliferation in colon cancer and retinoblastoma (a rare cancer that develops immature cells in the retina) cells.

Phytochemicals: Polysaccharides, Flavonoids, Lectin, Phenols.

Minerals: Calcium, Copper, Iron, Magnesium, Manganese, Potassium, Phosphorus, Selenium, Zinc.

Vitamins: Vitamin A, Vitamin C, Vitamin E, Vitamin K, Folic Acid, Pantothenic Acid, Pyridoxine, Riboflavin, and Thiamin.

Onions

About: Belongs to the Alliaceae family. The sulfur-containing compounds make onions a great anti-blood clotting food. Onions are a great source of antioxidants according to the latest research. Onions help boost the immune system thanks to the allicin.

Cancer & Disease Fighting: Research has shown onions to be an excellent source for the lowering of risk in certain cancers such as colorectal, laryngeal, and ovarian cancers. Try to include onions, leeks, and garlic in your meals daily. The allium group is a powerful group of vegetables against prostate cancer.

Phytochemicals: Flavonoids, Allicin, Fisetin, Isorhamnetin, Kaempferol, Quercetin.

Minerals: Calcium, Copper, Iron, Magnesium, Manganese, Potassium, Phosphorus, Zinc.

Vitamins: Vitamin C, Folic Acid, Pantothenic Acid, Pyridoxine, Riboflavin, and Thiamin.

Parsnips

About: Belongs to the Apiaceae family. Parsnips are a good source of vitamin C. Parsnips are a good source of fiber as well.

Cancer & Disease Fighting: Parsnips have been shown to be antiproliferative in leukemia and colon cancer cells in humans.

Phytochemicals: Bergapten, Falcarinol, Falcarindiol, Isopimpinellin, Myristicin, Psoralen, Umbelliferone, Xanthotoxin.

Minerals: Calcium, Copper, Iron, Magnesium, Manganese, Potassium, Phosphorus, Selenium, Zinc.

Vitamins: Vitamin C, Vitamin K, Folic Acid, Pantothenic Acid, Pyridoxine, Riboflavin, Thiamin.

Peppers "Bell"

About: Belongs to the Solanaceae family. Bell peppers are one of the best sources of vitamin C. Vitamin C is needed in the production of collagen. Peppers help fight free radicals. They are also low in calories.

Cancer & Disease Fighting: One study on nightshade plants such as peppers found a diet rich in peppers might play a role in lowering the risk of Parkinson's. More research is needed on the peppers.

Phytochemicals: Anthocyanins, Flavonoids, β-Carotene and α-Carotene, Cryptoxanthins, Lutein, Zeaxanthins.

Minerals: Calcium, Copper, Iron, Magnesium, Manganese, Potassium, Phosphorus, Zinc.

Vitamins: Vitamin A, Vitamin C, Vitamin E, Vitamin K, Folic Acid, Pantothenic Acid, Pyridoxine, Riboflavin, and Thiamin.

Potatoes

About: Belongs to the Solanaceae family. Potatoes have been shown to help keep blood sugars in a normal range. Potatoes are a great source of soluble and insoluble fiber. The potato skin is an excellent source of iron.

Cancer & Disease Fighting: Potatoes are shown to help fight colon cancer due to their fiber content and vitamin C levels. Vitamin C helps fight the free radicals in the body.

Phytochemicals: Alkaloidal Glycosides, Flavonoids, Carotenes, Quercetins, Zeaxanthins.

Minerals: Calcium, Iron, Magnesium, Manganese, Potassium, Phosphorus, Zinc.

Vitamins: Vitamin C, Vitamin K, Folic Acid, Pantothenic Acid, Pyridoxine, Riboflavin, and Thiamin.

Pumpkin

About: Belongs to the Cucurbitaceae family. Pumpkin seeds are a great source of monounsaturated fatty acids. Pumpkin seeds are also a good source of the amino acid tryptophan. Pumpkin is very low in calories.

Cancer & Disease Fighting: The healthy levels of vitamin A in pumpkin has been shown to protect against lung cancer as well as oral cavity cancers. The carotenoids have been found to reduce oxidative stress caused by free radicals.

Phytochemicals: Carotenoids, β-Carotene, and α-Carotene, Cryptoxanthins, Lutein, Zeaxanthins.

Minerals: Calcium, Copper, Iron, Magnesium, Manganese, Potassium, Phosphorus, Selenium, Zinc.

Vitamins: Vitamin A, Vitamin C, Vitamin E, Vitamin K, Folic Acid, Pantothenic Acid, Pyridoxine, Riboflavin, and Thiamin.

Radicchio

About: Belongs to the Asteraceae family. Radicchio is also called chicory. Radicchio is very low in calories, and a great source of vitamin K. Radicchio also has anti-inflammatory properties.

Cancer & Disease Fighting: The high vitamin K levels help to limit neuronal damage in the brain.

Phytochemicals: Flavonoids, Anthocyanidins, Carotenoids, Lutein, Zeaxanthins.

Minerals: Calcium, Copper, Iron, Magnesium, Manganese, Potassium, Phosphorus, Selenium, Sodium, Zinc.

Vitamins: Vitamin A, Vitamin C, Vitamin E, Vitamin K, Folic Acid, Pantothenic Acid, Pyridoxine, Riboflavin, and Thiamin.

Radish

About: Belongs to the Brassicaceae family. Radishes are a good source of vitamin C.

Cancer & Disease Fighting: The flavonoids and polyphenols inhibit cell proliferation and cause apoptosis in cancer cells.

Phytochemicals: Sulforaphane, Indoles, Carotenoids, β-Carotene, Lutein, Zeaxanthins.

Minerals: Calcium, Copper, Iron, Magnesium, Manganese, Potassium, Sodium, Zinc.

Vitamins: Vitamin C, Vitamin E, Vitamin K, Folic Acid, Pantothenic Acid, Pyridoxine, Riboflavin, and Thiamin.

Rhubarb

About: Belongs to the Polygonaceae family. Rhubard is a low-calorie vegetable. Rhubard has modest amounts of vitamin K that helps with bone formation.

Cancer & Disease Fighting: More research is needed on rhubarb.

Phytochemicals: Flavonoids.

Minerals: Calcium, Copper, Iron, Magnesium, Manganese, Phosphorus, Selenium, Potassium, Zinc.

Vitamins: Vitamin A, Vitamin C, Vitamin E, Vitamin K, Folic Acid, Pantothenic Acid, Pyridoxine, Riboflavin, and Thiamin.

Rutabaga

About: Belongs to the Brassicaceae family. Rutabaga carries the right amount of vitamin C.

Cancer & Disease Fighting: Research has stated that the plant sterol brassinolide has been shown to induce apoptosis in prostate cancer cells.

Phytochemicals: Indole-3-Carbinol, Brassinolide, Tocopherol, Cerebroside, Ceramide.

Minerals: Calcium, Copper, Iron, Magnesium, Manganese, Potassium, Zinc.

Vitamins: Vitamin C, Folic Acid, Pantothenic Acid, Pyridoxine, Riboflavin, Thiamin.

Shallots

About: Belongs to the Amaryllidaceae family. Shallots have been shown to decrease blood vessel stiffness due to nitric oxide (NO).

Cancer & Disease Fighting: Studies done on lab animals have shown anti-tumor effects. More research is needed on shallots.

Phytochemicals: Flavonoids, Kaempferol, Quercetin, Diallyl Disulfide, Diallyl Trisulfide, Allyl Propyl Disulfide.

Minerals: Calcium, Copper, Iron, Magnesium, Manganese, Potassium, Phosphorus, Sodium, Zinc.

Vitamins: Vitamin A, Vitamin C, Folic Acid, Pantothenic Acid, Pyridoxine, Riboflavin, and Thiamin.

Snap Peas

About: Belongs to the Fabaceae family. The high vitamin C levels help to combat the free radicals in the body and reduce inflammation.

Snap peas also contain ample amounts of vitamin A which is needed to maintain good skin and healthy eyesight.

Cancer & Disease Fighting: Snap peas contain porphyrins and lectins which have been shown to inhibit the growth of certain cancers such as colon, gastric, and liver cancers.

Phytochemicals: Flavonoids, Porphyrins, Lectins, Carotenoids, β-Carotene, Lutein, Zeaxanthins.

Minerals: Calcium, Copper, Iron, Magnesium, Manganese, Potassium, Zinc.

Vitamins: Vitamin A, Vitamin C, Vitamin E, Vitamin K, Folic Acid, Pantothenic Acid, Pyridoxine, Riboflavin, and Thiamin.

Spinach

About: Belongs to the Amaranthaceae family. Spinach is an excellent source of vitamin A and vitamin K. It also has high levels of iron and manganese. Spinach also contains small amounts of omega-3 fatty acids. Spinach also helps boost the immune system to help fight off infections.

Cancer & Disease Fighting: Spinach has long been associated with reducing the risk of multiple cancers such as the bladder, head, neck, gallbladder, liver, lung, ovarian, prostate, and stomach.

Phytochemicals: Flavonoids, Kaempferol, Quercetin, Lignans, Carotenoids, β-Carotene, Lutein, Zeaxanthins.

Minerals: Calcium, Copper, Iron, Magnesium, Manganese, Potassium, Sodium, Zinc.

Vitamins: Vitamin A, Vitamin C, Vitamin E, Vitamin K, Folic Acid, Pantothenic Acid, Pyridoxine, Riboflavin, and Thiamin.

Sweet Potatoes

About: Belongs to the Convolvulaceae family. Sweet potatoes contain vast amounts of vitamin A which is one of the highest of any root vegetable.

Cancer & Disease Fighting: Sweet potatoes have been known to prevent the growth of cancers such as liver and lung cancers. Researchers have also found that sweet potatoes have the ability to protect against cancers such as breast cancer, gallbladder cancer, kidney cancer, and leukemia.

Phytochemicals: Flavonoids, Carotenoids, β-Carotene.

Minerals: Calcium, Iron, Magnesium, Manganese, Phosphorus, Potassium, Sodium, Zinc.

Vitamins: Vitamin A, Vitamin C, Vitamin E, Vitamin K, Folic Acid, Pantothenic Acid, Pyridoxine, Riboflavin, and Thiamin.

Swiss Chard

About: Belongs to the Amaranthaceae family. Swiss chard is loaded with vitamin K which is known for preventing neuronal damage in the brain. Researchers have also stated that Swiss chard is great for maintaining bone health. Other research has found that the intake of Swiss chard has helped with the secretion of insulin. There has been research on the role Swiss chard plays with regard to Alzheimer's and Parkinson's disease; the results have not published as of yet. Swiss chard also helps boost the immune system due to the high levels of vitamin C.

Cancer & Disease Fighting: Researcher on Swiss chard has found that precancerous lesions in animals were significantly reduced following the intake of Swiss chard. More research involving humans is needed.

Phytochemicals: Flavonoids, Carotenoids, β-Carotene, α-Carotene, Lutein, Zeaxanthin

Minerals: Calcium, Copper, Iron, Magnesium, Manganese, Phosphorus, Potassium, Selenium, Sodium, Zinc.

Vitamins: Vitamin A, Vitamin C, Vitamin E, Vitamin K, Folic Acid, Pantothenic Acid, Pyridoxine, Riboflavin, and Thiamin.

Tomatoes

About: Belongs to the Solanaceae family. Tomatoes are very low in calories and have carotenoids such as lycopene that help protect our skin from ultraviolet (UV) rays. Tomatoes have high levels of β-Carotene that help boost the immune system.

Cancer & Disease Fighting: The antioxidant powers found in tomatoes have been shown to protect against breast cancer, colon cancer, endometrial cancer, lung cancer, and prostate cancer.

Phytochemicals: Flavonoids, Carotenoids, α-Carotene, β-Carotene, Lycopene, Lutein, Zeaxanthin, Chlorophyll.

Minerals: Calcium, Iron, Magnesium, Manganese, Phosphorus, Potassium, Zinc.

Vitamins: Vitamin A, Vitamin C, Vitamin E, Vitamin K, Folic Acid, Pantothenic Acid, Pyridoxine, Riboflavin, and Thiamin.

Turnips Greens

About: Belongs to the Brassicaceae family. Turnip greens carry all the nutrients, not the root. Turnips greens are a great source of vitamin A and vitamin K.

Cancer & Disease Fighting: Turnip greens have sulfur-containing glucosinolates that have been linked through research to prevent cell growth in the colon, gastric, and liver cancers as well as leukemia.

Phytochemicals: Carotenoids, β-Carotene, Lutein, Glucosinolates.

Minerals: Calcium, Copper, Iron, Magnesium, Manganese, Phosphorus, Potassium, Zinc.

Vitamins: Vitamin A, Vitamin C, Vitamin E, Vitamin K, Folic Acid, Pantothenic Acid, Pyridoxine, Riboflavin, and Thiamin.

Watercress

About: Belongs to the Brassicaceae family. Watercress is very low in calories.

Cancer & Disease Fighting: Watercress has been shown to help protect the body against lung cancer due to the Isothiocyanates.

Phytochemicals: Isothiocyanates, Carotenoids, β-Carotene, Lutein, Zeaxanthins, Glucosinolates.

Minerals: Calcium, Copper, Iron, Magnesium, Manganese, Phosphorus, Potassium, Selenium, Sodium, Zinc.

Vitamins: Vitamin A, Vitamin C, Vitamin E, Vitamin K, Folic Acid, Pantothenic Acid, Pyridoxine, Riboflavin, and Thiamin.

Zucchini Squash

About: Belongs to the Cucurbitaceae family. Zucchini squash has a modest amount of vitamin C which helps combat the attacks from free radicals.

Cancer & Disease Fighting: More research is needed on the squash family and its role in fighting cancer and diseases.

Phytochemicals: Carotenoids, β-Carotene, Lutein, Zeaxanthins.

Minerals: Calcium, Iron, Magnesium, Manganese, Phosphorus, Potassium, Zinc.

Vitamins: Vitamin A, Vitamin C, Vitamin K, Folic Acid, Pantothenic Acid, Pyridoxine, Riboflavin, and Thiamin.

Mushrooms

List of Commonly Used Mushrooms

Button (white, crimini, portabella)

About: Belongs to the Basidiomycetes family. There are three types of button mushrooms crimping, portabella, and white. Button mushrooms are loaded with antioxidants. They have more antioxidants than green peppers, pumpkins, carrots, tomatoes, and green beans. White button mushrooms contain trace amounts of vitamin B12; if you cook the mushrooms, you can cook the B vitamins out of the mushroom. The best is to steam the mushroom. The button mushrooms offer essential amino acids.

Cancer & Disease Fighting: Researchers have shown that button mushrooms have the ability to inhibit the activity of aromatase and suppress breast cancer cell proliferation. On MCF-7aro cells.

Phytochemicals: Flavonoids, Flavones, Isoflavones, β-Glucans, Polysaccharides, Ergocalciferol.

Minerals: Calcium, Copper, Iron, Magnesium, Manganese, Potassium, Phosphorus, Sodium, Zinc.

Vitamins: Vitamin C, Vitamin D, Vitamin B12, Folic Acid, Pantothenic Acid, Pyridoxine, Riboflavin, and Thiamin.

Enoki

About: Belongs to the Physalacriaceae family. The phytochemicals in enoki mushrooms have been shown to lower cholesterol.

Cancer & Disease Fighting: Enoki mushrooms have been shown to have anticancer properties to fight against melanoma.

Phytochemicals: Polysaccharides, Flammulin, Proflanin, β-Glucans.

Minerals: Copper, Iron, Magnesium, Manganese, Potassium, Phosphorus, Sodium, Zinc.

Vitamins: Vitamin D, Folic Acid, Pantothenic Acid, Pyridoxine, Riboflavin, and Thiamin.

Maitake

About: Belongs to the Meripilaceae family. The maitake mushroom is loaded with vitamin D which is essential for bone development. The maitake is also packed with niacin which is needed for DNA repair as well as in the role of metabolism with fats and carbohydrates. This mushroom has also been known to help boost the immune system. The high zinc levels help increase the white blood cells.

Cancer & Disease Fighting: Researchers have stated the phytochemical β-Glucans found in maitake mushrooms have been found to cause apoptosis in cancer cells. There has also been research on the maitake mushroom showing promise in breast cancer, lung cancer, and myelodysplastic syndrome (MDS).

Phytochemicals: Polysaccharides, β-Glucans.

Minerals: Copper, Iron, Magnesium, Manganese, Potassium, Phosphorus, Sodium, Zinc.

Vitamins: Vitamin D, Folic Acid, Pantothenic Acid, Pyridoxine, Riboflavin, and Thiamin.

Morels

About: Belongs to the Morchellaceae family. The morel mushroom is loaded with vitamin D. The morel also contains very high amounts of iron.

Cancer & Disease Fighting: The Morel mushroom has great antioxidant power that helps prevent heart disease and also works to help fight cancer.

Phytochemicals: Polysaccharides.

Minerals: Calcium, Copper, Iron, Magnesium, Manganese, Potassium, Phosphorus, Sodium, Zinc.

Vitamins: Vitamin D, Folic Acid, Pantothenic Acid, Pyridoxine, Riboflavin, and Thiamin.

Oyster Mushroom

About: Belongs to the Pleurotaceae family. Oyster mushrooms are a good source of protein.

Cancer & Disease Fighting: More research is needed on oyster mushrooms and cancer.

Phytochemicals: Polysaccharides, β-Glucans.

Minerals: Copper, Iron, Magnesium, Manganese, Potassium, Phosphorus, Sodium, Zinc.

Vitamins: Vitamin D, Folic Acid, Pantothenic Acid, Pyridoxine, Riboflavin, and Thiamin.

Shitake

About: Belongs to the Morchellaceae family. Shitake mushrooms are loaded with niacin, vitamins B5 and B6. Shitake is low in calories. There are modest amounts of vitamin D in this mushroom.

Cancer & Disease Fighting: Lentinan acts as an immune modulator that is known to inhibit tumor growth.

Phytochemicals: Eritadenin, Polysaccharides, Lentinan.

Minerals: Copper, Iron, Magnesium, Manganese, Potassium, Phosphorus, Sodium, Zinc.

Vitamins: Vitamin D, Folic Acid, Pantothenic Acid, Pyridoxine, Riboflavin, and Thiamin.

12

Legumes/Nuts/Seeds & Whole Grains

Legumes are a great source of non-animal protein as well as a great source of needed fiber. Legumes are an essential source of vitamins and minerals. Legumes have been shown to help prevent heart disease. The fiber in legumes is great for lowering cholesterol by bonding to the cholesterol and removing it from the body before it builds up in the blood vessel walls. The fiber in legumes helps to balance the pH levels in the gut. Legumes have a low glycemic index (GI).

Nuts and seeds are essential for the growth and development of your body and should be included in your diet on a daily basis. Nuts have been shown to play a role in reversing metabolic syndrome. According to a study in the New England Journal of Medicine stated that increased nut consumption has been associated with a reduced risk of major chronic diseases, including cardiovascular disease and type 2 diabetes mellitus. Research has proven that just four Brazilian nuts a month can reduce LDL cholesterol by as much as 45% and carry those values in the blood for 30 days. We only need about a handful of mixed nuts daily.

Whole grains are a great source of fiber and phytochemicals. Whole grains are digested slower than that of processed grains. When whole grains are processed slower it helps keep blood sugar and insulin levels low. The Nurse's study showed that women that 5 grams or more of whole grain fiber cereals had about a 30% less risk of getting type 2 diabetes than the ones who ate less than 2.5 grams of whole grain fiber per day.

Below is a list of Commonly Used Legumes, Nuts, Seeds, and Whole Grains.

Legumes

Legume: Adzuki Beans

About: Belongs to the Fabaceae family. Adzuki beans are loaded with fiber. The phytochemicalβ-Sitosterol helps to lower the cholesterol in the body.

Cancer & Disease Fighting: The adzuki beans contain fiber that binds to toxins in the colon and takes them out of the body, therefore, lowering the risk of cancer.

Phytochemicals: Flavonoids, Isoflavones, Pro-Anthocyanidin Dimers, Phytosterols, β-Sitosterol.

Minerals: Calcium, Copper, Iron, Magnesium, Manganese, Phosphorus, Potassium, Selenium, Zinc.

Vitamins: Vitamin A, Folic Acid, Pantothenic Acid, Pyridoxine, Riboflavin, Thiamin.

Legume: **Black Beans**

About: Belongs to the Fabaceae family. Black beans are a great source of dietary fiber. Black beans are also a great source of antioxidants that fight against free radicals.

Cancer & Disease Fighting: The black beans have been shown to lower the risk of colon cancer.

Phytochemicals: Flavonoids, Anthocyanins, Delphinidin, Petunien, Malvidin, Kaempferol, Quercetin.

Minerals: Calcium, Copper, Iron, Magnesium, Manganese, Phosphorus, Potassium, Selenium, Zinc.

Vitamins: Vitamin A, Folic Acid, Pantothenic Acid, Pyridoxine, Riboflavin, Thiamin.

Legume: **Chickpeas (garbanzo beans)**

About: Belongs to the Fabaceae family. Chickpeas are a great source of folates. Folates play an essential co-factor role in DNA synthesis.

Cancer & Disease Fighting: The isoflavones found in chickpeas have been shown to reduce the risk of certain cancers in post-menopausal women as well as osteoporosis. The high dietary fiber found in chickpeas helps lower the risk of colon cancer.

Phytochemicals: Flavonoids, Isoflavones, Biochanin-A, Glycitein, Genistein, Daidzein, Formononetin.

Minerals: Calcium, Copper, Iron, Magnesium, Phosphorus, Potassium, Sodium, Zinc.

Vitamins: Vitamin A, Vitamin C, Folic Acid, Pantothenic Acid, Pyridoxine, Riboflavin, Thiamin.

Legume: **Cowpeas (black-eye peas)**

About: Belongs to the Fabaceae family. Cowpeas are a great source of copper, iron, and folate. The high fiber levels have been shown to reduce blood cholesterol levels.

Cancer & Disease Fighting: The biochanin-A found in cowpeas is a phytoestrogen. Scientists have stated that biochanin-A plays an essential role in preventing certain cancers. Phytoestrogens like biochanin-A have been found to inhibit the growth of HCT-8 human colon cancer cells.

Phytochemicals: Flavonoids, Isoflavones, Biochanin-A.

Minerals: Calcium, Copper, Iron, Magnesium, Manganese, Phosphorus, Potassium, Selenium, sodium, Zinc.

Vitamins: Vitamin C, Vitamin E, Vitamin K, Folic Acid, Pantothenic Acid, Pyridoxine, Riboflavin, Thiamin.

Legume: **Kidney Beans (white and red)**

About: Belongs to the Fabaceae family. White kidney beans are also known as cannellini beans. !!!!! ALERT!!!!! Kidney beans must be soaked and cooked (boiled for 30 minutes) because of the high amounts of phytohemagglutinin. Kidney beans are high in fiber, and they are a great source of protein.

Cancer & Disease Fighting: The high fiber in kidney beans has been shown to help lower the risk of cardiovascular disease.

Phytochemicals: Flavonoids, Saponins, Phytic Acid.

Minerals: Calcium, Copper, Iron, Magnesium, Manganese, Phosphorus, Potassium, Selenium, Sodium, Zinc.

Vitamins: Vitamin C, Vitamin E, Vitamin K, Folic Acid, Pantothenic Acid, Pyridoxine, Riboflavin, Thiamin.

Legume: **Lentils**

About: Belongs to the Fabaceae family. Lentils are an excellent source of protein. Lentils help to lower cholesterol levels. Lentils are with folates and iron. Lentils are loaded with the amino acid arginine which is needed to help prevent high blood pressure, and it is crucial to the growth of tissue. Arginine is necessary for the development of young bodies. It is also needed for the production of nitric oxide. It opens the blood vessels for increased blood flow. Arginine also is required for hair growth.

Cancer & Disease Fighting: Lentils have been shown to lower the risk of breast cancer. Researchers have also found that a higher intake of lentils can reduce the risk of esophagus, throat, and larynx cancers. Researchers have also stated that lentils help lower the risk of cardiovascular disease. The fiber found in lentils has also been shown to reduce the risk of colon cancer.

Phytochemicals: Flavonoids, Isoflavones, Pro-Anthocyanidin Dimers, Glycosides, Catechin, Gallocatechin, Phytic Acid, Saponins, β-Sitosterol.

Minerals: Calcium, Copper, Iron, Magnesium, Phosphorus, Potassium, Zinc.

Vitamins: Vitamin A, Vitamin C, Folic Acid, Pantothenic Acid, Pyridoxine, Riboflavin, Thiamin.

Legume: **Lima Beans**

About: Belongs to the Fabaceae family. Lima beans are a great source of iron and folates. Lima beans are an excellent source of plant-based protein. The β-Sitosterol contained in the lima bean has been shown to help lower cholesterol.

Cancer & Disease Fighting: The fiber content of the lima beans helps to lower the risk of colon cancer according to the researchers. The isoflavones have been shown to inhibit breast cancer in laboratory animals. More research is needed in human trials.

Phytochemicals: Flavonoids, Isoflavones, Daidzein, Genistein, β-Sitosterol.

Minerals: Calcium, Copper, Iron, Magnesium, Manganese, Phosphorus, Potassium, Selenium, Sodium, Zinc.

Vitamins: Vitamin E, Vitamin K, Folic Acid, Pantothenic Acid, Pyridoxine, Riboflavin, Thiamin.

Legume: **Navy Bean**

About: Belongs to the Fabaceae family. Navy beans are an excellent source of needed minerals such as copper, iron, Magnesium, Manganese, Phosphorus, and Potassium.

Cancer & Disease Fighting: The navy bean is an excellent source of dietary fiber that researchers have stated helps to lower the risk of colon cancer.

Phytochemicals: Flavonoids, Isoflavones.

Minerals: Calcium, Copper, Iron, Magnesium, Manganese, Phosphorus, Potassium, Selenium, Zinc.

Vitamins: Folic Acid, Pantothenic Acid, Pyridoxine, Riboflavin, Thiamin.

Legume: **Pinto Bean**

About: Belongs to the Fabaceae family.

Cancer & Disease Fighting: The pinto bean is an excellent source of dietary fiber that researchers have stated helps to lower the risk of colon cancer.

Phytochemicals: Flavonoids, Isoflavones, Biochanin-A, Genistein, Daidzein, Kaempferol.

Minerals: Calcium, Copper, Iron, Magnesium, Manganese, Phosphorus, Potassium, Selenium, Zinc.

Vitamins: Vitamin C, Folic Acid, Pantothenic Acid, Pyridoxine, Riboflavin, Thiamin.

Legume: **Split Pea**

About: Belongs to the Fabaceae family. Split peas are great for helping stabilize blood sugar levels. Dried split peas are also loaded with fiber. Split peas have a high amount of both copper and manganese.

Cancer & Disease Fighting: Dried split peas are a great source of dietary fiber that researchers have stated to lower the risk of colon cancer. The isoflavone daidzein has been shown to help reduce the risk of prostate cancer.

Phytochemicals: Flavonoids, Isoflavones, Daidzein, Carotenoids, β-Carotene.

Minerals: Calcium, Copper, Iron, Magnesium, Manganese, Phosphorus, Potassium, Selenium, Sodium, Zinc.

Vitamins: Vitamin C, Vitamin K, Folic Acid, Pantothenic Acid, Pyridoxine, Riboflavin, Thiamin.

Nuts

Nut: **Almond**

About: Belongs to the Rosaceae family. Almonds are loaded with copper, manganese, magnesium, and phosphorus. Almonds are an excellent source of mono-unsaturated fatty acids such as oleic, and palmitoleic acids, that help raise HDL cholesterol and also lower the bad LDL cholesterol. Almonds are an excellent source of vitamin E that helps fight the free radicals in the body. Resveratrol a phytochemical found in almonds has been shown to cross the blood-brain barrier. Resveratrol has been shown to cause apoptosis in Hodgkin's lymphoma on cell line L-428.

Cancer & Disease Fighting: Almonds have been found to help reduce cancer cell proliferation in vitro. The mono-unsaturated fatty acid has been shown to help prevent coronary artery disease and strokes.

Phytochemicals: Flavonoids, Phytosterols, Proanthocyanidins, Protocatechuic-Acid, Methylquercetin, Catechin, Kaempferol, Resveratrol.

Minerals: Calcium, Copper, Iron, Magnesium, Manganese, Phosphorus, Potassium, Selenium, Zinc.

Vitamins: Vitamin E, Folic Acid, Pantothenic Acid, Pyridoxine, Riboflavin, Thiamin.

Nut: **Brazil**

About: Belongs to the Lecythidaceae family. Brazil nuts carry vast amounts of Selenium. Eating just a few Brazilian nuts each month can help lower the LDL levels in the body and research has shown that it can carry those levels for about 30 days. This study stated that these results were better than taking a statin and is a well-published study. Brazilian nuts carry large amounts of the amino acid arginine which is converted to nitric oxide in the body.

Cancer & Disease Fighting: Just a couple of Brazilian nuts each month can reduce the risk of coronary artery disease and strokes as well as liver cirrhosis. The high selenium levels also help in lowering the risk of cancer.

Phytochemicals: Phenols, Proanthocyanidins, Phytosterols.

Minerals: Calcium, Copper, Iron, Magnesium, Manganese, Phosphorus, Potassium, Selenium, Zinc.

Vitamins: Vitamin C, Vitamin E, Folic Acid, Pantothenic Acid, Pyridoxine, Riboflavin, Thiamin.

Nut: **Cashew**

About: Belongs to the Anacardiaceae family. Cashews are a great source of protein as well as monounsaturated fatty acids that help in the lowering of LDL (bad) cholesterol and increasing the HDL (good) cholesterol. Cashews are loaded with iron and copper.

Cancer & Disease Fighting: Some studies done on cancer and cashews showed that eating two or more servings per week of cashews showed a 46% lower risk of cancer returning.

Phytochemicals: Flavonoids, Phytosterols, Flavonols, Proanthocyanidins, Carotenoids, Lutein, Zeaxanthin.

Minerals: Calcium, Copper, Iron, Magnesium, Manganese, Phosphorus, Potassium, Selenium, Zinc.

Vitamins: Vitamin C, Vitamin E, Vitamin K, Folic Acid, Pantothenic Acid, Pyridoxine, Riboflavin, Thiamin.

Nut: **Chestnut**

About: Belongs to the Fagaceae family. Chestnuts are rich in vitamin C. Phytosterols have been shown to help reduce LDL cholesterol.

Cancer & Disease Fighting: The high vitamin C levels help fight against the free radicals that cause cell damage. The mono-unsaturated fatty acid has been shown to help prevent coronary artery disease and strokes.

Phytochemicals: Flavonoids, Phytosterols.

Minerals: Calcium, Copper, Iron, Magnesium, Manganese, Phosphorus, Potassium, Zinc.

Vitamins: Vitamin A, Vitamin C, Folic Acid, Pantothenic Acid, Pyridoxine, Riboflavin, Thiamin.

Nut: **Hazelnut (filberts)**

About: Belongs to the Betulaceae family. Hazelnuts are a great source of copper and manganese. Copper and manganese are cofactors for an antioxidant enzyme called superoxide dismutase. Superoxide dismutase is an excellent defense for all living cells that are exposed to oxygen. Hazelnuts are a great source of vitamin E.

Cancer & Disease Fighting: The α-Tocopherol from vitamin E has been shown to help lower the risk of bladder cancer by as much as 50%.

Phytochemicals: Flavonoids, Proanthocyanidins.

Minerals: Calcium, Copper, Iron, Magnesium, Manganese, Phosphorus, Potassium, Zinc.

Vitamins: Vitamin C, Vitamin E, Vitamin K, Folic Acid, Pantothenic Acid, Pyridoxine, Riboflavin, Thiamin.

Nut: **Macadamia**

About: Belongs to the Proteaceae Family. Macadamia is an excellent source of thiamin (B1).

Cancer & Disease Fighting: There has been research that shows β-Sitosterol works to block the production of dihydrotestosterone, which has proved to cause the growth of prostate cancer cells. In other studies, it has been shown to help prevent the growth of colon cancer.

Phytochemicals: Phenols, Phytosterols, β-Sitosterol.

Minerals: Calcium, Copper, Iron, Magnesium, Manganese, Phosphorus, Potassium, Selenium, Zinc.

Vitamins: Vitamin C, Vitamin E, Folic Acid, Pantothenic Acid, Pyridoxine, Riboflavin, Thiamin.

Nut: **Peanut**

About: Belongs to the Fabaceae family. Peanuts as well pistachios are known to have the phytochemicals found in the skin of red grapes "resveratrol." Resveratrol has been shown to cause apoptosis in Hodgkin's lymphoma on cell line L-428. Roasting peanuts or boiling them has been shown to increase the bioavailability of the phytochemicals, isoflavone, biochanin-A, and Genistein. Peanuts are loaded with the amino acid arginine which is needed to help prevent high blood pressure, and it is essential to the growth of tissue. Arginine is necessary for the development of young bodies. It is also needed for the production of nitric oxide. It opens the blood vessels for increased blood flow. Arginine also is required for hair growth.

Cancer & Disease Fighting: Resveratrol has been shown to cause apoptosis in Hodgkin's lymphoma on cell line L-428.

Phytochemicals: Stilbenes, Resveratrol, Isoflavone, Biochanin-A, Proanthocyanidins.

Minerals: Calcium, Copper, Iron, Magnesium, Manganese, Phosphorus, Potassium, Selenium, Zinc.

Vitamins: Vitamin E, Folic Acid, Pantothenic Acid, Pyridoxine, Riboflavin, Thiamin.

Nut: **Pecan**

About: Belongs to the Juglandaceae family. Pecans are a great source of copper and manganese. The pecan is loaded with antioxidant power. Pecans also help reduce the risk of gallstones.

Cancer & Disease Fighting: The mono-unsaturated fatty acids found in the pecan have been shown to help prevent coronary artery disease and strokes. Pecan is also a great source of the amino acid L-arginine that researchers have found to help treat male pattern baldness.

Phytochemicals: Flavonoids, Carotenoids, β-Carotene, Cryptoxanthin-β, Lutein, Zeaxanthin, Ellagic Acid, Tannins.

Minerals: Calcium, Copper, Iron, Magnesium, Manganese, Phosphorus, Potassium, Selenium, Zinc.

Vitamins: Vitamin A, Vitamin C, Vitamin E, Folic Acid, Pantothenic Acid, Pyridoxine, Riboflavin, Thiamin.

Nut: **Pine Nuts**

About: Belongs to the Pinaceae family. Pine nuts are a great source of copper and manganese. Pine nuts contain the omega-6 fatty acid pinolenic acid which researchers have found to help trigger the release of the enzyme CCK (cholecystokinin), and GLP-1 (glucan-like peptide-1) in the gut, which helps suppress hunger. Pine nuts also contain monounsaturated fatty acid oleic acid which has been shown to help lower LDL cholesterol.

Cancer & Disease Fighting: More research is needed on pine nuts role in cancer prevention.

Phytochemicals: Flavonoids, Phytosterols, Carotenoids, β-Carotene, Lutein, Zeaxanthin.

Minerals: Calcium, Copper, Iron, Magnesium, Manganese, Phosphorus, Potassium, Selenium, Zinc.

Vitamins: Vitamin A, Vitamin C, Vitamin E, Folic Acid, Pantothenic Acid, Pyridoxine, Riboflavin, Thiamin.

Nut: **Pistachio**

About: Belongs to the Anacardiaceae family. Pistachios are an excellent plant-based source of protein. Pistachios are also a great source of copper and manganese. Pistachios are a great source of vitamin E with y-tocopherol that helps maintain healthy skin.

Cancer & Disease Fighting: Pistachios are a rich source β-Carotene which helps protect against certain cancers.

Phytochemicals: Flavonoids, Phenols, Proanthocyanidins, Phytosterols, Stilbenes, Resveratrol, Carotenoids, β-Carotene.

Minerals: Calcium, Copper, Iron, Magnesium, Manganese, Phosphorus, Potassium, Selenium, Zinc.

Vitamins: Vitamin A, Vitamin C, Vitamin E, Folic Acid, Pantothenic Acid, Pyridoxine, Riboflavin, Thiamin.

Nut: **Walnut**

About: Belongs to the Juglandaceae family. Walnuts are a great source of vitamin E with y-tocopherol that helps maintain healthy skin. Walnuts are also an excellent source of copper and manganese. In the body, copper is used as a cofactor for enzymes that aid in the production of superoxide dismutase. Walnuts are loaded with the amino acid arginine which is needed to help prevent high blood pressure, and it is essential to the growth of tissue. Arginine is required for the development of young bodies. It is also needed for the production of nitric oxide. It opens the blood vessels for increased blood flow. Arginine also is necessary for hair growth.

Cancer & Disease Fighting: A study done on walnuts stated that they had seen a decrease in DNA damage. There are multiple studies done with animals that show that walnut phytochemicals have slowed or prevented the growth of breast and prostate cancers. Human trials have been started.

Phytochemicals: Flavonoids, Ellagic Acid, Proanthocyanidins, Carotenoids, β-Carotene, Lutein, Zeaxanthin, Melatonin.

Minerals: Calcium, Copper, Iron, Magnesium, Manganese, Phosphorus, Potassium, Selenium, Zinc.

Vitamins: Vitamin A, Vitamin C, Vitamin E, Folic Acid, Pantothenic Acid, Pyridoxine, Riboflavin, Thiamin.

Seeds

Seed: **Chia**

About: Belongs to the Labiatae family. Chia seeds are a good source of plant-based protein. Chia seeds are also high in antioxidants. The chia seed is very high in omega-3 fatty acids. Gram for gram chia seeds contains more omega-3s than salmon. Chia seeds help to lower LDL cholesterol.

Cancer & Disease Fighting: α-Linolenic acid has been shown to induce apoptosis in breast cancer and cervical cancer. There have been some studies that state if you have prostate cancer you might want to avoid chia seeds.

Phytochemicals: Flavonoids, Quercetin, Ferulic Acid, Caffein Acid, Phytoestrogens, Lignans, α-Linolenic Acid (ALA).

Minerals: Calcium, Copper, Iron, Magnesium, Manganese, Phosphorus, Potassium, Selenium, Sodium, Zinc.

Vitamins: Vitamin A, Vitamin C, Vitamin E, Vitamin K, Folic Acid, Riboflavin, Thiamin.

Seed: **Flax**

About: Belongs to the Linaceae family. Flax seeds are rich in oleic acid which is a monounsaturated fatty acid. Like chia seeds, flax seeds are an excellent source for plant-based proteins. Flax seeds are a great source of vitamin E which helps maintain healthy skin as well as help fight free radicals that do damage to our cells.

Cancer & Disease Fighting: Alpha Linolenic Acid has been shown to induce apoptosis in breast cancer and cervical cancer.

Phytochemicals: Flavonoids, Carotenoids, Lutein, Zeaxanthin, Phytoestrogens, Lignans, α-Linolenic Acid (ALA), Secoisolariciresinol Diglucoside.

Minerals: Calcium, Copper, Iron, Magnesium, Manganese, Potassium, Sodium, Zinc.

Vitamins: Vitamin C, Vitamin E, Vitamin K, Folic Acid, Pantothenic Acid, Pyridoxine, Riboflavin, Thiamin.

Seed: **Hemp**

About: Belongs to the Cannabaceae family. Hemp is a good source of vitamin E. Hemp is an excellent source of protein about the same as beef by weight. A plant-based complete protein is hard to find, which is due in part to the amino acid lysine which is located in hemp and quinoa. Lysine found in quinoa makes it a complete protein. Hemp has been found to reduce symptoms of PMS and menopause. Hemp has been shown to treat dry skin and help maintain healthy hair.

Cancer & Disease Fighting: More research is needed on hemp seeds and their role in cancer prevention.

Phytochemicals: Flavonoids, Prostaglandins, Gamma-Linolenic Acid (GLA), α-Linolenic Acid (ALA), Linoleic Acid.

Minerals: Calcium, Iron, Magnesium, Phosphorus, Potassium, Zinc.

Vitamins: Vitamin A, Vitamin C, Vitamin E, Folic Acid, Pantothenic Acid, Riboflavin, Thiamin.

Seed: **Poppy**

About: Belongs to the Papaveraceae family. Poppy seeds are loaded with minerals. Poppy seeds are rich in oleic acid and Linoleic acid which have been shown to help lower the LDL levels in the blood.

Cancer & Disease Fighting: The omega-3 and omega-6 values have been shown to help fight certain cancers such as breast, liver, skin, and stomach.

Phytochemicals: Flavonoids, Oleic Acid, Linoleic Acid.

Minerals: Calcium, Copper, Iron, Magnesium, Manganese, Phosphorus, Potassium, Selenium, Sodium, Zinc.

Vitamins: Vitamin C, Vitamin E, Folic Acid, Pantothenic Acid, Pyridoxine, Riboflavin, Thiamin.

Seed: **Pumpkin**

About: Belongs to the Cucurbitaceae family. Pumpkin seeds are rich in oleic acid and Linoleic acid which have been shown to help lower the LDL levels in the blood. Pumpkin seeds are a good source of the amino acid tryptophan and glutamate. Tryptophan is needed to convert into serotonin. Pumpkin seeds are mineral-rich. The pumpkin seeds contain a large amount of vitamin E which is required to maintain healthy skin as well as help fight free radicals. Pumpkin seeds are loaded with the amino acid arginine which is needed to help prevent high blood pressure, and it is essential to the growth of tissue. Arginine is required for the development of young bodies. It is also needed for the production of nitric oxide. It opens the blood vessels for increased blood flow. Arginine also is required for hair growth.

Cancer & Disease Fighting: Pumpkin seeds have been shown to help lower the risk of colon, lung, and stomach cancers. Pumpkin seeds have also been shown to reduce the growth of prostate cancer cells.

Phytochemicals: Flavonoids, β-Sitosterol, Carotenoids, β-Carotene, Cryptoxanthin-β, Lutein, Zeaxanthin.

Minerals: Calcium, Copper, Iron, Magnesium, Manganese, Phosphorus, Potassium, Selenium, Zinc.

Vitamins: Vitamin A, Vitamin C, Vitamin E, Folic Acid, Pantothenic Acid, Pyridoxine, Riboflavin, Thiamin.

Seed: **Quinoa**

About: Belongs to the Chenopodiaceae family. Quinoa is a seed of the Chenopodium (goosefoot) plant. A plant-based complete protein is hard to find that is due in part to the amino acid lysine which is found in hemp and quinoa. Lysine is also found in hemp making it a complete protein. Quinoa is high in antioxidants that help to fight the free radicals in the body that damage the cells.

Cancer & Disease Fighting: Quinoa has been shown to slow cancer cell proliferation. More research is needed on this powerhouse food.

Phytochemicals: Flavonoids, Saponin, Quercetin, Kaempferol, Oleic Acid, Linoleic Acid, Carotenoids, β-Carotene, Cryptoxanthin-β, Lutein, Zeaxanthin.

Minerals: Calcium, Copper, Iron, Magnesium, Manganese, Phosphorus, Potassium, Selenium, Zinc.

Vitamins: Vitamin A, Vitamin E, Folic Acid, Riboflavin, Thiamin.

Seed: **Sesame**

About: Belongs to the Pedaliaceae family. Sesame seeds are loaded with minerals. Sesame is great for monounsaturated fatty acids which help in the lowering of LDL cholesterol.

Cancer & Disease Fighting: The lignan sesamin has been found to reduce the growth of human breast tumors (MCF-7) at high levels of circulating estrogen in athymic mice. The phytochemical has also been shown to minimize the risk of mortality in breast cancer patients.

Phytochemicals: Flavonoids, Lignans, Sesamin, Carotenoids, β-Carotene, Sesamol, Sesaminol, Oleic Acid.

Minerals: Calcium, Copper, Iron, Magnesium, Manganese, Phosphorus, Potassium, Selenium, Zinc.

Vitamins: Vitamin E, Folic Acid, Pantothenic Acid, Pyridoxine, Riboflavin, Thiamin.

Seed: **Sunflower**

About: Belongs to the Asteraceae family. Sunflower seeds are rich in polyunsaturated fatty acids linoleic acid and monounsaturated oleic acid. The polyphenols help by removing the oxidant agents in the body that cause other substances in the body to lose their electrons.

Cancer & Disease Fighting: The selenium in the sunflower seeds helps to fight cancers. Sunflower seeds have also been shown to aid in DNA repair as well as slowing the growth of the cancer cell.

Phytochemicals: Flavonoids, Carotenoids, β-Carotene, Oleic Acid, Linoleic Acid, Polyphenols, Chlorogenic-Acid, Quinic Acid, Caffein Acids.

Minerals: Calcium, Copper, Iron, Magnesium, Manganese, Phosphorus, Potassium, Selenium, Sodium, Zinc.

Vitamins: Vitamin A, Vitamin C, Vitamin E, Folic Acid, Pantothenic Acid, Pyridoxine, Riboflavin, Thiamin.

Whole Grains

Common Whole Grains

Whole Grain: **Amaranth**

About: Belongs to the Amaranthus family. Amaranth is an excellent source of plant protein. Amaranth is strong in amino acid power with high levels of arginine, lysine, Isoleucine, leucine, threonine, tryptophan, and valine. Amaranth carries BCAAs (leucine, isoleucine, and valine). Amaranth has also been shown to boost the immune system as well as prevent premature graying.

Cancer & Disease Fighting: The antioxidants in amaranth have been shown to help prevent inflammation and help fight cancer.

Phytochemicals: Flavonoids, Carotenoids, β-Carotene, Lutein, Zeaxanthin.

Minerals: Calcium, Iron, Magnesium, Manganese, Phosphorus, Potassium, Selenium, Zinc.

Vitamins: Vitamin E, Folic Acid, Pantothenic Acid, Pyridoxine, Riboflavin, Thiamin.

Whole Grain: **Barley**

About: Belongs to the Poaceae family. Barley is loaded with fiber. Barley has also been shown to reduce LDL cholesterol. Barley has a high level of β-glucan that has been shown to play a role in insulin resistance.

Cancer & Disease Fighting: High selenium levels have been shown to help lower the risk of serval cancers. The high fiber also has been shown to reduce the risk of colon cancer.

Phytochemicals: Flavonoids, Flavanols, Lignans, Anthocyanins, Proanthocyanidins, Phytosterols, β-Carotene, Lutein, Zeaxanthin.

Minerals: Calcium, Copper, Iron, Magnesium, Manganese, Phosphorus, Potassium, Selenium, Zinc.

Vitamins: Vitamin A, Folic Acid, Pantothenic Acid, Pyridoxine, Riboflavin, Thiamin.

Whole Grain: **Buckwheat**

About: Belongs to the Polygonaceae family. The phytochemical rutin is a strong antioxidant that is known for fighting free radicals that damage healthy cells. Rutin is also essential for the increase of blood vessel elasticity.

Cancer & Disease Fighting: Buckwheat has been shown to have a cytotoxic effect on human breast, liver, and stomach cancer.

Phytochemicals: Flavonoids, Rutin, Quercetin, Orientin, Vitexin, Isovitexin, Isoorientin, Flavones, Flavanols, Flavanones, Phytosterols.

Minerals: Calcium, Copper, Iron, Magnesium, Manganese, Phosphorus, Potassium, Selenium, Zinc.

Vitamins: Folic Acid, Pantothenic Acid, Pyridoxine, Riboflavin, Thiamin.

Whole Grain: **Oats**

About: Belongs to the Poaceae family. Oats are an excellent food choice because it is low in saturated fat and very low in cholesterol.

Cancer & Disease Fighting: Studies have shown that oats help to fight cancer by the antioxidants. Other studies have shown that oats can lower the risk of colon cancer.

Phytochemicals: Flavonoids, Phytosterols, β-Sitostanol, Sitostanol, Campesterol, Campestanol, Carotenoids.

Minerals: Calcium, Copper, Iron, Magnesium, Manganese, Phosphorus, Potassium, Selenium, Zinc.

Vitamins: Vitamin E, Folic Acid, Pantothenic Acid, Pyridoxine, Riboflavin, Thiamin.

Whole Grain: **Rice (brown)**

About: Belongs to the Gramineae family. Brown rice is a low "glycemic index" food. The short-grain brown rice is healthier than the long grain. Brown rice has also been shown to lower cholesterol levels and help reduce the risk of heart disease. The folic acid levels aid in the development of new cells.

Cancer & Disease Fighting: The phytochemicals and minerals found in brown rice have been found to lower the risk of cancers. One phytochemical selenium has been shown to reduce the risk of colon cancer. Researchers have stated that brown rice can help lower the risk of type 2 diabetes.

Phytochemicals: Flavonoids, Carotenoids, Lutein, Zeaxanthin, Flavone, Flavonols, y-Oryzanol.

Minerals: Calcium, Copper, Iron, Magnesium, Manganese, Phosphorus, Potassium, Selenium, Zinc.

Vitamins: Vitamin E, Vitamin K, Folic Acid, Pantothenic Acid, Pyridoxine, Riboflavin, Thiamin.

Whole Grain: **Rye**

About: Belongs to the Poaceae family. Rye has high levels of dietary fiber which has been shown to help lower the risk of cardiovascular disease. One study found that when children consume low amounts of whole grains such as rye, had a direct correlation with a higher rate of asthma.

Cancer & Disease Fighting: The high levels of lignans found in rye have been shown to help lower the risk of breast cancer.

Phytochemicals: Flavonoids, Lignans, Benzoxazinoids, Phenolic Acids, Alkylresorcinols, Carotenoids, β-Carotene, Lutein, Zeaxanthin.

Minerals: Calcium, Copper, Iron, Magnesium, Manganese, Phosphorus, Potassium, Selenium, Zinc.

Vitamins: Vitamin A, Vitamin E, Vitamin K, Folic Acid, Pantothenic Acid, Pyridoxine, Riboflavin, Thiamin.

Whole Grain: **Wheat**

About: Belongs to the Poaceae family. Eating whole grains has been shown to lower the risk of heart attacks by helping to reduce blood pressure.

Cancer & Disease Fighting: The lignans which are converted in the gut to enterolactone and enterodiol have been shown to help play a protective role in cardiovascular death. Enterolactone has been shown to help protect against breast cancer in post-menopausal women.

Phytochemicals: Flavonoids, Lignans, Alkylresorcinols, Ferlic Acid, Saponins, Stanols, Carotenoids, β-Carotene, Lutein, Zeaxanthin,

Minerals: Calcium, Copper, Iron, Magnesium, Manganese, Phosphorus, Potassium, Selenium, Sodium, Zinc.

Vitamins: Vitamin A, Vitamin E, Vitamin K, Folic Acid, Pantothenic Acid, Pyridoxine, Riboflavin, Thiamin.

13

Fruits

Fruits, nature's exquisite gift, have been a cornerstone of human nutrition for centuries. Packed with essential vitamins, minerals, fiber, and antioxidants, fruits offer a delectable and nutritious way to promote overall health and well-being. This essay delves into the intricacies of how and why fruits are indispensable for the human body, examining their diverse array of nutrients and the myriad ways in which they contribute to our health.

Fruits are veritable storehouses of essential nutrients, each variety offering a unique blend of vitamins and minerals crucial for maintaining optimal health. Vitamin C, found abundantly in citrus fruits like oranges and grapefruits, is renowned for its immune-boosting properties. It plays a pivotal role in collagen synthesis, and wound healing, and acts as a potent antioxidant, neutralizing harmful free radicals that can damage cells.

Beyond vitamin C, fruits provide a rich tapestry of other vitamins, including vitamin A, essential for vision and immune function (found in fruits like mangoes and apricots), and vitamin K, vital for blood clotting and bone health (abundant in kiwi and berries). Moreover, the B-vitamin complex, found in bananas, avocados, and berries, is crucial for energy metabolism and the maintenance of a healthy nervous system.

Minerals such as potassium, magnesium, and folate are also prevalent in various fruits. Potassium, abundant in bananas and oranges, regulates blood pressure and supports proper heart function. Magnesium, found in avocados and figs, is essential for muscle and nerve function, while folate, present in citrus fruits and berries, is crucial for DNA synthesis and cell division, especially during pregnancy.

Fruits are an excellent source of dietary fiber, a component indispensable for digestive health. Soluble fiber, found in apples, pears, and citrus fruits, helps regulate blood sugar levels and lower cholesterol. On the other hand, insoluble fiber, abundant in the skins of fruits like grapes and kiwi, adds bulk to stool, preventing constipation and promoting a healthy digestive system.

The fiber content in fruits also aids in weight management by promoting satiety and reducing overall calorie intake. Regular consumption of fiber-rich fruits contributes to a feeling of fullness, discouraging overeating and supporting weight loss efforts. Additionally, fiber plays a role in maintaining a healthy gut microbiome, fostering the growth of beneficial bacteria that contribute to immune function and overall well-being.

Fruits are potent sources of antioxidants, compounds that combat oxidative stress in the body. Oxidative stress occurs when there is an imbalance between free radicals and antioxidants, leading to cellular damage and inflammation. Berries, such as blueberries, strawberries, and raspberries, are particularly rich in antioxidants like anthocyanins and quercetin, which have been linked to a reduced risk of chronic diseases, including heart disease and certain types of cancer.

The diverse array of antioxidants in fruits not only protects cells from damage but also supports skin health by neutralizing free radicals that contribute to premature aging. Vitamins like vitamin E, found in avocados and kiwi, work synergistically with other antioxidants to maintain the elasticity of the skin and protect it from environmental stressors.

Regular consumption of fruits has been associated with a decreased risk of several chronic diseases. The wealth of nutrients and bioactive compounds in fruits contributes to overall cardiovascular health by reducing blood pressure, lowering cholesterol levels, and improving blood vessel function. The potassium content in fruits helps regulate blood pressure, while the fiber and antioxidants contribute to cardiovascular well-being.

The anti-inflammatory properties of fruits play a pivotal role in preventing and managing inflammatory conditions such as arthritis. The polyphenols in fruits like cherries and citrus fruits have been shown to alleviate symptoms and reduce inflammation associated with arthritis and other inflammatory disorders.

Certain compounds in fruits have demonstrated anti-cancer properties, making them valuable in cancer prevention. For instance, the phytochemicals in berries, such as ellagic acid and resveratrol, have been linked to inhibiting the growth of cancer cells and reducing the risk of certain cancers. Citrus fruits, rich in vitamin C and flavonoids, have also shown promise in preventing cancers of the digestive and respiratory systems.

The fiber content in fruits further contributes to cancer prevention by promoting regular bowel movements and preventing the buildup of harmful substances in the colon. Additionally, antioxidants in fruits help neutralize free radicals, reducing the risk of DNA damage and the development of cancerous cells.

Fruits stand as nutritional powerhouses, offering a treasure trove of essential vitamins, minerals, fiber, and antioxidants that are vital for human health. From bolstering the immune system to supporting digestive health, preventing chronic diseases, and even contributing to cancer prevention, the benefits of incorporating fruits into one's diet are profound and diverse.

As we navigate the complexities of modern life, embracing the simplicity and goodness of nature's bounty in the form of fruits can be a transformative step toward achieving and maintaining optimal health. Whether enjoyed fresh, blended into smoothies, or incorporated into a variety of dishes, the vibrant colors and flavors of fruits not only tantalize the taste buds but also nourish the body from within, fostering a P53 Diet approach to well-being.

Common Fruit

Acai Berry

About: Belongs to the Arecaceae family. Acai berries have one of the highest antioxidant levels of most of the fruits in the super fruit category. It is because of the high levels of antioxidants that give Acai berries the power to help protect the body from bacteria and upper respiratory infections. Acai berries include healthy monounsaturated fats and omega-3, omega-6, and omega-9 fatty acids. These berries also contain essential amino acids. Acai berries contain reasonable amounts of fiber.

Cancer & Disease Fighting: Acai berry's high antioxidant levels have played an essential role in lowering the risk of certain cancers. More research is needed on cancer and the role acai berries play in cancer.

Phytochemicals: Flavonoids, Carotenoids, β-Stilbenes, Resveratrol, Anthocyanins, Ferulic Acid, Delphinidin, Cyanidin-3-galactoside, Ellagic Acid, β-sitosterol.

Minerals: Calcium, Iron, Magnesium, Phosphorus, Potassium, Zinc.

Vitamins: Vitamin A, Vitamin C, Vitamin E, Vitamin K, Folic Acid, Niacin, Pyridoxine, Riboflavin, Thiamin.

Apple

About: Belongs to the Rosaceae family. The old phrase "An apple a day keeps the doctor away" has a lot of truth to it, because of the phytochemicals in apples. The fiber in the apple is good for the colon. A study done in the U.K. showed that people in the study ate two apples a week had up to 32% lower risk of developing asthma than the people in the study who had no apples. The pectin in apples has also been shown to lower cholesterol. Researchers have also stated that apples have the ability to reduce the risk of heart disease due to the flavonols like quercetin found in the apples.

Cancer & Disease Fighting: Multiple studies done on the power of the apple on cancer have shown to help protect against breast, colon, liver, skin, stomach, and prostate cancers.

Phytochemicals: Flavonoids, Anthocyanins (red varieties), Dihydrochalcones, Flavonols, Kaempferol, Isoquercetin, Rutin, Reinstein, Hyperoside, Hydroxycinnamic Acids Derivatives.

Minerals: Calcium, Iron, Magnesium, Phosphorus, Potassium, Zinc.

Vitamins: Vitamin A, Vitamin C, Vitamin E, Vitamin K, Folic Acid, Pantothenic Acid, Pyridoxine, Riboflavin, Thiamin.

Apricot

About: Belongs to the Rosaceae family. Apricots are a great source of vitamin A which is needed to maintain healthy skin and help protect the lungs.

Cancer & Disease Fighting: The apricot is rich in β-Carotene and vitamins A and C which have been shown to help protect against cancers such as breast cancer, cervical cancer, colon cancer, lung, and prostate cancer.

Phytochemicals: Flavonoids, Carotenoids, β-Carotene, Lutein, Zeaxanthin, β-Cryptoxanthin, Glycoside.

Minerals: Calcium, Iron, Magnesium, Manganese, Phosphorus, Potassium, Zinc.

Vitamins: Vitamin A, Vitamin C, Vitamin K, Folic Acid, Pantothenic Acid, Pyridoxine, Riboflavin, Thiamin.

Avocado

About: Belongs to the Lauraceae family. Avocado has high-fat levels, but there are monounsaturated fats. Research has stated that higher levels of monounsaturated have been known to help reduce LDL cholesterol while increasing HDL cholesterol. The avocado is also a great source of potassium. There is a good number of antioxidants in avocados.

Cancer & Disease Fighting: There has been research done on avocados stating that there is anticancer activity fighting against breast, oral, and prostate cancer.

Phytochemicals: Flavonoids, Carotenoids, β-Carotene, Lutein, Zeaxanthin, β-Cryptoxanthin, Persin, Persenone A.

Minerals: Calcium, Copper, Iron, Magnesium, Manganese, Phosphorus, Potassium, Zinc.

Vitamins: Vitamin A, Vitamin C, Vitamin E, Vitamin K, Folic Acid, Pantothenic Acid, Pyridoxine, Riboflavin, Thiamin.

Banana

About: Belongs to the Musaceae family. Bananas are a great source of carbohydrates. They are also a good source of potassium. Bananas are a good source of pyridoxine (B6) that helps decrease homocysteine. Homocysteine plays a crucial role in coronary artery disease.

Cancer & Disease Fighting: Research has shown that bananas can help reduce the risk of breast and colorectal cancers and renal cell carcinoma.

Phytochemicals: Flavonoids, Carotenoids, α-Carotene, β-Carotene, Lutein, Zeaxanthin.

Minerals: Calcium, Copper, Iron, Magnesium, Manganese, Phosphorus, Potassium, Selenium, Zinc.

Vitamins: Vitamin A, Vitamin C, Vitamin E, Vitamin K, Folic Acid, Pantothenic Acid, Pyridoxine, Riboflavin, Thiamin.

Blackberry

About: Belongs to the Rosaceae family. Blackberries are packed full of antioxidants that help fight the damage caused by free radicals. Blackberries are a good source of vitamin C and vitamin K.

Cancer & Disease Fighting: The active compound found in blackberries through experiments has been shown to inhibit breast, colon, lung, skin, and prostate cancers.

Phytochemicals: Flavonoids, Anthocyanidins, Carotenoids,β-Carotene, Lutein, Zeaxanthin, Tannin, Kaempferol, Salicylic Acid, Ellagic Acid, Quercetin.

Minerals: Calcium, Copper, Iron, Magnesium, Manganese, Potassium, Selenium, Zinc.

Vitamins: Vitamin A, Vitamin C, Vitamin E, Vitamin K, Folic Acid, Pantothenic Acid, Pyridoxine, Riboflavin, Thiamin.

Black Raspberry

About: Belongs to the Rosaceae family. The black raspberry has been coined the king of the berries because of its high antioxidant levels.

Cancer & Disease Fighting: The black raspberry has been found by researchers to have prevention properties against certain cancers such as breast, cervical, colon esophageal, lung, oral, prostate, and skin cancers. As you can see black raspberries are wonderful for your body.

Phytochemicals: Flavonoids, Anthocyanins, Ellagic Acid, Carotenoids, α-Carotene, β-Carotene, Lutein, Zeaxanthin.

Minerals: Calcium, Copper, Iron, Magnesium, Manganese, Phosphorus, Potassium, Selenium, Sodium, Zinc.

Vitamins: Vitamin A, Vitamin C, Vitamin E, Vitamin K, Folic Acid, Pantothenic Acid, Pyridoxine, Riboflavin, Thiamin.

Blueberry

About: Belongs to the Ericaceae family. We all know blueberries are loaded with antioxidants that fight off the damage that free radicals cause. The chlorogenic acid in blueberries helps to lower blood glucose levels. Blueberries also work as a cofactor that helps metabolize carbohydrates, fats, and proteins.

Cancer & Disease Fighting: Multiple studies have shown that blueberries can help prevent the growth of selective cancer tumors in cervical, colon, lung, and prostate cancers as well as leukemia.

Phytochemicals: Flavonoids, Anthocyanins, Carotenoids, β-Carotene, Lutein, Zeaxanthin.

Minerals: Calcium, Iron, Magnesium, Manganese, Potassium, Zinc.

Vitamins: Vitamin A, Vitamin C, Vitamin E, Vitamin K, Folic Acid, Pantothenic Acid, Pyridoxine, Riboflavin, Thiamin.

Cherry

About: Belongs to the Rosaceae family. Cherries have been known to help treat gout. Cherries have also been known to reduce cholesterol oxidation. Researchers have also stated that cherries help to reduce muscle soreness.

Cancer & Disease Fighting: The consumption of cherries has been seen through research to help in the prevention of oral cancers.

Phytochemicals: Flavonoids, Anthocyanins, Carotenoids, β-Carotene, Lutein, Zeaxanthin.

Minerals: Calcium, Copper, Iron, Magnesium, Manganese, Phosphorus, Potassium, Zinc.

Vitamins: Vitamin A, Vitamin C, Folic Acid, Pantothenic Acid, Pyridoxine, Riboflavin, Thiamin.

Coconut

About: Belongs to the Palmaceae family. The coconut is very high in saturated fats.

Cancer & Disease Fighting: More research is needed to determine if coconut could help with the fight against cancer.

Phytochemicals: Flavonoids, Phytosterols, Cytokinins, Kinetin, Trans-Zeatin.

Minerals: Calcium, Copper, Iron, Magnesium, Manganese, Phosphorus, Potassium, Sodium, Zinc.

Vitamins: Vitamin C, Vitamin E, Folic Acid, Pantothenic Acid, Pyridoxine, Riboflavin, Thiamin.

Cranberry

About: Belongs to the Ericaceae family. Research has stated that cranberries have been found to protect against infections such as e.coli in the urinary tract. Cranberries are high in antioxidants. Cranberries can help prevent the formation of alkaline stones in the urinary tract. Cranberries have also been shown to reduce the levels of LDL cholesterol and increase the good cholesterol HDL.

Cancer & Disease Fighting: Research has shown that cranberries can cause apoptosis on multiple cancer cell lines such as breast, colon, lung, ovaries, and prostate.

Phytochemicals: Flavonoids, Myricetin, Cyanidin, Hydroxycinnamate, Quercetin, Peonidin, Proanthocyanidin, Carotenoids, β-Carotene, Lutein, Zeaxanthin.

Minerals: Calcium, Copper, Iron, Magnesium, Manganese, Phosphorus, Potassium, Zinc.

Vitamins: Vitamin A, Vitamin C, Vitamin E, Vitamin K, Pantothenic Acid, Pyridoxine, Riboflavin, Thiamin.

Dates

About: Belongs to the Arecaceae family. Dates are rich in dietary fiber called beta-D-glucan which decreases the body's ability to absorb cholesterol. Dates are also loaded with carbohydrates.

Cancer & Disease Fighting: Dates are rich in antioxidants which have been shown to aid in the prevention of certain cancers. More research is needed on dates to determine their role in cancer prevention such as breast, colon, endometrial, lung, pancreatic, and prostate cancers.

Phytochemicals: Flavonoids, Carotenoids, β-Carotene, Lutein, Zeaxanthin, Tannins.

Minerals: Calcium, Copper, Iron, Magnesium, Manganese, Phosphorus, Potassium, Zinc.

Vitamins: Vitamin A, Vitamin K, Folic Acid, Pantothenic Acid, Pyridoxine, Riboflavin, Thiamin.

Fig

About: Belongs to the Moraceae family. Figs are a great source of fiber. They also carry ample amounts of calcium. The chlorogenic acid in figs helps lower blood sugar levels.

Cancer & Disease Fighting: Figs have been shown to inhibit cancers such as breast, skin, and stomach cancers in controlled experiments.

Phytochemicals: Flavonoids, Catechin, Epicatechin, Rutin, Carotenoids, Carotenoids, β-Carotene, Lutein, Zeaxanthin, Gallic-Acid, Chlorogenic-Acid, Syringic Acid.

Minerals: Calcium, Copper, Iron, Magnesium, Manganese, Potassium, Zinc.

Vitamins: Vitamin A, Vitamin C, Vitamin E, Vitamin K, Folic Acid, Pantothenic Acid, Pyridoxine, Riboflavin, Thiamin.

Grapes

About: Belongs to the Vitaceae family. Resveratrol has also been shown to reduce the risk of stroke. The antioxidant power of grapes has been shown to help fight inflammation.

Cancer & Disease Fighting: Resveratrol from the skin of grapes has been shown to induce apoptosis in Hodgkin's Lymphoma-derived L-428 cells this depends on dosage, however in lower dosage resveratrol caused cell cycle arrest in the S-Phase of the cycle. There has been an array of studies that have shown to inhibit certain cancers such as bladder, brain, breast, colon, head & neck, lung, pancreatic, and skin cancers as well as leukemia.

Phytochemicals: Flavonoids, Anthocyanidins, Polyphenols, Resveratrol, Catechin, Gallic Acid, Chlorogenic Acid, Syringic Acid, Procyanidins.

Minerals: Calcium, Copper, Iron, Magnesium, Manganese, Potassium, Zinc.

Vitamins: Vitamin A, Vitamin C, Vitamin E, Vitamin K, Folic Acid, Pantothenic Acid, Pyridoxine, Riboflavin, Thiamin.

Grapefruit

About: Belongs to the Rutaceae family. Grapefruit is an excellent source of vitamin C as well as pectin. The grapefruit is also a great source of vitamin A.

Cancer & Disease Fighting: Grapefruit has been shown to inhibit colon cancer.

Phytochemicals: Flavonoids, Lycopene, Polyamine, Aspermidine.

Minerals: Calcium, Copper, Iron, Magnesium, Manganese, Phosphorus, Potassium, Zinc.

Vitamins: Vitamin A, Vitamin C, Vitamin E, Folic Acid, Pantothenic Acid, Pyridoxine, Riboflavin, Thiamin.

Guava

About: Belongs to the Myrtaceae family. It is native to Central America. Guava is an excellent source of vitamin C. Vitamin C is essential for collagen synthesis. Collagen is necessary for maintaining healthy tissues in the skin and organs. Guava carries almost twice the amount of lycopene as tomatoes. Lycopene helps protect the skin from UV rays.

Cancer & Disease Fighting: Guava has been shown to inhibit certain cancers such as lung and prostate cancers.

Phytochemicals: Flavonoids, Catechin, Lycopene, Gallic Acid, Gallocatechin, Guaijaverin, Leucocyanidin, Amritoside, Quercetin.

Minerals: Calcium, Copper, Iron, Magnesium, Manganese, Phosphorus, Potassium, Selenium, Zinc.

Vitamins: Vitamin A, Vitamin C, Vitamin E, Vitamin K, Folic Acid, Pantothenic Acid, Pyridoxine, Riboflavin, Thiamin.

Indian Gooseberry

About: Belongs to the Phyllanthaceae family.

Cancer & Disease Fighting: Gooseberries have been shown to inhibit certain cancers such as cervical, liver, lung, and oral cancers.

Phytochemicals: Flavonoids, Flavones, Anthocyanins, Tannins, Gallic Acid, Ellagic Acid, Kaempferol, Emblicanin A & B, Phyllanemblin, Punicafolin, Punigluconin.

Minerals: Calcium, Copper, Iron, Magnesium, Manganese, Phosphorus, Potassium, Zinc.

Vitamins: Vitamin A, Vitamin C, Folic Acid, Pantothenic Acid, Pyridoxine, Riboflavin, Thiamin.

Jackfruit

About: Belongs to the Moraceae family. It is native to the Asia area. Jackfruit is a good source of vitamin C. It also can be a replacement for BBQ pork sandwiches. It tastes so good you won't be able to tell the difference if done right.

Cancer & Disease Fighting: Jackfruit has been shown to inhibit breast cancer and skin cancer.

Phytochemicals: Flavonoids, Artocarpin, Isobutyl Isovalerate, 2-Methylbutanol, Butyl Isovalerate, Jacalin.

Minerals: Calcium, Copper, Iron, Magnesium, Manganese, Phosphorus, Potassium, Zinc.

Vitamins: Vitamin A, Vitamin C, Folic Acid, Pantothenic Acid, Pyridoxine, Riboflavin, Thiamin.

Kiwi

About: Belongs to the Actinidiaceae family. Kiwi is an excellent source of omega-3 fatty acids which help to reduce the risk of ADHD, autism, coronary heart disease, and stroke. Kiwi also is a good source of vitamin K which is known for controlling the neuronal damage in the brain that plays a role in Alzheimer's disease. Kiwi also has been found to improve laxation and digestion.

Cancer & Disease Fighting: Kiwifruit has been shown to inhibit the proliferation of pancreatic cancer cell lines.

Phytochemicals: Flavonoids, Carotenoids, β-Carotene, Lutein, Zeaxanthin.

Minerals: Calcium, Copper, Iron, Magnesium, Manganese, Phosphorus, Potassium, Zinc.

Vitamins: Vitamin A, Vitamin C, Vitamin E, Vitamin K, Folic Acid, Riboflavin, Thiamin.

Lemon

About: Belongs to the Rutaceae family. Lemons are a great source to fight against the free radicals in the body. Lemons are loaded with vitamin C power. Lemon contains citric acid that helps with the digestion process and also helps dissolve kidney stones.

Cancer & Disease Fighting: Research has stated that lemons have the ability to promote apoptosis on breast cancer cell lines. Lemons also have chemoprotective effects on cervical and colon cancers.

Phytochemicals: Flavonoids, Flavonone, Hesperetin, Naringin, Naringenin, Obacunone Glucoside, Deacetylnomilinic Acid, Limonene.

Minerals: Calcium, Copper, Iron, Magnesium, Manganese, Potassium, Zinc.

Vitamins: Vitamin A, Vitamin C, Vitamin E, Folic Acid, Pantothenic Acid, Pyridoxine, Riboflavin, Thiamin.

Lime

About: Belongs to the Rutaceae family. Limes carry the same properties as lemons. Limes are a great source to fight against the free radicals in the body. Lemons are loaded with vitamin C power. Limes contain citric acid that helps with the digestion process and also helps dissolve kidney stones.

Cancer & Disease Fighting: Research has stated that limes have the ability to promote apoptosis on breast cancer cell lines. Limes also have chemoprotective effects on cervical and colon cancers.

Phytochemicals: Flavonoids, Carotenoids, β-Carotene, Lutein, Zeaxanthin, Flavonone, Hesperetin, Naringin, Naringenin, Obacunone Glucoside, Deacetylnomilinic Acid.

Minerals: Calcium, Copper, Iron, Magnesium, Manganese, Potassium, Zinc.

Vitamins: Vitamin A, Vitamin C, Vitamin E, Folic Acid, Pantothenic Acid, Pyridoxine, Riboflavin, Thiamin.

Mango

About: Belongs to the Anacardiaceae family. Mango is loaded with high levels of vitamin A, and vitamin C. Mangos also have high levels of Pyridoxine (vitamin B6). Vitamin B6 helps control homocysteine levels in the blood.

Cancer & Disease Fighting: Mangos has been stated to be one of the best of any fruit or vegetable in the risk reduction of gallbladder cancer. In lab tests, mangos have also been shown to stop normal cells from turning into cancer cells.

Phytochemicals: Flavonoids, Carotenoids, β-Carotene, Lutein, β-Cryptoxanthin, Zeaxanthin, Flavonols, Quercetin.

Minerals: Calcium, Copper, Iron, Magnesium, Manganese, Potassium.

Vitamins: Vitamin A, Vitamin C, Vitamin E, Vitamin K, Folic Acid, Pantothenic Acid, Pyridoxine, Riboflavin, Thiamin.

Melon

About: Belongs to the Cucurbitaceae family. Melons are a great source of vitamin A. Melons like honeydew melons are a great source of vitamin C which is needed to help boost the immune system and help with the production of collagen. Vitamin C also helps fight free radicals in the body. Melon is also low in calories. Research has found that eating melons can help to cure kidney stones. The melons also are high in fiber help improve your gut health and help you stay hydrated. Melons are a good source of pyridoxine (vitamin B6) which is needed for brain development.

Cancer & Disease Fighting: Melons have been shown to have chemoprotective properties that can help healthy tissues. The melon has also been shown in many studies to help prevent brain, breast, and colon cancers.

Phytochemicals: Flavonoids, Cucurbitacin A&B, Lycopene, Carotenoids, β-Carotene, Lutein, Phytoene, Zeaxanthin,

Minerals: Calcium, Copper, Iron, Magnesium, Manganese, Phosphorus, Potassium, Selenium, Sodium, Zinc.

Vitamins: Vitamin A, Vitamin C, Vitamin K, Folic Acid, Pantothenic Acid, Pyridoxine, Riboflavin, Thiamin.

Nectarine

About: Belongs to the Rosaceae family. Nectarines have alkaline properties that help in digestion. Nectarines also help the colon walls by creating bonds with toxins and removing them from the body. Nectarines carry lutein which aids in promoting eye health.

Cancer & Disease Fighting: The phytochemicals in nectarines have been shown to help fight against colon cancer and lung cancer.

Phytochemicals: Flavonoids, Anthocyanins, Catechin, Chlorogenic-Acid, Quercetin, Didymin, Sinensetin, Carotenoids, β-Carotene, β-Cryptoxanthin, Lutein, Zeaxanthin.

Minerals: Calcium, Copper, Iron, Magnesium, Manganese, Phosphorus, Potassium, Zinc.

Vitamins: Vitamin A, Vitamin C, Vitamin E, Vitamin K, Folic Acid, Pantothenic Acid, Pyridoxine, Riboflavin, Thiamin.

Orange

About: Belongs to the Rutaceae family. Oranges are a great source of vitamin C. Vitamin C helps fight free radicals in the body. Oranges help to keep the immune system strong as well as maintain skin healthy by way of collagen. Hesperetin in oranges has been found to help lower high blood pressure and help keep cholesterol in check.

Cancer & Disease Fighting: Studies have shown that eating oranges helps inhibit breast, colon, and skin cancers.

Phytochemicals: Flavonoids, Hesperetin, Naringin, Naringenin, Carotenoids, β-Carotene, β-Cryptoxanthin, Lutein, Zeaxanthin.

Minerals: Calcium, Copper, Iron, Magnesium, Manganese, Potassium, Zinc.

Vitamins: Vitamin A, Vitamin C, Folic Acid, Pantothenic Acid, Pyridoxine, Riboflavin, Thiamin.

Papaya

About: Belongs to the Caricaceae family. Papayas have the enzyme papain that helps break down proteins. Papayas have high levels of vitamin C which helps fight the free radicals in the body that can damage healthy cells as well as promote healthy skin thanks to collagen. The high vitamin A levels help maintain healthy vision.

Cancer & Disease Fighting: Papayas help protect the body from lung and oral cancers thanks to the phytochemicals found in the carotenes.

Phytochemicals: Flavonoids, Carotenoids, β-Carotene, β-Cryptoxanthin, Lutein, Zeaxanthin.

Minerals: Calcium, Iron, Magnesium, Manganese, Phosphorus, Potassium, Sodium, Zinc.

Vitamins: Vitamin A, Vitamin C, Vitamin E, Vitamin K, Folic Acid, Pantothenic Acid, Pyridoxine, Riboflavin, Thiamin.

Peach

About: Belongs to the Rosaceae family. Both the peach and nectarine have alkaline properties that help in digestion. Peaches also help the colon walls by creating bonds with toxins and removing them from the body. Peaches carry lutein which aids in promoting eye health.

Cancer & Disease Fighting: The phytochemicals in peaches have been shown to help fight against colon cancer and lung cancer.

Phytochemicals: Flavonoids, Anthocyanins, Catechin, Chlorogenic-Acid, Quercetin, Didymin, Sinensetin, Carotenoids, β-Carotene, β-Cryptoxanthin, Lutein, Zeaxanthin.

Minerals: Calcium, Copper, Iron, Magnesium, Manganese, Phosphorus, Potassium, Zinc.

Vitamins: Vitamin A, Vitamin C, Vitamin E, Vitamin K, Folic Acid, Pantothenic Acid, Pyridoxine, Riboflavin, Thiamin.

Pear

About: Belongs to the Rosaceae family. Pears aid in weight loss and help digestion as well as regulate blood pressure levels. Pears also help in the repair of tissues. The immune system is boosted thanks to the phytochemicals in the pear.

Cancer & Disease Fighting: Pears help to lower the risk of certain cancers such as breast, lung, and stomach cancers.

Phytochemicals: Flavonoids, Quercetin, Hydroxycinnamic Acid, Carotenoids, β-Carotene, β-Cryptoxanthin, Lutein, Zeaxanthin.

Minerals: Calcium, Copper, Iron, Magnesium, Manganese, Phosphorus, Potassium, Zinc.

Vitamins: Vitamin A, Vitamin C, Vitamin E, Vitamin K, Folic Acid, Pantothenic Acid, Pyridoxine, Riboflavin, Thiamin.

Persimmon

About: Belongs to the Ebenaceae family. Persimmon has the ability to reduce oxidative stress on the cells and help with wrinkles, age sports muscle weakness, and premature aging thanks to the antioxidants.

Persimmons also help reduce macular degeneration, cataracts, and night vision.

Cancer & Disease Fighting: Research has shown that eating persimmons can reduce ear diseases and also fight cancer.

Phytochemicals: Flavonoids, Proanthocyanidins, Flavonoid Oligomers, Tannins, Phenolic Acid, Catechin, Gallocatechin, Betulinic Acid, Shibuol, Carotenoids, β-Carotene, β-Cryptoxanthin, Lutein, Zeaxanthin, Lycopene.

Minerals: Calcium, Iron, Magnesium, Manganese, Phosphorus, Potassium, Selenium, Sodium, Zinc.

Vitamins: Vitamin A, Vitamin C, Vitamin E, Vitamin K, Folic Acid, Pantothenic Acid, Pyridoxine, Riboflavin, Thiamin.

Pineapple

About: Belongs to the Bromeliaceae family. The pineapple has been well known to help with digestion and stomach-related issues. Pineapples have high levels of vitamin C which is needed for the production of collagen that helps maintain the structure of the blood vessels as well as the skin and bones. The pineapple contains bromelain a phytochemical that has been known to help reduce swelling and fight inflammation.

Cancer & Disease Fighting: The phytochemical bromelain has been known to inhibit the proliferation of both breast cancer and skin cancer.

Phytochemicals: Flavonoids, Bromelain, Carotenoids, β-Carotene.

Minerals: Calcium, Copper, Iron, Magnesium, Manganese, Phosphorus, Potassium, Sodium, Zinc.

Vitamins: Vitamin A, Vitamin C, Vitamin K, Folic Acid, Pantothenic Acid, Pyridoxine, Riboflavin, Thiamin.

Plum

About: Belongs to the Rosaceae family. Plums are rich in antioxidants that help protect healthy cells from free radical damage. The phytochemicals found in plums also help the digestion system.

Cancer & Disease Fighting: Plums are known to help prevent many cancers such as breast, colon, liver, and skin.

Phytochemicals: Flavonoids, Carotenoids, β-Carotene, β-Cryptoxanthin, Lutein, Zeaxanthin, Sorbitol, Isatin, Amygdalin.

Minerals: Calcium, Copper, Iron, Magnesium, Manganese, Phosphorus, Potassium, Selenium, Zinc.

Vitamins: Vitamin A, Vitamin C, Vitamin E, Vitamin K, Folic Acid, Pantothenic Acid, Pyridoxine, Riboflavin, Thiamin.

Pomegranate

About: Belongs to the Lythraceae family. Pomegranates have been shown to help reduce cholesterol and help to control weight.

Cancer & Disease Fighting: Pomegranates have been known to inhibit the proliferation of prostate cancer cells. Pomegranates also have been shown to be effective against lymphoma.

Phytochemicals: Flavonoids, Anthocyanins, Delphinidin-3-Glucoside, Cyanidin-3-Glucoside, Anthoxanthins, Gallic Acid, Ellagic Acid, Catechin, Ellagic Tannins.

Minerals: Calcium, Copper, Iron, Magnesium, Manganese, Phosphorus, Potassium, Selenium, Sodium, Zinc.

Vitamins: Vitamin C, Vitamin E, Vitamin K, Folic Acid, Pantothenic Acid, Pyridoxine, Riboflavin, Thiamin.

Quince

About: Belongs to the Rosaceae family.

Cancer & Disease Fighting: Quince contains 5-O-Caffeoylquinic Acid that has been known to inhibit the proliferation of certain cancer cell lines such as colon, kidney, liver, and lung cancers. Quince also helps the colon walls by creating bonds with toxins and removing them from the body.

Phytochemicals: Flavonoids, Tannins, Catechin, Epicatechin, Caffeoylquinic Acid, Procyanidin-B2, Oligomeric Procyanidin, Polymeric Procyanidin, 5-O-Caffeoylquinic Acid.

Minerals: Calcium, Copper, Iron, Magnesium, Phosphorus, Potassium, Selenium, Zinc.

Vitamins: Vitamin A, Vitamin C, Vitamin E, Vitamin K, Folic Acid, Pantothenic Acid, Pyridoxine, Riboflavin, Thiamin.

Raspberry

About: Belongs to the Rosaceae family.

Cancer & Disease Fighting: Ellagic Acid has been shown to inhibit tumor growth that is caused by carcinogens. Raspberries help to decrease the risk of cancer. The antioxidants found in raspberries help to protect DNA from damage caused by radiation. Raspberries are high in fiber. Epigallocatechin-3-gallute has been found to suppress the growth of esophangeal squamous cell carcinoma.

Phytochemicals: Cumaric Acid, Flavonoids, Anthocyanins, Ellagic Acid, Quercetin, Ferulic Acid, Gallotanins, Kaempferol, Salicylic Acid, Pelargonidin, Catechins, Epigallocatechin-3-gallute.

Minerals: Calcium, Copper, Iron, Magnesium, Manganese, Potassium, Zinc.

Vitamins: Vitamin A, Vitamin C, Vitamin E, Vitamin K, Folic Acid, Pyridoxine, Riboflavin.

Strawberry

About: Belongs to the Rosaceae family. Strawberries are loaded with high levels of vitamin C. Strawberries are rich in antioxidants that help protect healthy cells from free radical damage.

Cancer & Disease Fighting: A study was done that showed that 40 grams of dried strawberries daily over a period of months helped cause apoptosis in esophageal cancer cells. Strawberries have also been shown to inhibit cell proliferation in breast, cervical, colon, and prostate cancers.

Phytochemicals: Flavonoids, Anthocyanins, Ellagic Acid, Carotenoids, β-Carotene, β-Cryptoxanthin, Lutein, Zeaxanthin, Epigallocatechin-3-gallute.

Minerals: Calcium, Iron, Magnesium, Manganese, Potassium, Zinc.

Vitamins: Vitamin A, Vitamin C, Vitamin E, Vitamin K, Folic Acid, Pantothenic Acid, Pyridoxine, Riboflavin, Thiamin.

Tangerine

About: Belongs to the Rosaceae family. Tangerines are rich in vitamin A and vitamin C. The vitamin C in tangerines helps with the production of collagen which aids in healthy skin tissue wound healing, and arthritis.

Cancer & Disease Fighting: The antioxidants in tangerines help fight oxidative stress that can lead to cancer.

Phytochemicals: Flavonoids, Naringenin, Naringin, Hesperetin, Carotenoids, α-Carotene, β-Carotene, β-Cryptoxanthin, Lutein, Zeaxanthin, Lycopene.

Minerals: Calcium, Copper, Iron, Magnesium, Manganese, Potassium, Zinc.

Vitamins: Vitamin A, Vitamin C, Vitamin E, Folic Acid, Pantothenic Acid, Pyridoxine, Riboflavin, Thiamin.

Watermelon

About: Belongs to the Cucurbitaceae family. It helps maintain healthy skin and mucosa membranes.

Cancer & Disease Fighting: The phytochemicals Cucurbitacin E and Cucurbitacin B in watermelon help lower the risk of breast cancer. The high levels of antioxidants found in watermelons help protect against cancers such as breast, colon, endometrial, lung, and pancreatic cancers.

Phytochemicals: Flavonoids, Carotenoids, α-Carotene, β-Carotene, β-Cryptoxanthin, Lutein, Zeaxanthin, Cucurbitacin E, Cucurbitacin B.

Minerals: Calcium, Copper, Iron, Magnesium, Manganese, Potassium, Zinc.

Vitamins: Vitamin A, Vitamin C, Vitamin E, Folic Acid, Pantothenic Acid, Pyridoxine, Riboflavin, Thiamin.

14

Vitamins and Minerals

Understanding Nutrient Deficiency

Nutrient deficiency is a condition that occurs when the body lacks essential vitamins, minerals, and other vital nutrients necessary for optimal functioning. This condition can have widespread implications on health, affecting various physiological processes. I will delve into the causes, effects, and prevention strategies related to nutrient deficiency.

Several factors contribute to nutrient deficiency, and they can vary widely among individuals.

The most obvious cause of nutrient deficiency is an insufficient intake of essential nutrients through the diet. People who consume diets lacking in diversity, consisting primarily of processed and refined foods, are at a higher risk. Poor eating habits, such as skipping meals or relying on fast food, can also lead to nutrient imbalances.

Even with a nutrient-rich diet, malabsorption issues can prevent the body from absorbing and utilizing nutrients effectively. Conditions like celiac disease, Crohn's disease, and certain gastrointestinal disorders can impair nutrient absorption in the digestive tract, leading to deficiencies.

Certain life stages or conditions may increase the body's demand for specific nutrients. For instance, pregnancy, lactation, adolescence, and intense physical activity may require higher levels of certain vitamins and minerals. Failure to meet these increased demands can result in deficiencies.

Chronic illnesses, such as diabetes, kidney disease, and autoimmune disorders, can interfere with the body's ability to properly absorb and use nutrients. Additionally, some medications used to treat these conditions may contribute to nutrient depletion.

Environmental factors, including soil quality and food processing methods, can impact the nutrient content of foods. Poor soil quality may lead to lower nutrient levels in crops, affecting the nutritional value of the food we consume. Food processing methods, such as cooking and preservation, can also reduce nutrient content.

The effects of nutrient deficiency can manifest in various ways, impacting different systems within the body. The severity and specific symptoms depend on the type and extent of the deficiency. Here are some common effects associated with specific nutrient deficiencies:

Iron deficiency can lead to anemia, characterized by fatigue, weakness, and pale skin. In severe cases, it can affect cognitive function and immune response.

Inadequate vitamin D levels can result in weakened bones, leading to conditions like osteoporosis. It may also contribute to a weakened immune system and increased susceptibility to infections.

A deficiency in vitamin C can cause scurvy, characterized by fatigue, muscle weakness, joint and muscle aches, and bleeding gums.

Vitamin B12 deficiency can lead to anemia, neurological issues, and fatigue. Prolonged deficiency may result in irreversible nerve damage.

Insufficient calcium intake can lead to weakened bones, increasing the risk of fractures and osteoporosis. It can also affect blood clotting and muscle function.

Iodine deficiency can result in thyroid dysfunction, leading to goiter, hypothyroidism, and developmental issues in infants born to deficient mothers.

Zinc deficiency can impair immune function, wound healing, and growth. It may also affect cognitive function and reproductive health.

Magnesium deficiency can lead to muscle cramps, tremors, fatigue, and abnormal heart rhythms.

Preventing nutrient deficiency involves adopting a balanced P53 Diet that provides all essential nutrients in adequate amounts. Here are some strategies for preventing nutrient deficiency:

Consuming a diverse range of foods, including fruits, vegetables, nuts, seeds, and whole grains, ensures a balanced intake of essential nutrients. Nutrient-dense foods should be prioritized over processed and refined options. The P53 Diet website contains all the plant-based recipes to ensure your body gets the proper balance of nutrients. You can also get your daily nutrient totals including essential amino acids on the P53 Diet website.

Managing and treating underlying health conditions, such as digestive disorders or chronic illnesses, is essential for preventing nutrient deficiencies. This may involve, lifestyle changes.

Nutrient deficiency is a significant public health concern with wide-ranging implications for individual well-being and public health. Addressing this issue requires a multi-faceted approach, including promoting healthy dietary habits, monitoring nutrient levels, and addressing underlying health conditions. By understanding the causes, effects, and preventive measures associated with nutrient deficiency, individuals and healthcare professionals can work together to ensure optimal nutrition and overall health.

Now let's take a look at the vitamins and minerals your body needs on a daily basis according to the United States Government. Keep this book handy and use it as a reference guide for your nutritional health.

Vitamins

Vitamin: **A**

Benefits: There are two types of vitamin A, vitamin A (preformed) retinoids which is animal-based. The other is the β-carotene (provitamin A) carotenoids which is a whole plant precursor to vitamin A. β-carotene is an antioxidant like all the carotenoids. Remember that antioxidants help protect the cells in the body from free radicals as described in the chapter on "Amino Acids." Beta-carotene is converted in the liver and the intestine and needs alpha-carotene, beta-carotene, and β-cryptoxanthin to be converted to vitamin A. Beta-carotene is the red-orange pigment found in fruit and vegetables. I will only talk here about the provitamin A, not the preformed vitamin A. Higher intakes of carotenoids provitamin A have been linked to a decreased risk of lung cancer. High amounts of provitamin A are not associated with increased health risks; only the animal-based preformed vitamin A is according to research. Vitamin A is needed for good vision. It plays an essential role in the function and maintenance of the heart, lungs, kidneys, and other organs.

RDA: 900 micrograms (mcg) for men, 700 mcg for women

Best Sources: sweet potato, spinach, carrots, pumpkin, cantaloupe, red peppers, mangos, black-eyed peas, apricots, broccoli.

Vitamin: **B1 (THIAMIN)**

Benefits: Thiamin plays an essential role in energy metabolism and the growth, development, and function of cells. There has not been enough research on health risks from excessive consumption of thiamin.

RDA: 1.2 milligrams (mg) for men, 1.1 mg for women

Best Sources: rice, black beans, whole wheat bread, acorn squash, sunflower seeds, oatmeal, corn, barley, and some breakfast cereals.

Vitamin: **B2 (RIBOFLAVIN)**

Benefits: This vitamin is an essential component of two major coenzymes, flavin mononucleotide (FMN) and flavin adenine dinucleotide (FAD). These coenzymes play an indispensable role in energy production, growth and development, and metabolism of fats, drugs, and steroids.

RDA: 1.3 mg for men, 1.1 mg for women

Best Sources: some breakfast cereals, oats, mushrooms, almonds, quinoa, spinach, apples, whole wheat bread, kidney beans, sunflower seeds, tomatoes, and rice.

Vitamin: **B3 (NIACIN)**

Benefits: Researchers have found through studies that niacin has been shown to increase the levels of HDL (good) cholesterol as well as lowering triglycerides levels. Niacin has also been shown to help reduce atherosclerosis. A deficiency in niacin can lead to poor concentration, anxiety, fatigue, restlessness, apathy, and even depression. If you take too much niacin, it can cause skin rashes and dry skin. Niacin can be made in the body by the conversion of tryptophan. Try taking whole plant sources of niacin not supplements.

RDA: 16 mg for men, 14 mg for women

Best Sources: mushrooms, avocados, peanuts, brown rice, green peas, sweet potatoes, sweet yellow peppers, butternut squash, nectarines, jackfruit, edamame, red potatoes.

Vitamin: **B5 (PANTOTHENIC ACID)**

Benefits: Pantothenic acid plays a role in triglyceride synthesis and lipoprotein metabolism. Vitamin B5 is a component of coenzyme A (CoA). Pantothenic acid is absorbed in the intestine and delivered directly into the bloodstream.

RDA: Adequate Intake (AI): 5 mg

Best Sources: shiitake mushrooms, avocados, sunflower seeds, sweet potatoes, lentils, rye flour, cashews, garbanzo beans, broccoli, hazels nuts, brown rice, whole wheat flour, peanuts, oatmeal, cauliflower, kale, split peas, soybeans, pecans, brewer's yeast.

Vitamin: **B6 (PYRIDOXINE)**

Benefits: Pyridoxine is very important; it plays a role in more than 100 enzyme reactions. If you have a deficiency in vitamin B6 can lead to depression and confusion, as well as a weakened immune system. Deficiencies in B5 can also result from malabsorption syndromes, such as celiac disease, Crohn's disease, and ulcerative colitis.

RDA: 1.7mg for men and women

Best Sources: chickpeas, potatoes, some breakfast cereals, bananas, winter squash, raisins, onions, spinach, soybeans, lentils, kale, cauliflower, sweet potatoes, avocados, turnip greens, walnuts, navy beans, brown rice, sweet peppers, brussels sprouts.

Vitamin: **B12 (COBALAMIN)**

Benefits: Vitamin B12 is required for proper red cell blood cell formation. B12 also functions as a cofactor for methionine synthase catalyzes the conversion of homocysteine to methionine. Methionine is necessary for the creation of S-adenosylmethionine, a universal methyl donor for almost 100 different substrates, including DNA, RNA, hormones, proteins, and lipids. If you don't eat animal proteins, you will need to get your daily intake of B12 from another source; I take a B12 supplement. That is the only supplement I take.

RDA: 2.4 mcg

Best Sources: Nutritional yeast or B12 supplement

Vitamin: **B7 (BIOTIN)**

Benefits: Biotin is a cofactor for five carboxylases (propionyl-CoA carboxylase, pyruvate carboxylase, methylcrotonyl-CoA carboxylase MCC, acetyl-CoA carboxylase 1, and acetyl-CoA carboxylase 2) that catalyze critical steps in the metabolism of fatty acids, glucose, and amino acids. Biotin also plays a vital role in histone modifications, gene regulation (by modifying the activity of transcription factors), and cell signaling.

RDA: 30 mcg

Best Sources: brewer's yeast, soybeans, rice bran, walnuts, barley, pecans, almonds, oatmeal, spinach, apple, banana, broccoli, sunflower seeds, and sweet potatoes.

Vitamin: **Vitamin C (ASCORBIC ACID)**

Benefits: Humans cannot synthesize vitamin C. Vitamin C requires biosynthesis of collagen, L-carnitine, and certain neurotransmitters. Collagen is an essential component of connective tissue, which plays a vital role in wound healing. Vitamin C is also an essential physiological antioxidant and has been shown to regenerate other antioxidants within the body, including alpha-tocopherol (vitamin E). Ongoing research is examining whether vitamin C, is limiting the damaging effects of free radicals through its antioxidant activity, might help prevent or delay the development of certain cancers, cardiovascular disease, and other diseases in which oxidative stress plays a causal role. In addition to its biosynthetic and antioxidant functions, vitamin C plays an essential role in immune function and improves the absorption of non-heme iron, the form of iron present in plant-based foods. Insufficient vitamin C intake causes scurvy, which is characterized by fatigue or lassitude, widespread connective tissue weakness, and capillary fragility. Large doses of vitamin C have been known to induce apoptosis in specific cancer cells.

RDA: 90 mg for men, 75 mg for women

Best Sources: red peppers, oranges, kiwi, green pepper, broccoli, strawberries, Brussel sprouts, cantaloupe, turnip leaves, parsley, red cabbage, watercress, spinach, collard greens, guavas, kale leaves, green peas, papayas, mustard greens, mangoes, raspberries.

Vitamin: **CHOLINE**

Benefits: Choline is considered a part of the B vitamin. Choline can be made in the body from the amino acid methionine or serine. Choline is needed to make the neurotransmitter acetylcholine. Choline also plays an essential role in gene expression, cell membrane signaling, lipid transport, metabolism, and early brain development. Too much choline can be harmful.

RDA: 550mg for men, 425mg for women daily

Best Sources: soybeans, quinoa, Brussels sprouts, broccoli, cauliflower, sunflower seeds, brown rice, red potatoes, kidney beans, shiitake mushrooms, green peas, red cabbage, carrots, apples, kiwi, and tangerines.

Vitamin: **Vitamin D (CALCIFEROL)**

Benefits: When sunlight hits the skin in the form of ultraviolet rays, it triggers vitamin D synthesis. Vitamin D promotes calcium absorption in the gut and maintains adequate serum calcium and phosphate concentrations to enable normal mineralization of bone and to prevent hypocalcemic tetany.

RDA: 600 International Units (IU) for adults up to age 70, 800 IU for adults over 70

Best Sources: sunlight. GET OUTSIDE!

Vitamin: **Vitamin E (ALPHA-TOCOPHEROL)**

Benefits: Naturally occurring vitamin E exists in eight chemical forms (alpha-, beta-, gamma-, and delta-tocopherol and alpha-, beta-, gamma-, and delta-tocotrienol) that have varying levels of biological activity. Alpha- (or α-) tocopherol is the only form that is recognized to meet human requirements.

Serum concentrations of vitamin E (alpha-tocopherol) depend on the liver, which takes up the nutrient after the various forms are absorbed from the small intestine. The liver preferentially resecretes only alpha-tocopherol via the hepatic alpha-tocopherol transfer protein; the liver metabolizes and excretes the other vitamin E forms. As a result, blood and cellular concentrations of other forms of vitamin E are lower than those of alpha-tocopherol and have been the subjects of less research.

Antioxidants protect cells from the damaging effects of free radicals, which are molecules that contain an unshared electron. Free radicals damage cells and might contribute to the development of cardiovascular disease and cancer. Unshared electrons are highly energetic and react rapidly with oxygen to form reactive oxygen species (ROS). The body forms ROS endogenously when it converts food to energy, and antioxidants might protect cells from the damaging effects of ROS. The body is also exposed to free radicals from environmental exposures, such as cigarette smoke, air pollution, and ultraviolet radiation from the sun. ROS are part of signaling mechanisms among cells.

Vitamin E is a fat-soluble antioxidant that stops the production of ROS formed when fat undergoes oxidation. Scientists are investigating whether, by limiting free-radical production and possibly through other mechanisms, vitamin E might help prevent or delay the chronic diseases associated with free radicals.

RDA: 15 mg (22.4 IU) for men and women

Best Sources: wheat germ, sunflower seeds, almonds, hazelnuts, peanuts, spinach, broccoli, kiwi, tomatoes, and mangos.

Vitamin: **Vitamin B9 (FOLIC ACID)**

Benefits: Folate functions as a coenzyme or cosubstrate in single-carbon transfers in the synthesis of nucleic acids (DNA and RNA) and metabolism of amino acids. One of the most critical folate-dependent reactions is the conversion of homocysteine to methionine in the synthesis of S-adenosyl-methionine, a significant methyl donor. Another folate-dependent reaction, the methylation of deoxyuridylate to thymidylate in the formation of DNA, is required for proper cell division. An impairment of this reaction initiates a process that can lead to megaloblastic anemia, one of the hallmarks of folate deficiency.

When consumed, folates are hydrolyzed to the monoglutamate form in the gut before absorption by active transport across the intestinal mucosa. Passive diffusion also occurs when pharmacological doses of folic acid are consumed. Before entering the bloodstream, the enzyme dihydrofolate reductase reduces the monoglutamate form to THF and converts it to either methyl or formyl forms. The main form of folate in plasma is 5-methyl-THF.

The activity of dihydrofolate reductase varies significantly among individuals. When the capacity of dihydrofolate reductase is exceeded, unmetabolized folic acid can be present in the blood. Whether unmetabolized folic acid has any biological activity or can be used as a biomarker of folate status is not known. Folate is also synthesized by colonic microbiota and can be absorbed across the colon, although the extent to which colonic folate contributes to folate status is unclear. The total body content of folate is estimated to be 15 to 30 mg; about half of this amount is stored in the liver and the remainder in blood and body tissues.

Serum folate concentrations are commonly used to assess folate status; a value above 3 ng/mL indicates adequacy. This indicator, however, is sensitive to recent dietary intake, so it might not reflect long-term status. Erythrocyte folate concentrations provide a longer-term measure of folate intakes; a concentration above 140 ng/mL indicates adequate folate status.

RDA: 400 mcg (including from supplements); 600 mcg during pregnancy

Best Sources: spinach, black eye peas, asparagus, Brussels sprouts, romaine lettuce, avocado, rice, broccoli, green peas, kidney beans, mustard greens, peanuts, turnip greens, papaya, banana, cantaloupe.

Vitamin: **Vitamin K (PHYLLOQUINONE, MENADIONE)**

Benefits: "Vitamin K," the generic name for a family of compounds with a typical chemical structure of 2-methyl-1,4-naphthoquinone, is a fat-soluble vitamin that is naturally present in some foods and is available as a dietary supplement. These compounds include phylloquinone (vitamin K1) and a series of menaquinones (vitamin K2). Menaquinones have unsaturated isoprenyl side chains and are designated as MK-4 through MK-13, based on the length of their side chain. MK-4, MK-7, and MK-9 are the most well-studied menaquinones.

Phylloquinone is present primarily in green leafy vegetables and is the primary dietary form of vitamin K. Menaquinones, which are predominantly of bacterial origin, are present in modest amounts in various animal-based and fermented foods. Almost all menaquinones, in particular, the long-chain menaquinones, are also produced by bacteria in the human gut. MK-4 is unique in that the body produces it from phylloquinone via a conversion process that does not involve bacterial action.

Vitamin K functions as a coenzyme for vitamin K-dependent carboxylase, an enzyme required for the synthesis of proteins involved in hemostasis (blood clotting) bone metabolism, and other diverse physiological functions. Prothrombin (clotting factor II) is a vitamin K-dependent protein in plasma that is directly involved in blood clotting.

RDA: 120 mcg for men, 90 mcg for women

Best Sources: turnip greens, spinach, broccoli, soybeans, edamame, pine nuts, blueberries, grapes, cashews, carrots, figs, iceberg lettuce, and kale.

Minerals

Source: U.S. Department of Health and Human Services

Mineral: **CALCIUM**

Benefits: Calcium, the most abundant mineral in the body, is found in some foods, added to others, available as a dietary supplement, and present in some medicines (such as antacids). Calcium is required for vascular contraction and vasodilation, muscle function, nerve transmission, intracellular signaling, and hormonal secretion, though less than 1% of total body calcium is needed to support these critical metabolic functions. Serum calcium is very tightly regulated and does not fluctuate with changes in dietary intakes; the body uses bone tissue as a reservoir for, and source of calcium, to maintain constant concentrations of calcium in the blood, muscle, and intercellular fluids.

The remaining 99% of the body's calcium supply is stored in the bones and teeth where it supports their structure and function. The bone itself undergoes continuous remodeling, with constant resorption and deposition of calcium into new bone. The balance between bone resorption and deposition changes with age. Bone formation exceeds resorption in periods of growth in children and adolescents, whereas in early and middle adulthood both processes are relatively equal. In aging adults, particularly among postmenopausal women, bone breakdown exceeds formation, resulting in bone loss that increases the risk of osteoporosis over time.

RDA: 1000 mg for adults up to age 50, 1200 mg for adults over 50

Best Sources: soy milk, tofu, kale, almonds, cabbage, kale, broccoli, spinach, turnip greens, collard greens, brazil nuts, figs, watercress, sunflower seeds, olives, walnuts, sesame seeds, soybeans, pecans, romaine lettuce, green beans, carrots, cashews, celery, orange, pumpkin seeds, sweet potatoes, dates.

Mineral: **CHLORIDE**

Benefits: The body needs this negatively charged ion. This ion contains about 115 grams of chloride. Chloride is an electrolyte and along with potassium and sodium assists the body's electrical connections when dissolved in water. When chloride bonds with hydrogen in the stomach it makes hydrochloride acid a digestive enzyme that helps breakdown proteins. Chloride is essential to the function of the body. If the body did not have chloride, the fluid levels would not be able to be maintained and electrical connections to move muscles would not happen.

RDA: 2300 mg

Best Sources: kelp, olives, rye, tomatoes, lettuce, celery, and table salt.

Mineral: **CHROMIUM**

Benefits: Chromium is a mineral that humans require in trace amounts, although its mechanisms of action in the body and the amounts needed for optimal health are not well defined. It is found primarily in two forms: 1) trivalent (chromium 3+), which is biologically active and found in food, and 2) hexavalent (chromium 6+), a toxic form that results from industrial pollution. This fact focuses exclusively on trivalent (3+) chromium.

Chromium is known to enhance the action of insulin, a hormone critical to the metabolism and storage of carbohydrates, fat, and protein in the body. In 1957, a compound in brewers' yeast was found to prevent an age-related decline in the ability of rats to maintain normal levels of sugar (glucose) in their blood. Chromium was identified as the active ingredient in this so-called "glucose tolerance factor" in 1959.

Chromium also appears to be directly involved in carbohydrate, fat, and protein metabolism.

RDA: 35 mcg for men, 25 mcg for women

Best Sources: broccoli, garlic, basil, whole wheat bread, apples, bananas, green beans, potatoes, parsnips, carrots, navy beans, cabbage, blueberries, green peppers, spinach.

Mineral: **COPPER**

Benefits: Copper is essential in the body's different functions such as the manufacturing of hemoglobin and collagen structures, mainly in the arteries and the joints. Copper and zinc fight each other for absorption. If you have an abundance of zinc the amount of copper absorption will be decreased and vice versa. If your child is deficient in copper, the cholesterol levels can rise. Researchers have stated a link between copper deficiency to atherosclerosis.

RDA: 900 mcg

Best Sources: almonds, carrots, turnips, apples, green peas, papaya, molasses, garlic, barley, hazelnuts, brazil nuts, split peas, walnuts, ginger root, pecans, peanuts.

Mineral: **IODINE**

Benefits: Iodine is a trace element that is naturally present in some foods, added to others, and available as a dietary supplement. Iodine is an essential component of the thyroid hormones thyroxine (T4) and triiodothyronine (T3). Thyroid hormones regulate many important biochemical reactions, including protein synthesis and enzymatic activity, and are critical determinants of metabolic activity. They are also required for proper skeletal and central nervous system development in fetuses and infants.

Thyroid function is primarily regulated by thyroid-stimulating hormone (TSH), also known as thyrotropin. It is secreted by the pituitary gland to control thyroid hormone production and secretion, thereby protecting the body from hypothyroidism and hyperthyroidism. TSH secretion increases the thyroidal uptake of iodine and stimulates the synthesis and release of T3 and T4. In the absence of sufficient iodine, TSH levels remain elevated, leading to goiter, an enlargement of the thyroid gland that reflects the body's attempt to trap more iodine from the circulation and produce thyroid hormones.

Iodine may have other physiological functions in the body as well. For example, it appears to play a role in immune response and might have a beneficial effect on mammary dysplasia and fibrocystic breast disease.

The earth's soils contain varying amounts of iodine, which in turn affects the iodine content of crops. In some regions of the world, iodine-deficient soils are common, increasing the risk of iodine deficiency among people who consume foods primarily from those areas. Salt iodization programs, which many countries have implemented, have dramatically reduced the prevalence of iodine deficiency worldwide

RDA: 150 mcg

Best Sources: seaweed, corn, apple, bananas, prunes, green peas.

Mineral: **IRON**

Benefits: Iron is a mineral that is naturally present in many foods, added to some food products, and available as a dietary supplement. Iron is an essential component of hemoglobin, an erythrocyte protein that transfers oxygen from the lungs to the tissues. As a component of myoglobin, a protein that provides oxygen to muscles, iron supports metabolism. Iron is also necessary for growth, development, normal cellular functioning, and synthesis of some hormones and connective tissue.

Dietary iron has two primary forms: heme and non-heme. Plants and iron-fortified foods contain non-heme iron only, whereas meat, seafood, and poultry contain both heme and non-heme iron. Heme iron, which is formed when iron combines with protoporphyrin IX, contributes about 10% to 15% of total iron intakes in Western populations.

Most of the 3 to 4 grams of elemental iron in adults are in hemoglobin. Much of the remaining iron is stored in the form of ferritin or hemosiderin (a degradation product of ferritin) in the liver, spleen, and bone marrow or is located in myoglobin in muscle tissue. Humans typically lose only small amounts of iron in the urine, feces, gastrointestinal tract, and skin. Losses are more significant in menstruating women, because of blood loss. Hepcidin, a circulating peptide hormone, is the critical regulator of both iron absorption and the distribution of iron throughout the body, including in plasma.

Many different measures of iron status are available, and various measures are useful at different stages of iron depletion. Measures of serum ferritin can be used to identify iron depletion at an early stage. A reduced rate of delivery of stored and absorbed iron to meet cellular iron requirements represents a more advanced stage of iron depletion, which is associated with reduced serum iron, reticulocyte hemoglobin, and percentage transferrin saturation and with higher total iron binding capacity, red cell zinc protoporphyrin, and serum transferrin receptor concentration. The last stage of iron deficiency, characterized by iron-deficiency anemia (IDA), occurs when blood hemoglobin concentrations, hematocrit (the proportion of red blood cells in blood by volume), mean corpuscular volume and mean cell hemoglobin are low. Hemoglobin and hematocrit tests are the most commonly used measures to screen patients for iron deficiency, even though they are neither sensitive nor specific. Hemoglobin concentrations lower than 13 g/dL in men and 12 g/dL in women indicate the presence of IDA. Normal hematocrit values, which are generally three times higher than hemoglobin levels, are approximately 41% to 50% in males and 36% to 44% in females.

RDA: 8 mg for men, 18 mg for women (non-heme)

Best Sources: white beans, dark chocolate, lentils, spinach, tofu, kidney beans, chickpeas, tomatoes, potatoes, cashews, green beans, rice, raisins, pistachios, broccoli, cantaloupe, mushrooms, Swiss chard, black beans, pinto beans, beet greens, figs, sunflower seeds, sesame seeds, quinoa, turnip greens, apricots, blackstrap molasses.

Mineral: **MAGNESIUM**

Benefits: Magnesium, an abundant mineral in the body, is naturally present in many foods, added to other food products, available as a dietary supplement, and present in some medicines (such as antacids and laxatives). Magnesium is a cofactor in more than 300 enzyme systems that regulate diverse biochemical reactions in the body, including protein synthesis, muscle and nerve function, blood glucose control, and blood pressure regulation. Magnesium is required for energy production, oxidative phosphorylation, and glycolysis. It contributes to the structural development of bone and is required for the synthesis of DNA, RNA, and the antioxidant glutathione. Magnesium also plays a role in the active transport of calcium and potassium ions across cell membranes, a process that is important to nerve impulse conduction, muscle contraction, and normal heart rhythm.

An adult body contains approximately 25g of magnesium, with 50% to 60% present in the bones and most of the rest in soft tissues. Less than 1% of total magnesium is in blood serum, and these levels are kept under tight control. Normal serum magnesium concentrations range between 0.75 and 0.95 millimoles (mmol)/L. Hypomagnesemia is defined as a serum magnesium level of less than 0.75 mmol/L. Magnesium homeostasis is primarily controlled by the kidney, which typically excretes about 120 mg of magnesium into the urine each day. Urinary excretion is reduced when magnesium status is low.

Assessing magnesium status is difficult because most magnesium is inside cells or in bone. The most commonly used and readily available method for assessing magnesium status is the measurement of serum magnesium concentration, even though serum levels have little correlation with total body magnesium levels or concentrations in specific tissues. Other methods for assessing magnesium status include measuring magnesium concentrations in erythrocytes, saliva, and urine; measuring ionized magnesium concentrations in blood, plasma, or serum; and conducting a magnesium-loading (or "tolerance") test. No single method is considered satisfactory. Some experts but not others consider the tolerance test (in which urinary magnesium is measured after parenteral infusion of a dose of magnesium) to be the best method to assess magnesium status in adults. To comprehensively evaluate magnesium status, both laboratory tests and a clinical assessment might be required

RDA: 400-420 mg for men, 310-320 mg for women

Best Sources: almonds, spinach, cashews, peanuts, black beans, edamame, avocados, potatoes, brown rice, oatmeal, kidney beans, bananas, raisins, broccoli, apples, and carrots.

Mineral: **MANGANESE**

Benefits: Manganese is essential to your children's health even though you hear that much about it. Manganese is needed to help fight inflammation and sprains by increasing the levels of the enzyme superoxide dismutase. This mineral also plays a role in many chemical processes such as the processing of cholesterol, carbohydrates, and proteins. Researchers state that manganese can be helpful in the absorption of vitamins such as vitamin B and vitamin E. Some scientists have found it to relieve osteoarthritis and osteoporosis. Manganese is also a potent antioxidant to combat free radicals in the body. This mineral has also been found to help control epilepsy seizures.

RDA: 2.3 mg for men, 1.8 mg for women

Best Sources: pecans, Brazilian nuts, almonds, carrots, beet greens, oats, turnip greens, broccoli, split peas, spinach, raisins, brussels sprouts, rye, buckwheat, and whole wheat.

Mineral: **MOLYBDENUM**

Benefits: Molybdenum helps to play a part in preventing neurological damage in infants. Molybdenum also functions as a role in several enzymes.

RDA: 45mcg

Best Sources: brown rice, lentils, green peas, garlic, corn, potatoes, onions, cauliflower, oats, green beans, barley, split greens, molasses, cabbage, strawberries, whole wheat, and raisins.

Mineral: **PHOSPHORUS**

Benefits: Helps convert digested foods into energy. Phosphorus also helps play a role in carrying lipids in the blood and nutrients into and out of the body cells. This mineral helps build and protect bones and teeth.

RDA: 700 mg

Best Sources: lentils, almonds, peanuts, whole wheat bread.

Mineral: **POTASSIUM**

Benefits: Scientists are studying potassium to understand how it affects health. Here are some examples of what this research has shown.

High blood pressure is a significant risk factor for heart disease and stroke. People with low intakes of potassium have an increased risk of developing high blood pressure, especially if their diet is high in salt (sodium). Increasing the amount of potassium in your diet and decreasing the amount of sodium might help lower your blood pressure and reduce your risk of stroke.

Getting too little potassium can deplete calcium from bones and increase the amount of calcium in the urine. This calcium can form hard deposits (stones) in your kidneys, which can be very painful. Increasing the amount of potassium in your diet might reduce your risk of developing kidney stones.

People who have high intakes of potassium from fruits and vegetables seem to have stronger bones. Eating more of these foods might improve your bone health by increasing bone mineral density (a measure of bone strength).

Low intakes of potassium might increase blood sugar levels. Over time, this can increase the risk of developing insulin resistance and lead to type 2 diabetes. More research is needed to fully understand whether potassium intake affects blood sugar levels and the risk of type 2 diabetes.

Potassium from food has not been shown to cause any harm in healthy people who have normal kidney function. Excess potassium is eliminated in the urine.

However, people who have chronic kidney disease and those who use certain medications can develop abnormally high levels of potassium in their blood (a condition called hyperkalemia). Examples of these medications are angiotensin-converting enzyme inhibitors, also known as ACE inhibitors and potassium-sparing diuretics. Hyperkalemia can occur in these people even when they consume reasonable amounts of potassium from food.

Hyperkalemia can also develop in people with type 1 diabetes, congestive heart failure, liver disease, or adrenal insufficiency. Adrenal insufficiency is a condition in which the adrenal glands, located just above the kidneys, don't produce enough of certain hormones.

Even in healthy people, getting too much potassium from supplements or salt substitutes can cause hyperkalemia if they consume so much potassium that their bodies can't eliminate the excess.

RDA: AI 3400 mg for men, 2600 mg for women

Best Sources: avocados, acorn squash, banana, white beans, spinach, sweet potato, pomegranate.

Mineral: **SELENIUM**

Benefits: Selenium is a trace element that is naturally present in many foods, added to others, and available as a dietary supplement. Selenium, which is nutritionally essential for humans, is a constituent of more than two dozen selenoproteins that play critical roles in reproduction, thyroid hormone metabolism, DNA synthesis, and protection from oxidative damage and infection.

Selenium exists in two forms: inorganic (selenate and selenite) and organic (selenomethionine and selenocysteine). Both types can be good dietary sources of selenium. Soils contain inorganic selenites and selenates that plants accumulate and convert to organic forms, mostly selenocysteine and selenomethionine, and their methylated derivatives.

Most selenium is in the form of selenomethionine in animal and human tissues, where it can be incorporated nonspecifically with the amino acid methionine in body proteins. Skeletal muscle is the primary site of selenium storage, accounting for approximately 28% to 46% of the total selenium pool. Both selenocysteine and selenite are reduced to generate hydrogen selenide, which in turn is converted to selenophosphate for selenoprotein biosynthesis.

The most commonly used measures of selenium status are plasma and serum selenium concentrations. Concentrations in blood and urine reflect recent selenium intake. Analyses of hair or nail selenium content can be used to monitor longer-term intakes over months or years. Quantification of one or more selenoproteins (such as glutathione peroxidase and selenoprotein P) is also used as a functional measure of selenium status. Plasma or serum selenium concentrations of 8 micrograms (mcg)/dL or higher in healthy people typically meet needs for selenoprotein synthesis.

RDA: 55mcg

Best Sources: Brazilian nuts, brown rice, baked beans, oatmeal, spinach, cashews, bananas, potatoes, peaches, carrots, lettuce, green peas.

Mineral: **SODIUM**

Benefits: Most of the sodium found in the body is in the blood and around the cells. Sodium also plays an essential role in muscle contractions and nerve functions. Sodium helps the body maintain a healthy fluid balance.

RDA: 1500mg

Best Sources: avocados, spinach, oranges, tomatoes, potatoes, apricots, peaches, plums, cantaloupe, and strawberries.

Mineral: **ZINC**

Benefits: Zinc is an essential mineral that is naturally present in some foods, added to others, and available as a dietary supplement. Zinc is also found in many cold lozenges and some over-the-counter drugs sold as cold remedies.

Zinc is involved in numerous aspects of cellular metabolism. It is required for the catalytic activity of approximately 100 enzymes, and it plays a role in immune function, protein synthesis, wound healing, DNA synthesis, and cell division. Zinc also supports normal growth and development during pregnancy, childhood, and adolescence and is required for proper sense of taste and smell. A daily intake of zinc is required to maintain a steady state because the body has no specialized zinc storage system

RDA: 11 mg for men, 8 mg for women

Best Sources: baked beans, cashews, chickpeas, almonds, kidney beans, green peas, and oatmeal.

15

The P53 Lifestyle

Living a healthy lifestyle encompasses various facets, from dietary choices to personal hygiene practices. One key element is adopting a plant-based P53 Diet, which focuses on whole, unprocessed foods derived from plants. This dietary approach has gained popularity due to its potential health benefits.

A plant-based P53 Diet emphasizes fruits, vegetables, legumes, nuts, and seeds while eliminating animal products. These foods are rich in vitamins, minerals, fiber, and antioxidants, contributing to overall well-being. Research suggests that a plant-based diet may reduce the risk of chronic diseases such as heart disease, diabetes, and certain cancers.

The foundation of a plant-based P53 Diet lies in the consumption of a diverse range of plant foods. Colorful fruits and vegetables offer a spectrum of nutrients, and whole grains provide essential carbohydrates for energy. Legumes, such as beans and lentils, are excellent sources of protein and fiber. Nuts and seeds contribute healthy fats and additional nutrients.

Aside from dietary choices, personal hygiene is a crucial aspect of a healthy lifestyle. Many conventional hygiene products contain chemicals that may have adverse effects on health. Transitioning to natural and chemical-free hygiene products can contribute to a healthier lifestyle.

Chemical-free personal care products, including shampoo, soap, toothpaste, and deodorant, avoid potentially harmful substances like parabens, phthalates, and sulfates. These chemicals, found in numerous commercial products, have been linked to various health concerns, including hormonal disruptions and skin irritations.

Opting for natural alternatives can be beneficial for both personal health and the environment. Natural products often use plant-derived ingredients, essential oils, and other organic components. These substances can provide effective hygiene without the potential risks associated with synthetic chemicals.

In addition to dietary and personal care choices, regular physical activity is a cornerstone of a healthy lifestyle. Exercise contributes to cardiovascular health, weight management, and mental well-being. It is recommended to engage in a combination of aerobic activities, strength training, and flexibility exercises for overall fitness.

Adequate sleep is another vital component of a healthy lifestyle. Quality sleep plays a crucial role in physical and mental recovery, immune function, and overall resilience. Establishing a consistent sleep routine and creating a conducive sleep environment can promote restful and restorative sleep.

Managing stress is equally important for maintaining a healthy lifestyle. Chronic stress can have detrimental effects on both physical and mental health. Techniques such as meditation, deep breathing, and mindfulness can help manage stress levels. Finding activities that bring joy and relaxation, such as hobbies or spending time in nature, can also contribute to overall well-being.

Social connections and a supportive community are integral to a healthy lifestyle. Building and maintaining meaningful relationships provide emotional support and contribute to mental and emotional well-being. Connecting with others can also foster a sense of belonging and purpose.

Hydration is a simple yet often overlooked aspect of a healthy lifestyle. Drinking an adequate amount of water is essential for bodily functions such as digestion, circulation, and temperature regulation. Water intake varies based on individual needs, climate, and physical activity levels.

A healthy lifestyle encompasses various interconnected factors, including a plant-based diet, chemical-free personal care, regular physical activity, sufficient sleep, stress management, social connections, and proper hydration. Making conscious and informed choices in these areas can contribute to a holistic approach to health and well-being.

At the Grocery Store with Kids

Part of the healthy lifestyle is grocery shopping; this a great time to educate your children on why the whole plant is so crucial to their health. Get your kids excited about helping choose the fruit and vegetables always make this part fun for the younger kids. Have them pick different colored fruits and veggies. Eat the rainbow of colors.

Blue/Purple - These colors come from the phytochemical group of Anthocyanins and belong to the Flavonoids group. They give the dark blue pigments of fruit or vegetables like blueberry, raspberry, purple cauliflower, black rice, red cabbage, and more. Research has shown that Anthocyanins help reduce the risk of heart disease in women by decreasing blood pressure and preventing arterial stiffness. Anthocyanins have also been shown to lower LDL cholesterol. Studies have shown that

Anthocyanins play a role in inhibiting tumor growth in the esophagus. They also show promise in preventing the spread of certain cancers.

Green - This color comes from chlorophyll leafy green vegetables from the phytochemicals known as Isothiocyanates. Isothiocyanates are sulfur-containing phytochemicals. Isothiocyanates play an essential role in the war against cancer by helping to prevent esophageal cancer, and lung cancer cells from proliferation and can induce apoptosis in the cancer cells. Studies have shown that Isothiocyanates can also lower the risk of gastrointestinal cancer.

Green/Yellow - The green/yellow fruits and vegetables come from the Phytochemicals known as lutein which is a carotenoid. Lutein has been shown to block the damaging blue light that hits the eyes. Lutein has also been recognized for help in anti-aging such as macular degeneration.

Red - The red comes from lycopene. Lycopene has been found to help protect the skin and tissues. Research has also shown that lycopene can help to protect against prostate cancer.

Yellow/Orange - These colors come from carotenoids *β*-Carotene. Carotenoids have been shown to decrease the risk of certain cancers such as esophagus cancer, lung cancer, stomach cancer, as well as diseases of the eyes.

In America, there are a lot of people who do not eat a variety of colors in their food. Most of the food people eat nowadays is beige. This color mostly comes from foods that are processed. You need to eat different colored whole plant foods. There is not a pill on the market that can replace getting your nutrients from whole plant foods.

Each time I talked to young children about eating fruits and vegetables, I always made the fruit and veggies superheroes and explained to them that each one had powers to make them strong and healthy to fight off dangerous chemicals. As I stated earlier choosing organic over non-organic, is very important but again if there is not any organic fruit and vegetables available by the non-organic make sure to wash them. They still contain the phytochemicals that you need daily. When I buy fruit and veggies, I try to buy enough for five days. I also buy organic frozen fruit that I use for my daily fruit smoothie.

What do the stickers on fruit and vegetables mean?

These stickers are called "Price Look Up" (PLU) these contain the price and more.

If the sticker has a 4-digit number that means it was grown conventionally, indicating that the grower could have used pesticides and herbicides.

An example of a conventional navel orange PLU is 4012.

If there is number 9 in front of the 4-digit number that identifies the fruit or vegetable as being organic, meaning the grower cannot use antibiotics, pesticides, or herbicides on them.

An example of an organic navel orange PLU is 94012.

If there is number 8 in front of the 4-digit number that identifies the fruit or vegetable as being a genetically modified organism (GM0), it means scientists have genetically engineered the organism.

An example of a GMO navel orange PLU is 84012.

Eating Out Plant-Based Style

Eating out on a plant-based diet can be a delightful experience, as more restaurants are now offering diverse and creative plant-based options. Whether you're a committed plant-based eater or just exploring plant-based choices, navigating restaurant menus can be an enjoyable journey of discovery.

One of the key aspects of dining out on a plant-based diet is the increasing availability of plant-based alternatives. Many restaurants now incorporate plant-based proteins like tofu, tempeh, and seitan into their dishes, providing a satisfying and protein-rich substitute for traditional animal products. This shift reflects a growing awareness of dietary preferences and environmental concerns, making it easier than ever to find flavorful and fulfilling plant-based meals.

When perusing a menu, look for dishes that highlight a variety of vegetables, grains, and legumes. Salads, stir-fries, and grain bowls are often versatile options that can be customized to suit your taste and dietary preferences. Additionally, many restaurants now feature plant-based burgers made from ingredients like black beans, chickpeas, or mushrooms, offering a satisfying alternative to traditional meat burgers.

Don't hesitate to communicate your dietary preferences with the server or chef. Most restaurants are accommodating and willing to make adjustments to meet your needs. You might discover off-menu plant-based options or find that a non-vegetarian dish can be modified to suit your preferences.

Ethnic cuisines often provide a rich tapestry of plant-based choices. Mediterranean, Indian, Thai, and Mexican cuisines, for example, typically offer a variety of plant-centric dishes bursting with flavors. Dishes like falafel, vegetable curries, or bean-based tacos can be both delicious and nourishing.

When dining out, it's also essential to be mindful of hidden animal products in sauces, dressings, or broths. Ask about the ingredients or request alternatives to ensure your meal aligns with your plant-based choices. Additionally, be aware of cross-contamination in restaurant kitchens, especially if you follow a strict plant-based P53 diet.

Exploring local and independent eateries can often yield exciting plant-based finds. These establishments may be more willing to experiment with plant-based ingredients and offer unique dishes that cater to diverse dietary preferences. Supporting local businesses also aligns with the ethos of many plant-based enthusiasts, who often seek sustainability not only in their food choices but also in their overall lifestyle.

Eating out while on a plant-based diet has evolved significantly, with restaurants increasingly recognizing the demand for diverse and delicious plant-centric options. By exploring menus, communicating preferences, and being open to culinary exploration, you can enjoy a wide array of satisfying plant-based meals at various eateries. The growing availability of plant-based alternatives and the culinary creativity of chefs make dining out a rewarding experience for those embracing a plant-based lifestyle.

The P53 Food Carts

The P53 food carts were founded to give people with cancer and other ailments a safe place to eat outside their homes. The recipes that are served at the food carts are from the p53diet.com website. There are currently 3 p53 food carts licensed in the Portland, Oregon area, with more carts on the way. The early success of the P53 Food cart has come due to the great tasting 100% plant-based ingredients. The carts offer bowls, soups, salads, freshly squeezed juices, and smoothies. All sauces are scratch homemade daily. Since the P53 food carts do not allow any cooking oils, preservatives, or animal products the food is incredibly good for you. The P53 food carts have a cult-like following due to the great-tasting food items that provide the vitamins and minerals that the body craves. You can find P53 food carts at fairs, festivals school events, farmers markets, etc. Please check the p53diet.com website for the cart locations you can also learn more about p53 food carts at thep53.com The P53 Food carts have been featured multiple times on local KOIN TV. The reporter Kohr Harlan was quoted saying that *"the sauces were so good you could drink them."* If you are interested in licensing a P53 Cart in your area please check thep53.com website for more information.

The P53 Channel

The P53 Channel Podcast is for all things P53 from diet to food carts and much more. I will host the show each week and cover a wide base of issues on health and nutrition. The show will be uploaded every Thursday at noon. Some of the broadcasts will be live with live callers. Please check the website at thep53.com to see any updates. All aired broadcasts are FREE. Please stay tuned we plan to be fully up and running by the first of January 2024.

Plastic Food Containers

If you buy foods that are in plastic containers, make sure to check the number on the plastic.

Listed below are what the numbers represent.

Plastic #1 Polyethylene Terephthalate (PET) - PET is used in the making of bottles for sports drinks, soda drinks, and other products such as condiment containers. PET can leach the metal antimony which is toxic. PET is somewhat safe. According to scientists, plastic #1 is safer than #3, #6, and #7.

Plastic #2 High-Density Polyethylene (HDPE) - HDPE is used to make water bottles, juice bottles, and milk containers. HDPE has been shown to release estrogenic chemicals that disrupt the hormones in the body. According to scientists, plastic #2 is safer than #3, #6, and #7, but there are concerns because of the release of estrogenic chemicals.

Plastic #3 Polyvinyl Chloride (PVC) - PVC is used in the making of deli wraps, meat wraps, and shrink wrap as many other products such as toys and flooring.

Research has stated that PVC has been linked to asthma and autism.

STAY AWAY FROM #3.

Plastic #4 Low-Density Polyethylene (LDPE) - This is used in the milking of paper milk cartons as well as coffee cups. Most of the research has stated that LDPE is deemed safe but could leach estrogenic chemicals. According to scientists, plastic #4 is safer than #3, #6, and #7.

Plastic #5 Polypropylene (PP) - Polypropylene is used to make containers for takeout food. Polypropylene is unlikely to leach into the food due to its high heat tolerance. According to scientists, plastic #5 is safer than #3, #6, and #7.

Plastic #6 Polystyrene (PS) - Polystyrene is another name for Styrofoam. Polystyrene is used for making cups plates and other products. Polystyrene in food containers can leach into the food. This can occur when heated. Coffee is served in these styrofoam cups which is a bad idea. STAY AWAY FROM #6

Plastic #7 - This is a plastic not made of any of the plastics listed above. This number could represent a combination of plastics. This category of plastic could contain these endocrine disrupters BPA or BPS. Endocrine disrupters are chemicals that interfere with any system in the body. These endocrine disrupters have been known to cause cancer, learning disabilities, birth defects, and other developmental disorders. STAY AWAY FROM #7

My personal choice is #5; this choice is because of the high heat tolerance which should lower the chemical reaction that could leach chemicals into the food. Please, when choosing products at the grocery store look for those products that have been deemed safe. Remember ***STAY AWAY FROM #3, #6, #7.***

How To Read Nutrition Labels?

Source: fda.gov

The Nutrition Facts Label must list total fat, saturated fat, trans fat, cholesterol, sodium, total carbohydrate, dietary fiber, sugars, protein, vitamin A, vitamin C, calcium, and iron.

The Nutrition Facts Label may also list monounsaturated fat, polyunsaturated fat, soluble fiber, insoluble fiber, sugar alcohol, other carbohydrates, vitamins (such as biotin, folate, niacin, riboflavin, pantothenic acid, thiamin, vitamin B6, vitamin B12, vitamin D, vitamin E, and vitamin K) and minerals (such as chromium, copper, iodine, magnesium, manganese, molybdenum, phosphorus, potassium, selenium, and zinc).

The Serving Size

The first place to start when you look at the Nutrition Facts label is the serving size and the number of servings in the package. Serving sizes are standardized to make it easier to compare similar foods; they are provided in familiar units, such as cups or pieces, followed by the metric amount, e.g., the number of grams.

The size of the serving on the food package influences the number of calories and all the nutrient amounts listed on the top part of the label. Pay attention to the serving size, especially how many servings there are in the food package. Then ask yourself, "How many servings am I consuming"? (e.g., 1/2 serving, 1 serving, or more)

The Percent Daily Value (%DV)

The % Daily Values (%DVs) are based on the Daily Value recommendations for key nutrients but only for a 2,000-calorie, daily diet--not 2,500 calories. You, like most people, may not know how many calories you consume in a day. But you can still use the %DV as a frame of reference whether or not you consume more or less than 2,000 calories.

The %DV helps you determine if a serving of food is high or low in a nutrient. Note: a few nutrients, like trans-fat, do not have a %DV

Do you need to know how to calculate percentages to use the %DV? No, the label (the %DV) does the math for you. It helps you interpret the numbers (grams and milligrams) by putting them all on the same scale for the day (0-100%DV). The %DV column doesn't add up vertically to 100%. Instead, each nutrient is based on 100% of the daily requirements for that nutrient (for a 2,000 calorie, diet). This way you can tell high from low and know which nutrients contribute a lot, or a little, to your daily recommended allowance. 5%DV or less is low, and 20%DV or more is high.

%DV Not Listed

Trans Fat: Experts could not provide a reference value for trans fat, nor any other information that the FDA believes is sufficient to establish a Daily Value or %DV. Scientific reports link trans-fat (and saturated fat) with raising blood LDL ("bad") cholesterol levels, both of which increase your risk of coronary heart disease, a leading cause of death in the US.

Protein: A %DV is required to be listed if a claim is made for protein, such as "high in protein." Otherwise, unless the food is meant for use by infants and children under four years old, none is needed. Current scientific evidence indicates that protein intake is not a public health concern for adults and children over four years of age.

Sugars: No daily reference value has been established for sugars because no recommendations have been made for the total amount to eat in a day. Keep in mind, that the sugars listed on the Nutrition Facts label include naturally occurring sugars (like those in fruit and milk) as well as those added to a food or drink. Check the ingredient list for specifics on added sugars.

Using the %DV

Comparisons: The %DV also makes it easy for you to make comparisons. You can compare one product or brand to a similar product. Just make sure the serving sizes are similar, especially the weight (e.g., gram, milligram, ounces) of each product. It's easy to see which foods are higher or lower in nutrients because the serving sizes are generally consistent for similar types of foods, (see the comparison example at the end) except in a few cases like cereals.

Nutrient Content Claims: Use the %DV to help you quickly distinguish one claim from another, such as "reduced fat" vs. "light" or "nonfat." Just compare the %DVs for Total Fat in each food product to see which one is higher or lower in that nutrient--there is no need to memorize definitions. This works when comparing all nutrient content claims, e.g., less, light, low, free, more, high, etc.

Dietary Trade-Offs: You can use the %DV to help you make dietary trade-offs with other foods throughout the day. You don't have to give up a favorite food to eat a healthy diet. When a food you like is high in fat, balance it with foods that are low in fat at other times of the day. Also, pay attention to how much you eat so that the total amount of fat for the day stays below 100%DV.

Calories (and Calories from Fat)

Calories provide a measure of how much energy you get from a serving of this food. Many Americans consume more calories than they need without meeting recommended intakes for a number of nutrients. The calorie section of the label can help you manage your weight (i.e., gain, lose, or maintain.)

Remember: the number of servings you consume determines the number of calories you eat (your portion amount).

The calories from Fat section of the label also shows the total calories.

General Guide to Calories

40 Calories is low

100 Calories is moderate

400 Calories or more is high

The General Guide to Calories provides a general reference for calories when you look at a Nutrition Facts label. This guide is based on a 2,000 calorie, diet.

Eating too many calories per day is linked to overweight and obesity.

Please refer to the chapter on "Carbohydrates & Fiber" for more information.

Fat

The total fat is broken out into the kinds of fats and on the right side of the label is the % of Daily Value. As stated above % of daily values do not exist for Trans-fat, Polyunsaturated, and Monounsaturated Fats. The fats are listed in grams per serving size.

Total Fat - Total

Saturated Fat - Try to limit saturated fats

Trans Fat - Trans fats are known to increase the risk of cancer

Polyunsaturated Fat - Healthy

Monounsaturated Fat - Healthy

Cholesterol

The cholesterol is measured in milligrams. Only animal food products contain cholesterol. If you are eating the right way this should be zero and the percent of daily value should be zero as well.

Sodium

Sodium is measured in milligrams. Most of the sodium found in the body is in the blood and around the cells. Sodium also plays a vital role in muscle contractions and nerve functions. Sodium helps the body maintain a healthy fluid balance. You as parents need to keep the sodium levels in your children's diet at a healthy level. As stated in earlier chapters too much sodium is not healthy for the body. Please refer to the chapter on "Vitamins & Minerals" for the recommended daily allowance for children.

Total Carbohydrate

Total carbohydrates are measured in grams. This includes all carbs even simple carbs and sugars. You also need to check both fiber and sugar.

Dietary Fiber

Fiber comes in both soluble and insoluble. Soluble fiber can be found in foods like dried beans, and oatmeal. Soluble fiber is known to help lower cholesterol. Insoluble fiber can be found in fruit, whole grains, and vegetables. Insoluble fibers can protect against bowel issues and help with digestion. Please refer to the chapter *"The Basics of the P53 Diet & Lifestyle"* for the recommended daily allowance.

Sugars

These are simple sugars such as glucose, dextrose, fructose, and galactose. There is hardly any nutritional value in these sugars. Sugars are found in almost everything. Make sure you keep the sugar and the added sugars very low.

Protein

Proteins are measured in grams.

Vitamins and Minerals

This part of the label lists the vitamins and minerals based on 2,000 calories a day.

Ingredients

The ingredients here are listed in order of quantity. I encourage you to use the chapter on "Toxins" to make sure there are not any dangerous chemicals in the food you are purchasing for consumption.

Supplemental Vitamins & Minerals

The Supplemental Vitamins and minerals are listed below the proteins and are chosen and provided by the food producer.

Please remember this is a lifestyle, not a temporary diet. Take the time to read the labels while at the grocery store. This means looking at the ingredients as well as the sugar, sodium, and other nutrition facts. The ingredients list can also match the list of known carcinogens in this book. I know that reading the labels adds more time to your shopping day. Please take that time for the sake of your health.

Excessive Exercise and Oxidative Stress

Excessive exercise, while generally beneficial for overall health, can indeed lead to a phenomenon known as oxidative stress. This occurs when the body's antioxidant defenses are overwhelmed by an excess of free radicals generated during intense physical activity. Free radicals are highly reactive molecules that can damage cells, proteins, and DNA, contributing to a range of health issues.

During moderate exercise, the body produces free radicals as natural byproducts of metabolism. Antioxidants, which the body produces or obtains from the diet, usually neutralize these free radicals. However, when exercise intensity and duration exceed the body's capacity to manage oxidative stress, the balance is disrupted, leading to potential harm.

Intensive and prolonged physical activity increases oxygen consumption, resulting in higher production of free radicals. This heightened oxidative state may outpace the body's ability to scavenge these radicals, allowing them to accumulate and cause damage to cellular structures. Organs such as the heart, lungs, and muscles, which are heavily involved in exercise, are particularly vulnerable to oxidative stress.

Oxidative stress has been associated with various negative health outcomes, including inflammation, muscle fatigue, and impaired recovery. It can compromise the integrity of cell membranes and disrupt cellular functions. Moreover, oxidative damage to DNA may contribute to the development of chronic conditions and accelerate the aging process.

One key factor in managing oxidative stress is the body's endogenous antioxidant defense system. This system includes enzymes like superoxide dismutase, catalase, and glutathione peroxidase. Regular exercise enhances the activity of these enzymes, reinforcing the body's ability to counteract oxidative stress. However, extreme exercise can overwhelm this defense system, leading to a state of chronic oxidative stress.

Athletes engaged in prolonged and intense training regimens, such as endurance runners or professional athletes, may be at a higher risk of experiencing oxidative stress. The paradox here is that while exercise is crucial for health, excessive training can tip the balance, turning a beneficial activity into a potential health risk.

It is essential for individuals engaging in intense exercise to adopt strategies that mitigate oxidative stress. Adequate nutrition plays a pivotal role in this regard. Consuming a diet rich in antioxidants, including vitamins C and E, as well as minerals like selenium, can help support the body's defense mechanisms. Additionally, proper hydration is crucial for flushing out toxins and supporting overall metabolic processes.

Balancing high-intensity workouts with sufficient rest and recovery is equally important. Overtraining syndrome, characterized by persistent fatigue, decreased performance, and increased susceptibility to illness, may be a manifestation of chronic oxidative stress. Recognizing the signs of overtraining and adjusting exercise routines accordingly can prevent long-term health consequences.

While exercise is a cornerstone of a healthy lifestyle, it is crucial to recognize the potential drawbacks of excessive physical activity. Striking a balance between challenging workouts and adequate recovery, along with maintaining a well-rounded, nutrient-rich diet, is key to reaping the benefits of exercise without subjecting the body to undue oxidative stress.

16

Recipes & Meal Planning

RECIPES

Orzo, Sweet Potato, Ginger

Servings 5 | Prep Time 30 mins | Total Time 1 hr
Calories 150.7 | Carbohydrates 30.3 | Fat 3g | Protein 4.8g

INGREDIENTS

- 1 tsp Salt
- 1 1/2 cup Orzo Uncooked
- 1 3/4 cups Sweet Potato, diced
- 2 cups White Onion, diced
- 2 tbsp Fresh Garlic, minced
- 1 tbsp Fresh Ginger, grated
- 1/2 cup Shitake Mushrooms, stems removed, dice caps
- 1 tbsp Balsamic Vinegar
- 3 tbsp Soy Sauce, Gluten-Free, Low Sodium, NO SODIUM BENZOATE!
- 2 cups Spinach, remove stems, finely chopped

DIRECTIONS

1. In a large pot boil water and salt add orzo and cook for 5 minutes. Drain and rinse with cold water. Set aside.
2. In a large skillet, add a thin layer of water. Heat to medium-high and medium-high potatoes. Cook for 3-4 minutes on each side.
3. Reduce heat to medium and stir in the onions, garlic and ginger. Saute for 1-2 minutes.
4. Add the shitake mushrooms and cook for 1 minute then flip and cook for 1 minute more.
5. Mix in the balsamic vinegar and the soy mix to prevent sticking. Cook for 3 minutes.
6. Turn the heat back to medium-high and add the orzo gradually, stirring constantly cook for 5 minutes.
7. Add the spinach and cook for about 1 minute or until the spinach has softened.

Vegetable Broth

Servings 6 | Prep Time 1hr | Total Time 1h 7mins
Calories 18.77 | Carbohydrates 4.32g | Fat 0.09g | Protein 0.64g

INGREDIENTS

- 1 whole Yellow Onion, chunks
- 3 cloves Garlic, cut in half
- 3 stalks Celery with leaves, cut into chunks
- 1 tsp Black Peppercorns

- 1 tsp Sea Salt
- 10 cups Water
- 1/2 tsp Basil dried
- 1/2 tsp Sage dried
- 1/2 tsp Thyme dried

DIRECTIONS

- Place water in large cooking pot
- Add all ingredients
- Bring to boil
- Reduce to simmer for 1 hour
- Strain vegetables. (use as compost)
- This will reduce to about 6 cups

Lisa's Rustic White Bean, Mushrooms and Quinoa

Servings 6 | Prep Time 30 mins | Total Time 2 hrs
Calories 254.54 | Carbohydrates 53.87g | Fat 2.54g | Protein 11.94

INGREDIENTS

- 3 15oz cans Cannellini Beans, drain and rinse
- 3 cups Portebella Mushroom, steamed and diced
- 6 cups Vegetable Broth
- 1/2 cup Quinoa
- 4 cups Baby Spinach, chopped
- 1/2 tsp Liquid Smoke, Brand: Wright's
- 1 tsp Paprika
- 2 tsp Sea salt

- 2 tsp Rosemary, dried
- 2 tbsp Lemon Juice, freshly squeezed
- 1/4 tsp Black Pepper
- 2 cloves Fresh Garlic, minced
- 1 large Onion, diced small pieces

DIRECTIONS

- Stir in mushrooms into a large pot. Cook til soft, about 4 minutes. Remove mushrooms from the pot, then set aside.
- Add the other 1/2 tbsp to the large pot, and slowly add the onions while stirring. Cook for about 15 minutes or until they start to caramelize. Stir in the garlic at the 10-minute mark.
- Add vegetable broth, beans, liquid smoke, and all spices, bring to a boil on high heat, then reduce heat to medium and simmer for 30 minutes.
- Stir in mushrooms and quinoa for about 20 minutes.
- Remove from heat, stir in spinach, and add the lemon juice. Until the spinach is wilted.
- Serve

Dave's Quick Black Bean Burger

Servings 4 | Prep Time 15 mins | Total Time 20 mins
Calories 189.5 | Carbohydrates 38.03g | Fat 3.12g| Protein 9.95g

INGREDIENTS

- 15 oz can Black Beans, drained
- 3 tbsp Onions, minced
- 3/4 tsp Salt

- 1 1/2 tsp Garlic Powder
- 2 tsp Parsley
- 1 tsp Chili Powder
- 2/3 cup Whole Wheat Flour, no bleached flour

DIRECTIONS

- Using the food processor or blender, blend the black beans until halfway smashed. Transfer to a large bowl.
- Mix in the onions, salt, garlic powder, parsley, and chili powder. Mash with a fork to combine.
- Slowly add in the flour to form a sticky mixture. You may not need or use all the flour.
- Form the mixture into patties and fry in the pan. Use a tbsp of water in the pan if needed. Fry until the middle is no longer mushy, about 4 minutes on each side.

Dave's Pico

Servings 10 | Prep Time 30 mins | Total Time 30 mins
Calories 59.8 | Carbohydrates 11.9g | Fat 0.4g | Protein 3.24g

INGREDIENTS

- 1 whole White Onion, diced
- 1 tsp Garlic, fresh, chopped
- 2 large Tomatoes, fresh, diced
- 1 15oz can Black Beans, low sodium, no additives, drain and rinse
- 1 4oz can Green Chilies, mild, drain
- 2 tbsp Lime Juice, freshly squeezed
- 1/4 cup Cilantro, freshly chopped

- 1 large Red Pepper, washed and diced
- 1 tbsp Cumin
- 1/4 tsp Black Pepper
- 1/8 tsp Cayenne
- 1 tbsp Sea Salt

DIRECTIONS

- Dice onion, red pepper, and tomatoes and place in a large bowl.
- Chop garlic and cilantro and place in a bowl with other ingredients.
- Drain and rinse black beans and add to bowl.
- Drain green chilies and add to bowl
- Add 2 tbsp of lime juice to the bowl.
- Add chopped cilantro to bowl.
- Add cumin, black pepper, cayenne, and sea salt to the bowl.
- Mix all ingredients well and serve

9 Cup Salad

Servings 9 | Prep Time 25 mins| Total Time 25 mins
Calories 109.8 | Carbohydrates 10.8g | Fat 5.7g | Protein 5.5g

INGREDIENTS

- 1 cup Broccoli, chopped fine
- 1 cup Cauliflower, diced
- 1/2 cup Yellow Bell Pepper, diced
- 1/2 cup Red Bell Pepper, diced
- 1 cup Radishes, sliced
- 1 cup Carrots, diced
- 1 cup Celery, diced
- 1 cup White Onion, diced

- 1 cup Green Peas
- 1/2 cup Cranberries, dried, chopped
- 1/2 cup Pumpkin Seeds, raw roasted

DIRECTIONS

- Chop all ingredients
- Place in Large Bowl

Italian Seasoning

Servings 10 | Prep Time 5 mins | Total Time 5 mins
Calories 4.96 | Carbohydrates 1.39g | Fat 0.07g | Protein 0.33g

INGREDIENTS

- 1 tsp Garlic Powder
- 1 tbsp Parsley, dried
- 1 tbsp Red Chili Flakes
- 1 tbsp Thyme, dried
- 2 tbsp Basil, dried
- 2 tbsp Oregano, dried
- 1 tbsp Rosemary, dried

DIRECTIONS

Just mix together.

Italian Dressing

Servings | Prep Time | Total Time
Calories 12.6 | Carbohydrates 1.96g | Fat 0.02g | Protein 0.12g

INGREDIENTS

- 1/4 cup Apple Cider Vinegar
- 1 /2 cup Water
- 1 tbsp Dijon Mustard
- 1 large Garlic Clove

DIRECTIONS

To get started right away, just tap any placeholder text (such as this) and start typing.

Cucumber and Kale Green Juice

Servings 2 | Prep Time 10 mins | Total Time 10 mins
Calories 160.9 | Carbohydrates 37.95g | Fat 1g | Protein 3.15g

INGREDIENTS

- 2 cups Cucumbers
- 2 cups Honeydew Melon, peeled and seeded
- 1 whole Apple, cored

- 5 large Kale Leaves
- 1/2 cup Fresh Mint Leaves
- 1/4 cup Lemon Juice, freshly squeezed, with no added sugar or preservatives

DIRECTIONS

- Juice the cucumbers, melon, apple, kale, and mint.
- Transfer to the shaker cup and add the lemon juice. Shake well.

Butter Bean Veggie Soup

Servings 12 | Prep Time 6 mins | Total Time 31 mins
Calories 114.38 | Carbohydrates 20.91g | Fat 0.42g | Protein 7.12g

INGREDIENTS

- 6 cups Vegetable Broth
- 3 stalks Celery, diced fine
- 1 15oz can Lentils, rinse and drain
- 1 15oz can Butter Beans, rinse and drain
- 1 cup Green Beans, cut and diced
- 1 cup Peas, frozen is ok
- 1 cup Carrots, diced, frozen is ok
- 1 tsp Cumin
- 1 1/2 tsp Onion Powder
- 1 tsp Garlic Powder

DIRECTIONS

- Place vegetable broth soup pot.
- Add all ingredients.

- Bring to a boil.
- Reduce heat and simmer for 10 minutes.

Red Cabbage and Pineapple Salad

Servings 6 | Prep Time 20 mins | Total Time 20 mins
Calories 98.56 | Carbohydrates 19.47g | Fat 2.55g | Protein 1.67g

INGREDIENTS

- 4 cups Red Cabbage, chopped
- 1/8 tsp Sea Salt, to taste
- 2 cups Pineapple, cubed
- 2 tbsp Apple Juice, no added sugar or preservatives
- 1 tbsp Apple Cider Vinegar
- 2 tbsp Fresh Chives, chopped
- 1/2 tsp Cumin
- 1/8 tsp Black Pepper, to taste

DIRECTIONS

- In a large bowl, add the chopped cabbage and salt and allow to rest for 2-3 minutes. Add in the pineapple.
- In a small bowl, mix the remaining ingredients. Pour over the cabbage mixture and mix well.

Mushroom and Farro Stew

Servings 4 | Prep Time 1hr | Total Time 1hr
Calories 401.51 | Carbohydrates 75.48g | Fat 6.3g | Protein 14.16g

INGREDIENTS

- 4 cups Vegetable Broth
- 1 1/2 cups Farro
- 1 tsp Salt
- 1 tsp Black Pepper, freshly cracked
- 2 cups Mushrooms Portobello Caps, sliced 1/2' wide
- 1 cup Mushrooms, assorted, trimmed, quartered
- 1 cup Onion, chopped fine
- 3 cloves Garlic, minced
- 1 tsp Thyme, fresh, minced
- 14.5oz can Tomatoes, drained, diced, fire-roasted
- 2 tbsp Parsley, fresh, minced

DIRECTIONS

- Bring broth and farro to simmer in a large saucepan and cook until farro is tender and creamy about 22-25 minutes. Season with salt and pepper to taste, cover, and keep warm.
- Combine the Portobello and assorted mushrooms in a covered bowl and microwave until tender about 6-8 minutes.
- Heat a tablespoon of water in the Dutch oven over medium-high heat then sauté the onions for about 7 minutes. Stir in the mushrooms and cook another 5 minutes until browned
- Mix in the garlic, thyme, and tomatoes; continue to cook for another 8 minutes until the sauce thickens.
- Remove pot from the heat, stir in parsley then serve atop farro. Enjoy!

Edamame and Roasted Red Pepper Barley Pilaf

Servings 6 | Prep Time 15 mins | Total Time 15 mins
Calories 315 | Carbohydrates 56.9g | Fat 4.41g | Protein 15.39g

INGREDIENTS

- 2 cups Edamame, frozen shelled, thawed, and drained
- 2 cups Barley, cooked
- 1/3 cups Red Peppers, roasted, chopped
- 2/3 cup Green Pea, frozen, thawed and drained
- 2/3 cup corn, frozen, thawed and drained
- 1 1/2 tbsp Dijon Mustard
- 2 tbsp Lemon Juice, freshly squeezed, no added sugar or preservatives
- 3/4 tsp Garlic Powder
- 1/8 tsp Salt
- 1/4 tsp Black Pepper
- 1/4 cup Cilantro, fresh, chopped

DIRECTIONS

- In a large bowl, add the edamame, cooked barley, roasted peppers, peas, and corn. Set aside.
- In a small bowl, mix the mustard, lemon juice, and garlic powder. Whisk well, then drizzle over the edamame and barley mixture. Gently toss.
- Season with salt and pepper and garnish with cilantro and avocado.

Cranberry and Apricot Quinoa

Servings 4 mins | Prep Time 10 mins | Total Time 30 mins
Calories 327.62 | Carbohydrates 59.22g | Fat 8.54g | Protein 7.25g

INGREDIENTS

- 1 cup Quinoa
- 2 cups Apple Juice, freshly squeezed, no added sugar, no preservatives
- 1 cup Water
- 1/2 cup Onion, diced
- 2 cups Celery, diced
- 1/2 tsp Nutmeg
- 1/2 tsp Cinnamon
- 1/4 tsp Cloves
- 1/2 cup Cranberries, dried, no added sugar
- 1/2 cup Apricots, dried, chopped
- 1 tsp Parsley
- 1/4 tsp Salt

DIRECTIONS

- In a large stock pot with a lid, add the quinoa, apple juice, and water. Bring to a slow simmer, cover, and cook for 15 minutes or until the quinoa is done.
- While the quinoa is cooking, in a large skillet, sauté the onion and celery in a tbsp of water until veggies are soft. Stir often.
- Add the onion mixture to the quinoa and add the remaining ingredients. Gently toss and heat through.

Spicy Cucumber Spinach Juice

Servings 1 | Prep Time 10 mins | Total Time 10 mins
Calories 128.8 | Carbohydrates 29.9g | Fat 1.18g | Protein 4.9g

INGREDIENTS

- 1 cup Cucumber, unpeeled
- 1 cup Green Apple, unpeeled, sliced
- 2 cups Spinach, stalks removed
- 1 tbsp Ginger Root, unpeeled
- 1 cup Parsley
- 4 tbsp Lemon Juice, freshly squeezed, no sugar added or preservatives
- 1 tsp Cayenne Pepper, ground

DIRECTIONS

- Juice together the cucumber, apple, spinach, and ginger. When pushing through the parsley, drizzle in the lemon juice to allow for easier juicing.
- Sprinkle cayenne juice into juice and mix well.
- Drink immediately or pour into an airtight container and keep in the refrigerator for up to 12 hours. Enjoy!

Artichoke and Basil Spaghetti

Servings 6 | Prep Time 10 mins | Total Time 25 mins
Calories 161 | Carbohydrates 29.25g | Fat 3.17g | Protein 5.16g

INGREDIENTS

- 12 oz Tinkyada Brown Rice Spaghetti Noodles, cooked
- 6 oz Artichoke Hearts, fresh, drained, chopped

- 2 large Tomatoes, chopped
- 1/2 cup Basil, fresh, chopped
- 1/2 cup Black Olives, sliced
- 1/2 tsp Rosemary
- 2 tbsp Nutritional Yeast
- 1/8 tsp Salt, to taste
- 1/8 tsp Black Pepper, to taste

DIRECTIONS

- Prepare the Tinkyada pasta according to package instructions.
- In a separate stock pot, combine all remaining ingredients except the salt and pepper. Heat through, stirring often. Add in cooked pasta and serve.

Caribbean Red Beans and Rice

Servings 4 | Prep Time 15 mins | Total Time 1hr
Calories 214.71 | Carbohydrates 45.51g | Fat 1.59g | Protein 8.84g

INGREDIENTS

- 3 cloves Garlic
- 3/4 cup Onion, chopped
- 1 1/4 cups Celery, chopped
- 2 tbsp Parsley, fresh, chopped
- 1 3/4 cups Vegetable Broth
- 1/2 tsp Rosemary
- 1/2 tsp Thyme
- 1/4 tsp Cloves
- 15 oz can Kidney Beans, drained, rinsed
- 1 1/2 cups Water
- 2 bay Leaves

- 1 1/2 cups Brown Rice, uncooked
- 1/8 tsp Salt, to taste
- 1/8 tsp Black Pepper, to taste

DIRECTIONS

- Using a food processor, add garlic, onion, celery, and parsley. Process until finely grated or minced.
- In a large stock pot with a lid, pour enough of the broth to cover the bottom of the pan. Heat to medium-high and add the onion mixture. Sauté until soft, stirring often. Add rosemary, thyme, cloves, and beans. Stir well. Heat for 2 more minutes.
- Reduce heat to medium and mix in the remaining vegetable broth, water, bay leaves, and rice. Bring to a low simmer, cover, and cook for 30 minutes.
- Lower heat to low, uncover and cook for 10 more minutes or until rice is done and when the liquid is almost absorbed. Remove bay leaves and season with salt and pepper.

Dave's Everyday Smoothie

Servings 2.5 | Prep Time 5 mins | Total Time 5 mins
Calories 92.4 | Carbohydrates 23.64g | Fat 0.27g | Protein 1.36g

INGREDIENTS

- 1 cup Pineapple, frozen
- 1/2 medium Banana, peeled
- 1/2 medium Grapefruit, peeled
- 1/2 large Orange, peeled

DIRECTIONS

- Place all ingredients into a blender and blend until smooth.

Beet Carrot Juice

Servings 1 | Prep Time 10 mins | Total Time 10 mins
Calories 220 | Carbohydrates 51.9g | Fat 0.9g | Protein 5.7g

INGREDIENTS

- 2 cups Carrots, peeled
- 1 cup Beets, with greens, peeled, washed well
- 1 cup Green Apple, unpeeled, sliced
- 1 cup Watercress

DIRECTIONS

- Juice first the carrots, then the beets with their greens, and finish off with the apple and watercress. Make sure to stir the juice between each new addition.
- Drink immediately or place in an airtight container in the refrigerator for up to 12 hours. Enjoy!

Dave's Quiche Chickpea Veggie Muffins

Servings 9 | Prep Time 30 mins | Total Time 30 mins
Calories 121.66 | Carbohydrates 19.19g | Fat 2.89g | Protein 5.68g

INGREDIENTS

- 1 1/2 tbsp Earth Balance Butter, used to grease the pan
- 1 1/2 cups Garbanzo Fava Flour, Brand: Bob's Red Mill
- 1 1/2 cups Water, best if water is warm
- 1 tsp Baking Powder, NO ALUMINUM Brand: Bob's Red Mill
- 2 tsp Salt
- 1/2 tsp Black Pepper, fresh, cracked
- 1 1/2 cups Peas, frozen, small diced
- 1 1/2 cups Carrots, frozen, small diced

DIRECTIONS

- Preheat the oven to 425 degrees and coat a 12-cup muffin tin with a 1/2 tbsp Earth Balance Butter.
- In a large bowl, stir together the flour, water, baking powder, salt and pepper. The batter will be lumpy and that's fine. Set aside while you prepare the veggies.
- In a large skillet, heat the remaining plant-based butter over medium to high heat. Add the frozen veggies and allow them to cook till heated through.
- Give the batter another whisk and try to get most of the remaining lumps out. Add the veggies to the batter; fill the coated muffin tin with the batter to the top. Bake for 15 minutes, or until tops are set. Toothpick tests the muffins to check that are cooked through.
- Let cool in the tin for 5 minutes, then pop them out to cool on a wire rack. Serve while still warm. Enjoy!

Veggie Mexican Rice

Servings 4 | Prep Time 45 mins | Total Time 45 mins
Calories 321.69 | Carbohydrates 53.87g | Fat 9.15g | Protein11.92g

INGREDIENTS

- 1 cup Long Grain Brown Rice, uncooked
- 1 cup Tomato, roughly chopped
- 1/2 cup Red Onion, roughly chopped
- 2 clove Garlic, minced
- 1 tbsp Cumin
- 1 1/2 tsp Chili Powder
- 1 tsp Oregano, dried
- 1 cup Red Bell Pepper, diced small
- 1 cup Zucchini, diced very small
- 1 cup Corn, frozen
- 15.5 oz can Black Beans, drained and rinsed
- 2 tsp Salt
- 1 cup Vegetable Broth
- 1/2 Lime, fresh-squeezed
- 1 cup Avocado, peeled, pitted, diced

DIRECTIONS

- Follow the instructions on the brown rice package on how to cook.
- Meanwhile, when rice is cooking, combine the tomato, onion, and garlic into a blender. Puree until liquefied. If the result is less than 1 cup of liquid, add a bit of vegetable broth.

- Once the rice is completed, move the rice to a large 3qt pot. Add the cumin, chili powder, oregano, salt, bell pepper, zucchini, corn, black beans, tomato puree, and stock to the pot. Bring to a simmer, cover, and reduce heat, cooking for approximately 15 minutes, stirring often.
- Remove the pot from the heat and fluff the rice with a fork. If all of the liquid has been absorbed but the rice is a bit underdone, leave it to stand, covered, for another 5 minutes.
- Add squeezed lime juice, and mix well.
- Top with avocado.

Zucchini Pomodoro Sauce with Fresh Basil

Servings 4 | Prep Time 10 mins | Total Time 20 mins
Calories 301.2 | Carbohydrates 56.37g | Fat 6.92g | Protein 6.84g

INGREDIENTS

- 2 1/2 cups Zucchini, sliced
- 4 cloves Garlic, minced
- 4 large Tomatoes, fresh, diced
- 1/3 cup Basil, chopped
- 2 cups Tinkyada Brown Rice Spaghetti Noodles, prepared per package instructions
- 1/8 tsp Salt, to taste
- 1/8 tsp Black Pepper, to taste

DIRECTIONS

- In a large saucepan over low heat, heat zucchini and garlic add in tbsp of water until zucchini is lightly softened. Add in the tomatoes and cook for an additional 5 minutes.
- Stir in basil and pasta. Salt and pepper to taste.

Meal Planning

Meal planning is a crucial component of maintaining a healthy lifestyle, and this holds especially true for individuals following a plant-based diet. Adopting a plant-based diet involves prioritizing fruits, vegetables, whole grains, legumes, nuts, and seeds while minimizing or eliminating animal products. Proper meal planning not only ensures that individuals meet their nutritional needs but also contributes to the overall success and sustainability of a plant-based lifestyle.

One of the key advantages of meal planning in a plant-based diet is the ability to achieve nutritional balance. Plant-based diets can provide all the essential nutrients the body needs, but careful planning is essential to avoid potential deficiencies. By including a variety of plant foods in different colors and textures, individuals can ensure they receive a broad spectrum of vitamins, minerals, and antioxidants. For instance, leafy greens offer calcium, legumes provide protein, nuts and seeds supply healthy fats, and a rainbow of vegetables delivers diverse nutrients.

Meal planning also helps individuals meet their protein requirements, a common concern for those new to plant-based eating. By strategically incorporating protein-rich foods such as beans, lentils, tofu, tempeh, and edamame into meals, individuals can easily achieve their protein goals without relying on animal products. Planning meals with a balance of plant proteins ensures that the body receives all essential amino acids, promoting muscle health and overall well-being.

Meal planning can contribute to better digestion and nutrient absorption. Plant-based diets, often high in fiber, support a healthy digestive system. Planning meals that include a mix of soluble and insoluble fiber from various plant sources can help prevent constipation, promote gut health, and support a diverse microbiome. Additionally, pairing certain foods together, such as combining vitamin C-rich foods with iron sources, can enhance the absorption of key nutrients.

For those concerned about meeting their energy needs on a plant-based diet, effective meal planning can address this apprehension. Including complex carbohydrates like whole grains, quinoa, and sweet potatoes provides a sustained release of energy, preventing energy dips and supporting overall vitality. Combining carbohydrates with healthy fats and proteins in meals creates a balanced and satisfying eating experience, reducing the likelihood of cravings or overeating.

Meal planning also contributes to financial savings and reduced food waste. Planning meals in advance allows individuals to create a shopping list based on their specific needs, reducing the likelihood of impulse purchases. Buying in bulk and using ingredients across multiple meals can be both cost-effective and environmentally friendly. By having a plan in place, individuals can make the most of their ingredients, minimizing the chances of items going to waste.

Meal planning plays a pivotal role in the success and sustainability of a plant-based diet. It ensures that individuals receive a diverse range of nutrients, meet their protein requirements, support digestion, and maintain energy levels. Furthermore, effective meal planning can contribute to financial savings and reduce food waste. By taking the time to thoughtfully plan plant-based meals, individuals can enjoy the numerous health benefits associated with this lifestyle while promoting overall well-being and longevity. Please check out the meal planning on the P53 Diet website https://p53diet.com/samples-of-the-diet/ for samples of meal planning.

A SAMPLE OF MY MEAL PLAN

Day 1 *(This is a sample of what I eat in a day)*

Breakfast

Frozen Fruit Smoothie - Organic fruit

1/4 cup raspberries - 16 calories, 0.02g fat, 0.37g protein, 3.67g carbohydrates, 2g fiber, 0.25mg sodium.

1/4 cup pineapple - 18.5 calories, 0.48g fat, 0.21g protein, 4.9g carbohydrates, 0.55g fiber, 0.5mg sodium.

1/4 cup orange - 21.25 calories, 0.06g fat, 0.42g protein, 5.29g carbohydrates, 1.08g fiber, 0mg sodium.

2 tbsp flaxseed (ground) - 70 calories, 4.5g fat, 3g protein, 4g carbohydrates, 3g fiber, 0mg sodium.

Oatmeal -

1 cup -166 calories, 3.6g fat, 5.9g protein, 28.1 carbohydrates, 4g fiber 9.4 sodium.

Morning Snack

Fruit - 1/2 cup of grapes - 60 calories, 0g fat, 1g protein, 14g carbohydrates, 1g fiber, 0mg sodium.

Lunch

Lentil Soup -

1 cup cooked lentils - 323 calories, 0.32g fat, 16.4g protein, 36.71g carbohydrates, 14.5g fiber, 431mg sodium.

Salad

2 cups - baby chard, baby kale, baby spinach, 14 calories, 0g fat, 3g protein, 3g carbohydrates, 1g fiber, 200mg sodium.

1/4 cup edamame - 50 calories, 1.5g fat, 4g protein, 5g carbohydrates, 2.5g fiber, 5mg sodium.

1/4 cup peeled cucumbers - 4 calories, 0.05g fat, 0.20g protein, 0.72g carbohydrates, 0.02g fiber, 0.74mg sodium.

1/4 cup celery - 15 calories, 0.99g fat, 0.32g protein, 1.52g carbohydrates, 0.58g fiber, 119mg sodium.

Dinner

Spaghetti

2oz brown rice Spaghetti noodles - 210 calories, 2g fat, 4g protein, 44g carbohydrates, 3g fiber, 0mg sodium.

1/2 cup organic spaghetti sauce - 50 calories, 1g fat, 2g protein, 10g carbohydrates, 2g fiber, 480mg sodium.

1 slice of whole grain bread with roasted garlic rubbed on

8 calories, 0.04g fat, 0.38g protein, 1.98g carbohydrates, 0.02g fiber, 2mg sodium.

Totals for Day 1

Calories = 1,025

Fats = 14.51

Proteins = 41.2 grams

Carbohydrates =165.89 grams

Fiber = 35.25 grams

Sodium = 1,247 milligrams

This is a sample of what I eat in a day, I get daily exercise, my daily dose of vitamin D, and sleep 8 hours, I also drink plenty of water *(more alkaline than acidic),* and I get all the essential amino acids this way. I also get the phytochemicals my body needs daily. If you and or your children choose to eat the way I do, you will need to make sure to take a vitamin B12 supplement as explained in a previous chapter. If you are a subscriber to the p53diet.com website all the daily totals will be done for you.

Attention, All Items listed below contain no animal proteins.

Monday

Breakfast:

Oatmeal w/Almond Milk, cinnamon

Whole Grain Toast w/sunflower butter

¼ Cup of Fruit

Snack:

Handful of Mixed Nuts

Lunch:

Brown Rice Pasta w/Spaghetti Sauce, Mushrooms, Olives, Garlic

Small Salad - Spinach, Romaine, Cucumbers, Chopped Walnuts, Sliced Almonds, Carrots, Bell Peppers

Snack:

Fruit Kabobs – Pineapple, Kiwi, Strawberry, Orange, Granny Smith Apple

Dinner:

Veggie Pitas

Healthy Dessert:

Slice of Carrot Cake

Tuesday

Breakfast:

Pancakes

Strawberry& Pineapple Smoothie

Snack:

Red Pepper Hummus

Lunch:

Black Bean Burrito

Chips & Salsa

Snack:

Handful of Mixed Nuts

Dinner:

Pizza (plant-based) with Low Sodium Crust

Healthy Dessert:

Oatmeal Raisin Cookies

Wednesday

Breakfast:

Fresh Strawberries

French Toast

12oz Glass of Almond Milk *(No sugar, No preservatives)*

Snack:

Celery Sticks with Sunflower Butter

Lunch:

Salad- Spinach, Romaine, Cucumbers, Chopped Walnuts, Carrots, Bell Peppers, Cherry Tomatoes

Cup of Chili w/Cornbread

Snack:

A handful of Mix Nuts

Dinner:

Mashed Potatoes with Non-Dairy Butter

¼ Cup of Cooked Peas

Healthy Dessert:

Ginger Spice Cookies

Thursday

Breakfast:

Fruit Smoothie

Oatmeal w/Blueberries

Snack:
¼ Cup of Fruit
Handful of Mixed Nuts
Lunch:
Tacos using Jackfruit as Meat Replacement
Snack:
Hummus Dip with Carrot Stick
Dinner:
Brown Rice Bowl w/Steamed Veggies
Healthy Dessert:
Coconut Pumpkin Bread

Friday
Breakfast:
Whole Grain Toast w/sunflower butter
Fruit Smoothie
Snack:
Celery Sticks with Sunflower Butter
Lunch:
Lentil Soup
Salad- Spinach, Romaine, Cucumbers, Chopped Walnuts, Carrots, Bell Peppers, Cherry Tomatoes
Snack:
Handful of Mixed Nuts
Dinner:
Garlic Pasta
Whole Grain Bread Slices
Healthy Dessert:
Sugar-Free Cocoa Balls

Saturday

Breakfast:
Whole Grain Waffle w/Strawberries
Oatmeal w/Almond Milk
Snack:
Handful of Mixed Nuts
Lunch:
Black Beans over Brown Rice
Fruit Smoothie
Snack:
Hummus Dip with Carrot Stick
Dinner:
Mashed Potatoes
Portabella Mushroom w/Steamed Veggies
Healthy Dessert:
Slice of Chocolate Cake

Sunday
Breakfast:
Whole Grain Toast w/Avocado Slices
Fruit Smoothie
Snack:
¼ Cup of Grapes
Lunch:
Hummus Vegetable Sandwich
¼ Cup of Strawberries and Blueberries
Iced Green Tea
Snack:
A handful of Mixed Nuts
Dinner:
Brown Rice Pasta w/Broccoli & Peas with Healthy Sauce
Whole Grain Toasted Bread w/garlic
Fresh Lemonade Low or No Added Sugar

Healthy Dessert:
Slice of Pumpkin Pie

In summary, now that you understand the damage that is caused to the body by bad chemistry, it should be easy to keep toxins out of your body. After reading this book you also understand which plant-based nutrients to put in your body. I hope you enjoyed this book. This is the way I control my health it has worked for me and others. I hope you get control of your health by joining the P53 Diet at p53diet.com

REFERENCES

Skorski, I., A. Bellacosa, M. Nieborowska-Skorska, R. Martinez, J.K. Choi, R.Trotta, P. Wodarski, D. Perrotti, T. O. Chan, M.A. Wasik, P.N. Tsichlis, and B.Calabretta, Transformation of hematopoietic cells by BCR/ABL requires activation of a P1-3k/Akt-dependent pathway, EMBO J 16(20): 6151-6161 (1997a).

Gonzales JF, Barnard ND, Jenkins DJ, et al. Applying the precautionary principle to nutrition and cancer. J Am Coll Nutr. 2014;33(3):239-246. 7

Tsou, M.F., H.F. Lu, S.C. Chen, L.T. Wu, Y.S. Chen, H.M. Kuo, S.S. Lin, and J.G.Chung, Involvement of Bax, Bc-2, Ca?+ and caspase-3 in capsaicin-induced apoptosis of human leukemia HI-60 cells, Anticancer Res 26(3A): 1965-1971(2006).

L-arginine. Facts & Comparisons eAnswers. https://www.wolterskluwercdi.com/facts-comparisons-online/. Accessed Dec. 20, 2020.

Treatment of Erectile Dysfunction with Pycnogenol and L-arginine R. STANISLAVOV & V. NIKOLOVA Pages 207-213 | Published online: 30 Nov 2010 https://doi.org/10.1080/00926230390155104

Arginine hydrochloride. IBM Micromedex. https://www.micromedexsolutions.com. Accessed Dec. 10, 2020.

L-arginine. Natural Medicines. https://naturalmedicines.therapeuticresearch.com. Accessed Dec. 20, 2020.

Teresa T. Fung, ScD, et al., "Low Carbohydrate Diets and All Cause and Cause Specific Mortality: Two Cohort Studies," Annals of Internal Medicine 153 (5) (2010): 289 298; A. Trichopoulou et al., "Low Carbohydrate-High Protein Diet and Long Term Survival in a General Population Cohort," European Journal of Clinical Nutrition 61 (5) (2007): 575-581; Hiroshi Noto, Atsushi Goto, Tetsuro Tsujimoto, Mitsuhiko Noda, "Low Carbohydrate Diets and All Cause Mortality: A Systematic Review and Meta Analysis of Observational Studies," PLOS ONE 8 (1) e55030, 2013.

Noto, Atsushi Goto, Tetsuro Tsujimoto, Mitsuhiko Noda, "Low Carbohydrate Diets and All Cause Mortality: A Systematic Review and Meta Analysis of Observational Studies," PLOS ONE 8 (1) e55030, 2013.

Kim, K.W., C.H. Choi, T.H. Kim, C.H. Kwon, J.S. Woo, and Y.K. Kim, Silibinin inhibits glioma cell proliferation via Ca?+/ROS/MAPK-dependent mechanism in vitro and glioma tumor growth in vivo, Neurochem Res 34(8): 1479-1490 (2009).

Scrimshaw NS, Murray EB. The acceptability of milk and milk products in populations with a high prevalence of lactose intolerance. Am J Clin Nutr. 1988;48(4 Suppl):1079-1159.

Freedman, N.D., Y. Park, A.F. Subar, A.R. Hollenbeck, M.F. Leitzmann, A. Schatzkin, and C.C. Abnet, Fruit and vegetable intake and esophageal cancer in a large prospective cohort study, Int J Cancer 121(12): 2753-2760 (2007).

Kumar, V., A.K. Abbas, N. Fausto, and J. Aster, Robbins e Cotran Pathologic Basis of Disease (8th Edn.), Elsevier (2010).

Front Cell Infect Microbiol. 2020; 10: 572912. Published online 2020 Nov 24. doi: 10.3389/fcimb.2020.572912 PMCID: PMC7732679 PMID: 33330122 Antibiotics as Major Disruptors of Gut Microbiota Jaime Ramirez, Francisco Guarner, * Luis Bustos Fernandez, Aldo Maruy, Vera Lucia Sdepanian, and Henry Cohen

Rajat Kr Sachdeva* Dental Institute, India *Corresponding Author: Rajat Kr Sachdeva, Dental Institute, India. Received: May 31, 2019; Published: july 08, 2019DOI: 10.31080/ASOR.2019.02.0076

Daube M. Alcohol's evaporating health benefits. BMJ. 2015;350:h407.

Adv Nutr. 2019 Nov; 10(Suppl 4): S296–S303. Published online 2019 Nov 15. doi: 10.1093/advances/nmz026 PMCID: PMC6855941 PMID: 31728493 Plant-Rich Dietary Patterns, Plant Foods and Nutrients, and Telomere Length Marta Crous-Bou,1,2,4 José-Luis Molinuevo,1,2 and Aleix Sala-Vila1,3,5

E. L. Richman, S. A. Kenfield, M. J. Stampfer, E. L. Giovannucci, J. M. Chan. Egg, red meat, and poultry intake and risk of lethal prostate cancer in the prostate-specific antigen-era: Incidence and survival. Cancer Prev Res (Phila) 2011 4(12):2110 - 2121.

Kresty, L.A., M.A. Morse, C. Morgan, P.S. Carlton, J. Lu, A. Gupta, M. Blackwood, and G.D. Stoner, Chemoprevention of esophageal tumorigenesis by dietary administration of lyophilized black raspberries, Cancer Res 61(16): 6112-6119 (2001).

Zaini, R., M.R. Clench, and C.L. Le Maitre, Bioactive chemicals from carrot (Daucus carota) juice extracts for the treatment of leukemia, / Med Food14(11): 1303-1312 (2011).

Common Side Effects from Antibiotics, and Allergies and Reactions. https://www.drugs.com/article/antibiotic-sideeffects-allergies-reactions.html
Medically reviewed by Leigh Ann Anderson, PharmD. Last updated on Sep 28, 2023.

.

Nicola M. McKeown et al., "Whole and Refined Grain Intakes Are Differentially Associated with Abdominal Visceral and Subcutaneous Adiposity in Healthy Adults: the Framingham Heart Study," American Journal of Clinical Nutrition 92 (5) (2010): 1165-1171.

E. Ackerstaff, B. R. Pflug, J. B. Nelson, Z. M. Bhujwalla. Detection of increased choline compounds with proton nuclear magnetic resonance spectroscopy subsequent to malignant transformation of human prostatic epithelial cells. Cancer Res. 2001 61(9):3599 - 3603.

Can, G., Z. Cakir, M. Kartal, U. Gunduz, and Y. Baran, Apoptotic effects of resveratrol, a grape polyphenol, on imatinib-sensitive and resistant K562 chronic myeloid leukemia cells, Anticancer Res 32(7): 2673-2678 (2012).

Michael Lefevre and Satya Jonnalagadda, "Effect of Whole Grains on Markers of Subclinical Inflammation," Nutrition Reviews 70 (7) (2012): 387-396, doi: 10.1111/j.1753 4887.2012.00487.

Chen, D., K.G. Daniel, M.S. Chen, D.J. Kuhn, K.R. Landis-Piwowar, and Q.P. Dou, Dietary flavonoids as proteasome inhibitors and apoptosis inducers in human leukemia cells, Biochem Pharmacol 69(10): 1421-1432 (2005).

Jennifer J. Otten, Jennifer Pitzi Hellwig, and Linda D. Meyers, eds., National Academy Dietary reference intakes: the essential guide to nutrient requirements, Washington DC: The National Academies Press, 2006) 144.

Parkin DM. International variation. Oncogene. 2004;23(38):6329-6340.

Dalla-Favera, R. and G. Gaidano, Molecular biology of lymphomas, De Vita, V.T. Jr, S. Hellman, and S.A. Rosenberg (Eds.), in Cancer: Principles and Practice of Oncology, Philadelphia: Lippincott Williams, and Wilkins (2001), pp. 2215-2235.

E. L. Richman, M. J. Stampfer, A. Paciorek, J. M. Broering, P. R. Carroll, J. M. Chan. Intakes of meat, fish, poultry, and eggs and risk of prostate cancer progression. Am. J. Clin. Nutr. 2010 91(3):712 - 721.

Tsubaki, M., M. Komai, T. Itoh, M. Imano, K. Sakamoto, H. Shimaoka, N. Ogawa, K . Mashimo, D. Fujiwara, I. Takeda, J. Mukai, K. Sakaguchi, I. Satou, and S. Nishida, Inhibition of the tumor necrosis factor-alpha autocrine loop enhances the sensitivity of multiple myeloma cells to anticancer drugs, Eur / Cancer 49(17): 3708-3717 (2013).

Hu, Y., C.Y. Sun, J. Huang, L. Hong, L. Zhang, and Z.B. Chu, Antimyeloma effects of resveratrol through inhibition of angiogenesis, Chin Med I (Engl) 120(19): 1672-1677 (2007).

Barch, D.H. and C.C. Fox, Selective inhibition of methylbenzylnitrosamine-induced formation of esophageal 06-methylguanine by dietary ellagic acid in rats, Cancer Res 48(24 Pt. 1): 7088-7092 (1988).

E. L. Richman, S. A. Kenfield, M. J. Stampfer, E. L. Giovannucci, S. H. Zeisel, W. C. Willett, J. M. Chan. Choline intake and risk of lethal prostate cancer: Incidence and survival. Am. J. Clin. Nutr. 2012 96(4):855 - 863.

World Cancer Research Fund International/American Institute for Cancer Research, "Food, Nutrition, Physical Activity, and the Prevention of Cancer: A Global Perspective," Washington, D.C.: AICR, 2007.

Harrison S, Lennon R, Holly J, et al. Does milk intake promote prostate cancer initiation or progression via effects on insulin-like growth factors (IGFs)? A systematic review and meta-analysis. Cancer Causes Control. 2017;28(6):497-528.

Tatman, D. and H. Mo, Volatile isoprenoid constituents of fruits, vegetables, and herbs cumulatively suppress the proliferation of murine B16 melanoma and human HL-60 leukemia cells, Cancer Lett 175(2): 129-139 (2002).

Tang, Q., G. Li, X. Wei, J. Zhang, J.E. Chiu, D. Hasenmayer, D. Zhang, and H. Zhang, Resveratrol-induced apoptosis is enhanced by inhibition of autophagy in esophageal squamous cell carcinoma, Cancer Lett 336(2): 325-337 (2013).

Nowell, P. and D. Hungerford, A minute chromosome in human chronic granulocytic leukemia, Science 132: 1497 (1960).

Lee, W.J., Y.R. Chen, and T.H. Tseng, Quercetin induces FasL-related apoptosis, in part, through promotion of histone H3 acetylation in human leukemia HI-60 cells, Oncol Rep 25(2): 583-591 (2011).

Venter C, Pereira B, Grundy J, Clayton CB, Arshad SH, Dean T. Prevalence of sensitization reported and objectively assessed food hypersensitivity amongst six-year-old children: a population-based study. *Pediatr Allergy Immunol.* 2006 Aug;17(5):356-63.

Kim, S., M.W. Gaber, J.A. Zawaski, F. Zhang, M. Richardson, X.A. Zhang, and Y. Yang, The inhibition of glioma growth in vitro and in vivo by a chitosan/ ellagic acid composite biomaterial, Biomaterials 30(27): 4743-4751 (2009).

Hashimoto, N., M. Tachibana, D.K. Dhar, H. Yoshimura, and N. Naga-sue, Expression of p53 and RB proteins in squamous cell carcinoma of the esophagus: Their relationship with clinicopathologic characteristics, Ann Surg Oncol 6(5): 489-494 (1999).

Kitagawa, I., M. Ueda, N. Ando, S. Ozawa, N. Shimizu, and M. Kitajima, Further evidence for prognostic significance of epidermal growth factor receptor gene amplification in patients with esophageal squamous cell carcinoma, Clin Cancer Res 2(5): 909-914 (1996).

Kellen, E., M. Zeegers, A. Paulussen, M. Van Dongen, and F. Buntinx, Fruit consumption reduces the effect of smoking on bladder cancer risk. The Belgian case control study on bladder cancer, Int J Cancer 118(10): 2572-2578 (2006).

M. Johansson, B. Van Guelpen, S. E. Vollset, J. Hultdin, A. Bergh, T. Key, O. Midttun, G. Hallmans, P. M. Ueland, P. Stattin. One-carbon metabolism and prostate cancer risk: Prospective investigation of seven circulating B vitamins and metabolites. Cancer Epidemiol. Biomarkers Prev. 2009 18(5):1538 - 1543.

Tang, L. and Y. Zhang, Mitochondria are the primary target in isothiocy-anate-induced apoptosis in human bladder cancer cells, Mol Cancer Ther 4(8): 1250-1259 (2005).

Ishii, N., D. Maier, A. Merlo, M. Tada, Y. Sawamura, A.C. Diserens, and E.G. Van Meir, Frequent co-alterations of TP53, p16/CDKN2A, p14ARF, PTEN tumor suppressor genes in human glioma cell lines, Brain Pathol 9(3): 469-479 (1999).

Lamm, D.L. and D.R. Riggs, Enhanced immunocompetence by garlic: Role in bladder cancer and other malignancies, J Nutr 131(3s): 1067S-1070S (2001).

Grana, X. and E.P. Reddy, Cell cycle control in mammalian cells: Role of cyclins, cyclin dependent kinases (CDKs), growth suppressor genes and cyclin-dependent kinase inhibitors (KIs), Oncogene 11(2): 211-219 (1995).

Dietary Reference Intakes for Energy, Carbohydrate, Fiber, Fat, Fatty Acids, Cholesterol, Protein, and Amino Acids, National Academies of Sciences, https://www.nationalacademies.org/hmd/Reports/2002/Dietary

Reference Intakes for Energy Carbohydrate Fiber Fat Fatty Acids Cholesterol Protein and Amino Acids. aspx.

Meyer, A.N., C.W. McAndrew, and D.J. Donoghue, Nordihydroguaiaretic acid inhibits an activated fibroblast growth factor receptor 3 mutant and blocks downstream signaling in multiple myeloma cells, Cancer Res 68(18): 7362-7370 (2008).

Schmitz, R., J. Stanelle, M.L. Hansmann, and R. Küppers, Pathogenesis of classical and lymphocyte-predominant Hodgkin lymphoma, Annu Rev Pathol 4: 151-174 (2009).

Han, X, T. Zheng, E. Foss, T.R. Holford, S. Ma, P. Zhao, M. Dai, C. Kim, Y. Zhang, Y. Bai, and Y. Zhang, Vegetable and fruit intake and non-Hodgkin lymphoma survival in Connecticut women, Leuk Lymphoma 51(6): 1047-1054 (2010).

Hosgood, H.D., D. Baris, S.H. Zahm, T. Zheng, and A.J. Cross, Diet and risk of multiple myeloma in Connecticut women, Cancer Causes Control 18(10): 1065-1076 (2007).

Chiu, B.C., S. Kwon, A.M. Evens, T. Surawicz, S.M. Smith, and D.D. Weisenburger, Dietary intake of fruit and vegetables and risk of non-Hodgkin lymphoma, Cancer Causes Control 22(8): 1183-1195 (2011).

Jakubikova, J., D. Cervi, M. Ooi, K. Kim, S. Nahar, S. Klippel, D. Cholujo-va, M. Leiba, J.F. Daley, J. Delmore, J. Negri, S. Blotta, D.W. McMillin, T. Hideshima, P.G. Richardson, J. Sedlak, K.C. Anderson, and C.S. Mitsiades, Anti-tumor activity, and signaling events triggered by the isothiocyanates, sulforaphane, and phenethyl isothiocyanate, in multiple myeloma, Haemato-logica 96(8): 1170-1179 (2011).

Saleem, A., M. Husheem, P. Härkönen, and K. Pihlaja, Inhibition of cancer cell growth by crude extract and the phenolics of Terminalia chebula retz. fruit, J Ethnopharmacol 81(3): 327-336 (2002).

Bunin, G.R., L.H. Kushi, P.R. Gallagher, L.B. Rorke-Adams, M.L. McBride, and A. Cnaan, Maternal diet during pregnancy and its association with medulloblastoma in children: A children's oncology group study (United States), Cancer Causes Control 16(7): 877-891 (2005).

Pasin, E., D.Y. Josephson, A.P. Mitra, R.J. Cote, and J.P. Stein, Superficial bladder cancer: An update on etiology, molecular development, classifica-tion, and natural history, Rev Urol 10(1): 31-43 (2008).

Health, United States, 2015: With Special Feature on Racial and Ethnic Health Disparities, National Center for Health Statistics, http://www.cdc.gov/nchs/data/hus/hus15.pdf#056.

C. Nanni, E. Zamagni, M. Cavo, D. Rubello, P. Tacchetti, C. Pettinato, M. Farsad, P. Castellucci, V. Ambrosini, G. C. Montini, A. Al-Nahhas, R. Franchi, S. Fanti. 11C-choline vs. 18F-FDG PET/CT in assessing bone involvement in patients with multiple myeloma. World J Surg Oncol 2007 5:68.

Yoo, C.B., K.T. Han, K.S. Cho, J. Ha, H.J. Park, J.H. Nam, U.H. Kil, and K.T. Lee, Eugenol isolated from the essential oil of Eugenia caryophyllata induces a reactive oxygen species-mediated apoptosis in HL-60 human promyelocytic leukemia cells, Cancer Lett 225(1): 41-52 (2005).

Tatetsu, H., S. Ueno, H. Hata, Y. Yamada, M. Takeya, H. Mitsuya, D.G. Tenen, and Y. Okuno, Down-regulation of PU.1 by methylation of distal regulatory elements and the promoter is required for myeloma cell growth, Cancer Res 67(11): 5328-5336 (2007).

Munday, R., P. Mhawech-Fauceglia, C.M. Munday, J.D. Paonessa, L. Tang, J.S. Munday, C. Lister, P. Wilson, J.W. Fahey, W. Davis, and Y. Zhang, Inhibition of urinary bladder carcinogenesis by broccoli sprouts, Cancer Res 68(5): 1593-1600 (2008).

Hu,]., C. La Vecchia, E. Negri, L. Chatenoud, C. Bosetti, X. Jia, R. Liu, G. Huang, D. Bi, and C. Wang, Diet and brain cancer in adults: A case-con-trol study in northeast China, Int J Cancer 81(1): 20-23 (1999).

A. Rubio Tapia, J.P. Ludvigsson, T.L. Brantner, J.A. Murray, J.E. Everhart,, "The Prevalence of Celiac Disease in the United States," American Journal of Gastroenterology, 107 (10) (2012):1538 44 doi: 10.1038/ ajg.2012.219.

Sawyers, C.I., J. McLaughlin, and O.N. Witte, Genetic requirement for Kas in the transformation of fibroblasts and hematopoetic cells by the Bc-Abl oncogene, J Exp Med 181(1): 303-313 (1995).

Kweon, S.H., J.H. Song, and T.S. Kim, Resveratrol-mediated reversal of doxorubicin resistance in acute myeloid leukemia cells via downregulation of MRP1 expression, Biochem Biophys Res Commun 395(1): 104-110 (2010).

Wu, S.B., J.J. Su, L.H. Sun, W. .Wang, Y. Zhao, H. Li, S.P. Zhang, G.H. Dai, C.G. Wang, and J.F. Hu, Triterpenoids and steroids from the fruits of Melia toosendan and their cytotoxic effects on two human cancer cell lines, J Nat Prod 73(11): 1898-1906 (2010).

Park, S.Y., N.J. Ollberding, C.G. Woolcott, L.R. Wilkens, B.E. Henderson, and L.N. Kolonel, Fruit and vegetable intakes are associated with lower risk of bladder cancer among women in the multiethnic cohort study, J Nutr 143(8): 1283-1292 (2013).

Svedberg J, de Haas J, Leimenstoll G, Paul F, Teschemacher H. Demonstration of beta-casomorphin immunoreactive materials in in vitro digests of bovine milk and in small intestine contents after bovine milk ingestion in adult humans. Peptides. 1985 Sep-Oct;6(5):825-30.

Broadhead, M.L., J.C.M. Clark, D.E. Myers, C.R. Dass, and P.F.M. Choong, The molecular pathogenesis of osteosarcoma: A review, Sarcoma doi: dx.doi. org/10.1155/ 2011/959248 2011).

Simon, R., K. Struckmann, P. Schraml, U. Wagner, I. Forster, H. Moch, A. Fijan, J. Bruderer, K. Wilber, M.J. Mihatsch, T. Gasser, and G. Sauter, Amplification pattern of 12q13-q15 genes (MDM2, CDK4, GLI) in urinary bladder cancer, Oncogene 21(16): 2476-2483 (2002).

Mathas, S., M. Janz, F. Hummel, M. Hummel, B. Wollert-Wulf, S. Lusatis, I. Anagnostopoulos, A. Lietz, M. Sigvardsson, F. Jundt, K. Jöhrens, K. Bom-mert, H. Stein, and B. Dörken, Intrinsic inhibition of transcription factor E2A by HLH proteins ABF-1 and Id2 mediates reprogramming of neoplastic B cells in Hodgkin lymphoma, Nat Immunol 7(2): 207-215 (2006).

Johnson JR, Kuskowski MA, Smith K, O'bryan TT, Tatini S. Antimicrobial-resistant and extraintestinal pathogenic Escherichia coli in retail foods. J Infect Dis. 2005;191(7):1040-9.

Pathak, A.K., M. Bhutani, A.S. Nair, K.S. Ahn, A. Chakraborty, H. Kadara, S. Guha, G. Sethi, and B.B. Aggarwal, Ursolic acid inhibits STAT3 activation pathway leading to suppression of proliferation and chemosensitization of human multiple myeloma cells, Mol Cancer Res 5(9): 943-955 (2007).

Abbaoui, B., K.M. Riedl, R.A. Ralston, J.M. Thomas-Ahner, S.]. Schwartz, S.K. Clinton, and A. Mortazavi, Inhibition of bladder cancer by broccoli isothiocyanates sulforaphane and erucin: Characterization, metabolism, and interconversion, Mol Nutr Food Res 56(11): 1675-1687 (2012).

Ishitsuka, K., T. Hideshima, M. Hamasaki, N. Raje, S. Kumar, H. Hideshima, N. Shiraishi, H. Yasui, A.M. Roccaro, P. Richardson, K. Podar, S. Le Gouill, D. Chauhan, K. Tamura, J. Arbiser, and K.C. Anderson, Honokiol overcomes conventional drug resistance in human multiple myeloma by induction of caspase-dependent and -independent apoptosis, Blood 106(5): 1794-1800(2005).

WHO definition of health. www.who.int/about/mission/en BMA founding principle. www.bma.org.uk Bae YH, Park K. Targeted drug delivery to tumors: myths, reality and possibility. J Control Release. 2011 Aug 10;153(3):198-205. doi: 10.1016/j jconrel.2011.06.001. Epub 2011 Jun 6. PMID: 21663778; PMCID: PMC3272876.

Troncoso, M.E., V.A. Biron, S.A. Longhi, L.A. Retegui, and C. Wolfenstein-Todel, Peltophorum dubium and soybean Kunitz-type trypsin inhibitors induce human Jurkat cell apoptosis, Int Immunopharmacol 7(5): 625-636 (2007).

Möller, F., O. Zierau, A. Jandausch, R. Rettenberger, M. Kaszkin-Bettag, and G. Vollmer, Subtype-specific activation of estrogen receptors by a special extract of Rheum rhaponticum (ERr 731), its aglycones and structurally related compounds in U2OS human osteosarcoma cells, Phytomedicine 14(11): 716-726 (2007).

Hou, Z., S. Sang, H. You, M.J. Lee, J. Hong, K.V. Chin, and C.S. Yang, Mechanism of action of (-)-epigallocatechin-3-gallate: Auto-oxidation-depen-dent inactivation of epidermal growth factor receptor and direct effects on growth inhibition in human esophageal cancer KYSE 150 cells, Cancer Res 65(17): 8049-8056 (2005).

Kost NV, Sokolov OY, Kurasova OB, Dmitriev AD, Tarakanova JN, Gabaeva MV, Zolotarev YA, Dadayan AK, Grachev SA, Korneeva EV, Mikheeva IG, Zozulya AA. Beta-casomorphins-7 in infants on different type of feeding and different levels of psychomotor development. Peptides. 2009 Oct;30(10):1854-60.

Gary Null et al - Death by Medicine www.webdc.com/pdfs/deathbymedicine.pdf

Allerberger F. Poultry and human infections. Clin Microbiol Infect. 2016;22(2):101-102.

Darmadi Blackberry et al., "Legumes: The Most Important Dietary Predictor of Survival in Older People of Different Ethnicities" Asia Pacific Journal of Clinical Nutrition 3 (2) (2004): 217-220.

Ruiz i Altaba, A., B. Stecca, and P. Sánchez, Hedgehog-Gli signaling in brain tumors: Stem cells and para developmental programs in cancer, Cancer Lett 204(2): 145-157 (2004).

Remer T. Potential renal acid load of foods and its influence on urine pH. *J Am Diet Assoc.* 1995 Jul;95(7):791-7.

Kilonzo-nthenge A, Brown A, Nahashon SN, Long D. Occurrence and antimicrobial resistance of enterococci isolated from organic and conventional retail chicken. J Food Prot. 2015;78(4):760-6.

Review on Antimicrobial Resistance https://amr-review.org/home.html

Spencer H, Norris C, Derler J, Osis D. Effect of oat bran muffins on calcium absorption and calcium, phosphorus, magnesium and zinc balance in men. *J Nutr.* 1991 Dec;121(12):1976-83.

Shimada, Y, M. Imamura, G. Watanabe, S. Uchida, H. Harada, T. Makino, and M. Kano, Prognostic factors of oesophageal squamous cell carcinoma from the perspective of molecular biology, Br | Cancer 80(8): 1281-1288 (1999).

Stein, J.P., D.A. Ginsberg, G.D. Grossfeld, S.J. Chatterjee, D. Esrig, M.G. Dickinson, S. Groshen, C.R. Taylor, P.A. Jones, D.G. Skinner, and R.J. Cote, Effect of p21WAF1/CIP1 expression on tumor progression in bladder cancer, J Natl Cancer Inst 90(14): 1072-1079 (1998).

Nordstrom L, Liu CM, Price LB. Foodborne urinary tract infections: a new paradigm for antimicrobial-resistant foodborne illness. Front Microbiol. 2013;4:29.

Liu, Q., X Chen, G Yang, X Min, and M. Deng, Apigenin inhibits cell migration through MAPK pathways in human bladder smooth muscle cells, Biocell 35(3): 71-79 (2011).

Colborn T. Neurodevelopment and endocrine disruption. Environ Health Perspect. 2004 Jun; 112(9):944-9. doi: 10.1289/ehp.6601. PMID: 15198913; PMCID: PMC1247186.

Park HR, Lee JM, Moon HE, Lee DS, Kim BN, Kim J, Kim DG, Paek SH. A Short Review on the Current Understanding of Autism Spectrum Disorders. Exp Neurobiol. 2016 Feb;25(1):1-13.

Zhang, X., Z. Liu, B. Xu, Z. Sun, Y. Gong, and C. Shao, Neferine, an alkaloid ingredient in lotus seed embryo, inhibits proliferation of human osteosarcoma cells by promoting p38 MAPK-mediated p21 stabilization, Eur I Pharmacol 677(1-3): 47-54 (2012).

Pouliquen, D., C. Olivier, E. Hervouet, F. Pedelaborde, L. Debien, M.T. Le Cabellec, C. Gratas, T. Homma, K. Meflah, EM. Vallette, and J. Menanteau, Dietary prevention of malignant glioma aggressiveness, implications in oxidant stress and apoptosis, Int J Cancer 123(2): 288-295 (2008).

Yamaji, T., M. Inoue, S. Sasazuki, M. Iwasaki, N. Kurahashi, T. Shimazu, S. Tsugane; and Japan Public Health Center-based Prospective Study Group, Fruit and vegetable consumption and squamous cell carcinoma of the esophagus in Japan: The JPHC study, Int] Cancer 123(8): 1935-1940 (2008).

Lukic, M., A. Segec, I. Segec, L. Pinotic, K. Pinotic, B. Atalic, K. Solic, and A. Viev, The impact of the vitamins A, C and E in the prevention of gastroesophageal reflux disease, Barrett's oesophagus and oesophageal adenocarcinoma, Coll Antropol 36(3): 867-872 (2012).

Zhang, W., K. Murao, X. Zhang, K. Matsumoto, S. Diah, M. Okada, K. Miyake, N. Kawai, Z. Fei, and T. Tamiya, Resveratrol represses YKL-40 expression in human glioma U87 cells, BMC Cancer 10: 593 2010). Chen, J.C., Y. Chen, J.H. Lin, J.M.

Wu, and S.H. Tseng, Resveratrol suppresses angiogenesis in gliomas: Evaluation by color Doppler ultrasound, Anticancer Res 26(2A): 1237-1245 (2006).

Millman JM, Waits K, Grande H, et al. Prevalence of antibiotic-resistant E. coli in retail chicken: comparing conventional, organic, kosher, and raised without antibiotics. F1000Res. 2013;2:155.

Shousha A, Awaiwanont N, Sofka D, et al. Bacteriophages Isolated from Chicken Meat and the Horizontal Transfer of Antimicrobial Resistance Genes. Appl Environ Microbiol. 2015;81(14):4600-6.

Cieślińska A, Sienkiewicz-Szłapka E, Wasilewska J, Fiedorowicz E, Chwała B, Moszyńska-Dumara M, Cieśliński T, Bukało M, Kostyra E. Influence of candidate polymorphisms on the dipeptidyl peptidase IV and μ-opioid receptor genes expression in aspect of the β-casomorphin-7 modulation functions in autism. Peptides. 2015 Mar;65:6-11.

Liu, M.J., Z. Wang, Y. Ju, R.N. Wong, and Q.Y. Wu, Diosgenin induces cell cycle arrest and apoptosis in human leukemia K562 cells with the disruption of Ca?+ homeostasis, Cancer Chemother Pharmacol 55(1): 79-90 (2005).

Skorski. T, P. Kanakaraj, M. Nieborowska-Skorska, M.Z. Ratajczak, S.C. Wen, G. Zon, A.M. Gewirtz, B. Perussia, and B. Calabretta, Phosphatidylinositol-3 kinase activity is regulated by BCR/ABL and is required for the growth of Philadelphia chromosome-positive cells, Blood 86(2): 726-736 (1995).

D.V. DiGiacomo, C.A. Tennyson, P.H. Green, R.T. Demmer, "Prevalence of Gluten Free Diet Adherence Among Individuals Without Celiac Disease in the USA: Results from the Continuous National Health and Nutrition Examination Survey 2009 2010", Scandinavian Journal of Gastroenterology, 48 (8) (2013):921 5. doi: 10.3109/00365521.2013.809598.

Asledottir T, Le TT, Petrat-Melin B, Devold T, Larsen L, Vegarud GE. Identification of bioactive peptides and quantification of β-casomorphin-7 from bovine β-casein A1, A2 and I after ex vivo gastrointestinal digestion. International Dairy Journal. 2017;71:98-106.

Torlakovic, E., A. Tierens, H.D. Dang, and J. Delabie, The transcription factor PU.1, necessary for B-cell development is expressed in lymphocyte predominance, but not classical Hodgkin's disease, Am J Pathol 159(5): 1807-1814 (2001).

Frazzi, R., R. Valli, I. Tamagnini, B. Casali, N. Latruffe, and F. Merli, Resveratrol-mediated apoptosis of Hodgkin lymphoma cells involves SIRT1 inhibition and FOXO3 hyperacetylation, Int I Cancer 132(5): 1013-1021 (2013).

Samant SS, Crandall PG, O'bryan C, Lingbeck JM, Martin EM, Seo HS. Sensory impact of chemical and natural antimicrobials on poultry products: a review. Poult Sci. 2015;94(7):1699-710.

Cade R, Privette M, Fregly M, Rowland N, Sun Z, Zele V, Wagemaker H, Edelstein C. Autism and Schizophrenia: Intestinal Disorders. Nutr Neurosci. 2000;3(1):57-72.

Side effects of antibiotics https://www.nhs.uk/conditions/antibiotics/side-effects/

Johnson JR, Porter SB, Johnston B, et al. Extraintestinal Pathogenic and Antimicrobial-Resistant Escherichia coli, Including Sequence Type 131 (ST131), from Retail Chicken Breasts in the United States in 2013. Appl Environ Microbiol. 2017;83(6).

Scheeren, F.A., S.A. Diehl, L.A. Smit, T. Beaumont, M. Naspetti, R.J. Bende, B. Blom, K. Karube, K. Ohshima, C.J. van Noesel, and H. Spits, IL-21 is expressed in Hodgkin lymphoma and activates STAT5; evidence that activated STAT5 is required for Hodgkin lymphomagenesis, Blood 111(9): 4706 4715 (2008).

D. Aune et al.,"Whole Grain Consumption and Risk of Cardiovascular Disease, Cancer, and All Cause and Cause Specific Mortality: Systematic Review and Dose Response Meta Analysis of Prospective Studies" BMJ 353 (i2716) (2016). doi: 10.1136/bmj.i2716.

Rim KT, Koo KH, Park JS. Toxicological evaluations of rare earths and their health impacts to workers: a literature review. Saf Health Work. 2013 Mar; 4(1):12-26. doi:10.5491/SHAW.2013.4.1.12. Epub 2013 Mar 11. PMID: 23516020; PMCID: PMC3601293.

Mitra, A.P., H. Lin, R.J. Cote, and R.H. Datar, Biomarker profiling for cancer diagnosis, prognosis, and therapeutic management, Natl Med J India 18(6): 304-312 (2005).

Xing, E.P., G.Y. Yang, L.D. Wang, S.T. Shi, and C.S. Yang, Loss of heterozygosity of Rb gene correlates with PRb protein expression and associates with p53 alteration in human esophageal cancer, Clin Cancer Res 5(5): 1231-1240 (1999).

Clarke A, Trivedi M. Bovine Beta Casein Variants: Implications to Human Nutrition and Health. IPCBEE. 2014;67(3):11-17.

Michaud, D.S., D. Spiegelman, S.K. Clinton, E.B. Rimm, W.C. Willett, and E.L. Giovannucci, Fruit and vegetable intake and incidence of bladder cancer in a male prospective cohort, I Natl Cancer Inst 91(7): 605-613 (1999).

Ma, L., J.M. Feugang, P. Konarski, J. Wang, J. Lu, S. Fu, B. Ma, B. Tian, C. Zou, and Z. Wang, Growth inhibitory effects of queretin on bladder cancer cell, Front Biosci 11: 2275-2285 (2006).Capodanno, A.-M., Bone: Osteosarco. Atlas Genet Cytogenet Oncol Haematol (2002). From http://AtlasGeneticsOncology.org/Tumors/OsteosarcID5043.html.

Rational Principles of Psychopharmacology for Therapists, Healthcare Providers and Clients www.breggin.com/wp-content/uploads/2008/06/Breggin2016_RationalPrinciples.pdf

Zhang, X., W.E. Zhao, L. Hu, L. Zhao, and J. Huang, Carotenoids inhibit proliferation and regulate expression of peroxisome proliferators-activated receptor gamma (PPARy) in K562 cancer cells, Arch Biochem Biophys 512(1): 96-106 (2011).

McLaughlin RW, Vali H, Lau PC, Palfree RG, De Ciccio A, Sirois M, Ahmad D, Villemur R, Desrosiers M, Chan EC. Are there naturally occurring pleomorphic bacteria in the blood of

4775.2002. PMID: 12454193; PMCID: PMC154583.

Chabance B, Marteau P, Rambaud JC, Migliore-Samour D, Boynard M, Perrotin P, Guillet R, Jollès P, Fiat AM. Casein peptide release and passage to the blood in humans during digestion of milk or yogurt. Biochimie. 1998 Feb;80(2):155-65.

Johnson JR, Porter S, Thuras P, Castanheira M. The Pandemic 30 Subclone of Sequence Type 131 (ST131) as the Leading Cause of Multidrug-Resistant Infections in the United States (2011-2012). Open Forum Infect Dis. 2017;4(2):ofx089.

Mullighan, C.G., S. Goorha, I. Radtke, C.B. Miller, E. Coustan-Smith, J.D. Dalton, K. Girtman, S. Mathew, J. Ma, S.B. Pounds, X. Su, C.H. Pui, M.V. Relling, W.E. Evans, S.A. Shurtleff, and J.R. Downing, Genome-wide analysis of genetic alterations in acute lymphoblastic leukemia, Nature 446(7137): 758-764 (2007).

Melnik BC, John SM, Carrera-Bastos P, Cordain L. The impact of cow's milk-mediated mTORC1-signaling in the initiation and progression of prostate cancer. Nutr Metab (Lond). 2012;9(1):74.

Low Levels of Ionizing Radiation May Cause Harm http://www8.nationalacademies.org/onpinews/newsitem.asp?RecordID=11340

Yaseen, A., S. Chen, S. Hock, R. Rosato, P. Dent, Y. Dai, and S. Grant, Resveratrol sensitizes acute myelogenous leukemia cells to histone deacetylase inhibitors through reactive oxygen species-mediated activation of the extrinsic apoptotic pathway, Mol Pharmacol 82(6): 1030-1041 (2012).

Nicolas-chanoine MH, Bertrand X, Madec JY. Escherichia coli ST131, an intriguing clonal group. Clin Microbiol Rev. 2014;27(3):543-74.

Food Irradiation: A Gross Failure https:// www.centerforfoodsafety.org/issues/1039/food-irradiation/reports/1398/food-irradiation-a-gross-failure

Calin, G.A. and C.M. Croce, Genomics of chronic lymphocytic leukemia microRNAs a new player with clinical significance, Semin Oncol 33(2): 167-173 (2006).

Jemal, A., F. Bray, M.M. Center, J. Ferlay, E. Ward, and D. Forman, Global cancer statistics, CA-Cancer I Clin 61(2): 69-90 (2011). Il. Mitra, A.P. and R.J. Cote, Molecular pathogenesis and diagnostics of bladder cancer, Annu Rev Pathol 4: 251-285 (2009).

Zhou, H.B., Y. Yan, Y.N. Sun, and J.R. Zhu, Resveratrol induces apoptosis in human esophageal carcinoma cells, World J Gastroenterol 9(3): 408-411 (2003).

Zeng,]., Y. Sun, K. Wu, L. Li, G. Zhang, Z. Yang, Z. Wang, D. Zhang, Y. Xue, Y. Chen, G. Zhu, x. Wang, and D. He, Chemopreventive and chemotherapeutic effects of intravesical silibinin against bladder cancer by acting on mitochondria, Mol Cancer Ther 10(1): 104-116 (2011).

Raitano, A.B, J.R. Halpern, T.M. Hambuch, and C.I. Sawyers, The Bcr-Abl leukemia oncogene activates Jun kinase and requires Jun for transformation, Proc Natl Acad Sci USA 92(25): 11746-11750 (1995).

Trivedi MS, Hodgson NW, Walker SJ, Trooskens G, Nair V, Deth RC. Epigenetic effects of casein-derived opioid peptides in SH-SY5Y human neuroblastoma cells. Nutr Metab (Lond). 2015 Dec 9;12:54.

Adhikari PA, Cosby DE, Cox NA, Lee JH, Kim WK. Effect of dietary bacteriophage supplementation on internal organs, fecal excretion, and ileal immune response in laying hens challenged by Salmonella Enteritidis. Poult Sci. 2017;96(9):3264-3271.

Synergy: The Big Unknowns of Pesticide Exposure https://beyondpesticides.org/assets/media/documents/infoservices/pesticidesandyou/Winter%2003-04/Synergy.pdf

Na, K. Y., I.W. Kim, and Y.K. Park, Mitogen-activated protein kinase pathway in osteosarcoma, Pathology 44(6): 540-546 (2012).

Uranishi, M., S. Lida, T. Sanda, T. Ishida, E. Tajima, M. Ito, H. Komatsu, H. Inagaki, and R. Ueda, Multiple myeloma oncogene 1 (MUM1)/interferon regulatory factor 4 (IRF4) upregulates monokine induced by interferon-gamma (MIG) gene expression in B-cell malignancy, Leukemia 19(8): 1471-1478 (2005).

Jang, K.Y., S.J. Jeong, S.H. Kim, J.H. Jung, J.H. Kim, W. Koh, C.Y. Chen, and S.H. Kim Activation of reactive oxygen species/AMP-activated protein kinase signaling mediates fistin'-induced apoptosis in multiple myeloma U266 cells, Cancer Lett 319(2): 197-202 (2012).

Jones TF, Schaffner W. New perspectives on the persistent scourge of foodborne disease. J Infect Dis. 2005;191(7):1029-31.

Effects of rare earth elements on the environment and human health: A literature review Rim, KT. Toxicol. Environ. Health Sci. (2016) 8: 189. https://doi.org/10.1007/s13530-016-
0276-y

Choi, S.H., H.R. Kim, H.J. Kim, I.S. Lee, N. Kozukue, C.E. Levin, and M. Friedman, Free amino acid and phenolic contents and antioxidative and cancer cell-inhibiting activities of extracts of 11 greenhouse-grown tomato varieties and 13 tomato-based foods, J Agric Food Chem 59(24): 12801-12814 (2011).

Gadde U, Kim WH, Oh ST, Lillehoj HS. Alternatives to antibiotics for maximizing growth performance and feed efficiency in poultry: a review. Anim Health Res Rev. 2017;18(1):26-45.

Ren, L., H.Y. Yang, H.I. Choi, K.J. Chung, U. Yang, I.K. Lee, H.J. Kim, D.S. Lee, B.J. Park, and T.H. Lee, The role of peroxiredoxin V in (-)-epigallocatechin 3-gallate-induced multiple myeloma cell death, Oncol Res 19(8-9): 391-398 (2011).

Zhu, J., L. Zhang, X. Jin, X. Han, C. Sun, and J. Yan, Beta-ionone-induced apoptosis in human osteosarcoma (U2OS) cells occurs via a p53-dependent signaling pathway, Mol Biol Rep 37(6): 2653-2663 (2010).

Antibiotic link to bowel cancer precursor' http://www.bbc.co.uk/news/health-39495192

P. Tighe et al., "Effect of Increased Consumption of Whole Grain Foods on Blood Pressure and Other Cardiovascular Risk Markers in Healthy Middle Aged Persons: A Randomized Controlled Trial," American Journal of Clinical Nutrition 92 (4) (2010): 733-40, doi: 10.3945/ajcn.2010.29417.

Robert A. Vogel et al., "Effect of a Single High Fat Meal on Endothelial Function in Healthy Subjects," American Journal of Cardiology 79 (3) (1997): 350-354; Jukka Montonen et al., "Consumption of Red Meat and Whole Grain Bread in Relation to Biomarkers of Obesity, Inflammation, Glucose Metabolism and Oxidative Stress," European Journal of Nutrition 52 (1) (2013): 337-345.

Aune D, Lau R, Chan DS, et al. Dairy products and colorectal cancer risk: a systematic review and meta-analysis of cohort studies. Ann Oncol. 2012;23(1):37-45.

Itakura, I., H. Sasano, C. Shiga, Y. Furukawa, K. Shiga, S. Mori, and H. Nagura, Epidermal growth factor receptor overexpression in esophageal carcinoma. An immunohistochemical study correlated with clinicopathologic findings and DNA amplification, Cancer 74(3): 795-804 (1994).

Zhang, S.M., D.J. Hunter, B.A. Rosner, E.L. Giovannucci, G.A. Colditz, F.E. Speizer, and W.C. Willett, Intakes of fruits, vegetables, and related nutrients and the risk of non-Hodgkin's lymphoma among women. Cancer Epidemiol Biomarkers Prev 9(5): 477-485 (2000).

Jundt, F., O. Acikgöz, S.H. Kwon, R. Schwarzer, I. Anagnostopoulos, B. Wiesner, S. Mathas, M. Hummel, H. Stein, H.M. Reichardt, and B. Dörken, Aberrant expression of Notchl interferes with the B-lymphoid phenotype of neoplastic B cells in classical Hodgkin lymphoma, Leukemia 22(8): 1587-1594 (2008).

Ornish D, Weidner G, Fair WR, et al. Intensive lifestyle changes may affect the progression of prostate cancer. J Urol. 2005;174(3):1065-1069.

de Magistris L, Familiari V, Pascotto A, Sapone A, Frolli A, Iardino P, Carteni M, De Rosa M, Francavilla R, Riegler G, Militerni R, Bravaccio C. Alterations of the intestinal barrier in patients with autism spectrum disorders and in their first-degree relatives. J Pediatr Gastroenterol Nutr. 2010 Oct;51(4):418-24.

Hixson E, Muma MH. Effect of Benzene Hexachloride on the Flavor of Poultry Meat. Science. 1947;106(2757):422-3.

Ito, K., I. Nakazato, K. Yamato, Y. Miyakawa, T. Yamada, N. Hozumi, K. Segawa, Y. Ikeda, and M. Kizaki, Induction of apoptosis in leukemic cells by homovanillic acid derivative, capsaicin, through oxidative stress: Implication of phosphorylation of p53 at Ser-15 residue by reactive oxygen species, Cancer Res 64(3): 1071-1078 (2004).

Toman, I., J. Loree, A.C. Klimowicz, N. Bahlis, R. Lai, A. Belch, L. Pilarski, and T. Reiman, Expression and prognostic significance of Oct2 and Bobl in multiple myeloma: Implications for targeted therapeutics, Leuk Lymphoma 52(4): 659-667 (2011).

Castino, R., A. Pucer, R. Veneroni, F. Morani, C. Peracchio, T.T. Lah, and C. Isidoro, Resveratrol reduces the invasive growth and promotes the acquisition of a long-lasting differentiated phenotype in human glioblastoma cells, J Agric Food Chem 59(8): 4264 4272 (2011).

Fiorentino M, Sapone A, Senger S, Camhi SS, Kadzielski SM, Buie TM, Kelly DL, Cascella N, Fasano A. Blood-brain barrier and intestinal epithelial barrier alterations in autism spectrum disorders. Mol Autism. 2016 Nov 29;7:49.

Tang, L., G.R. Zirpoli, K. Guru, K.B. Moysich, Y. Zhang, C.B. Ambrosone, and S.E. McCann, Consumption of raw cruciferous vegetables is inversely associated with bladder cancer risk, Cancer Epidemiol Biomarkers Prev 17(4): 938-944 (2008).

Brondino N, Fusar-Poli L, Rocchetti M, Provenzani U, Barale F, Politi P. Complementary and Alternative Therapies for Autism Spectrum Disorder. Evid Based Complement Alternat Med. 2015;2015:258589.

Lead Poisoning http://rachel.org/files/document/Lead_Poisoning.pdf

Susanna C. Larsson and Nicola Orsini,"Red Meat and Processed Meat Consumption and All CauseMortality: A Meta Analysis," American Journal of Epidemiology 179 (3) (2014): 282-289, doi: 10.1093/aje/ kwt261.

Li, T., W. Wang, and T. Li, Regulatory effect of resveratrol on JAK1/STAT3 signal transduction pathway in leukemia, Zhongguo Shi Yan Xue Ye Xue Za Zhi 16(4): 772-776 (2008).

Collins, C.D., Problems monitoring response in multiple myeloma, Cancer Imaging 5 (Spec. No. A): S119-S126 (2005).

U.S. Department of Agriculture, Agricultural Research Service. 2008. Nutrient Intakes from Food: Mean Amounts and Percentages of and Alcohol, One Day, 2005 2006. Available: https://www.ars.usda.gov/

Zhao, M., J. Ma, H.Y. Zhu, X.H. Zhang, Z.Y. Du, Y.J. Xu, and X.D. Yu, Apigenin inhibits proliferation and induces apoptosis in human multiple myeloma cells through targeting the trinity of CK2, Cdc37, and Hsp90, Mol Cancer 10:104 (2011).

Morris, S.W., M.N. Kirstein, M.B. Valentine, K.G. Dittmer, D.N. Shapiro, D.L. Saltman, and AT. Look, Fusion of a kinase gene, ALK, to a nucleolar protein gene, NPM, in NHL, Science 267(5196): 316-317 (1995).

Misso, G., S. Zappavigna, M. Castellano, G. De Rosa, M.T. Di Martino, P. Tagliaferri, P. Tassone, and M. Caraglia, Emerging pathways as individualized therapeutic target of multiple myeloma, Expert Opin Biol Ther (Suppl. 1): S95-S109 (2013).

Frattaroli J, Weidner G, Dnistrian AM, et al. Clinical events in prostate cancer lifestyle trial: results from two years of follow-up. Urology. 2008;72(6):1319-1323.

Siegel, R., D. Naishadham, and A. Jemal, Cancer statistics, 2013. CA-Cancer]Clin 63(1): 11-30 (2013).

Fuchs, O., Targeting of NF-kappaB signaling pathway, other signaling pathways and epigenetics in therapy of multiple myeloma, Cardiovasc Hematol Disord Drug Targets 13(1): 16-34 (2013).

Tang, L., G.R. Zirpoli, K. Guru, K.B. Moysich, Y. Zhang, C.B. Ambrosone, and S.E. McCann, Intake of cruciferous vegetables modifies bladder cancer survival, Cancer Epidemiol Biomarkers Prev 19(7): 1806-1811 (2010).

David Katz, "Humanity's Fishy Origins," Huffington Post, September 8, 2016, http://www.huffingtonpost.com/entry/humanitys fishy origins or the paleo elephant in_us_57d1b6394b0183117071735.

Mollenkopf DF, Cenera JK, Bryant EM, et al. Organic or antibiotic-free labeling does not impact the recovery of enteric pathogens and antimicrobial-resistant Escherichia coli from fresh retail chicken. Foodborne Pathog Dis. 2014;11(12):920-9.

The Global Problem of Lead Arsenate Pesticides http://www.lead.org.au/lanv10n3/lanv10n3-7.html

Veettil SK, Ching SM, Lim KG, Saokaew S, Phisalprapa P, Chaiyakunapruk N. Effects of calcium on the incidence of recurrent colorectal adenomas: A systematic review with meta-analysis and trial sequential analysis of randomized controlled trials. Medicine (Baltimore). 2017;96(32):e7661.

Geng Zong, Alisa Gao, Frank B. Hu, and Qi Sun, "Whole Grain Intake and Mortality from All Causes, Cardiovascular Disease, and Cancer," Circulation 133 (24) (2016): 2370-2380.

Renné, C., K. Willenbrock, R. Küppers, M.L. Hansmann, and A. Bräuninger, Autocrine and paracrine activated receptor tyrosine kinases in classical Hodgkin lymphoma, Blood 105(10): 4051-4059 (2005).

Tang, L. and Y. Zhang, Dietary isothiocyanates inhibit the growth of human bladder carcinoma cells, J Nutr 134(8): 2004-2010 (2004).

Hussain, A.R., S. Uddin, R. Bu, O.S. Khan, S.O. Ahmed, M. Ahmed, and K.S. Al-Kuraya, Resveratrol suppresses constitutive activation of AKT via generation of ROS and induces apoptosis in diffuse large B cell lymphoma cell lines, PLoS One 6(9): e24703 (2011).

Lin, X., G. Wu, W.Q. Huo, Y. Zhang, and ES. Jin, Resveratrol induces apoptosis associated with mitochondrial dysfunction in bladder carcinoma cells, Int J Urol 19(8): 757-764 (2012).

Gokbulut, A.A., E. Apohan, and Y. Baran, Resveratrol and quercetin-induced apoptosis of human 232B4 chronic lymphocytic leukemia cells by activation of caspase-3 and cell cycle arrest, Hematology 18(3): 144-150 (2013).

How many chemicals are in use today? https://cen.acs.org/articles/95/ig/chemicals-use-TCSA Chemical Substance Inventory https:// www.epa.gov/tsca-inventory

Ghoneum, M. and S. Gollapudi, Synergistic apoptotic effect of arabinoxylan rice bran MGN-3/Biobran) and curcumin (turmeric) on human multiple myeloma cell line U266 in vitro, Neoplasma 58(2): 118-123 (2011).

Ornish D, Magbanua MJ, Weidner G, et al. Changes in prostate gene expression in men undergoing an intensive nutrition and lifestyle intervention. Proc Natl Acad Sci USA. 2008;105(24):8369-8374.

Renné, C., J.I. Martin-Subero, M. Eickernjäger, M.L. Hansmann, R. Küppers, R. Siebert, and A. Bräuninger, Aberrant expression of ID2, a suppressor of B-cell-specific gene expression, in Hodgkin's lymphoma, Am] Pathol 169(2): 655-664 (2006).

Aune D, Navarro Rosenblatt DA, Chan DS, et al. Dairy products, calcium, and prostate cancer risk: a systematic review and meta-analysis of cohort studies. Am J Clin Nutr. 2015;101(1):87-117.

Cheng, L., Q. Wu, Z. Huang, O.A. Guryanova, Q. Huang, W. Shou, J.N. Rich, and S. Bao, LICAM regulates DNA damage checkpoint response of glioblastoma stem cells through NBS1, EMBO J 30(5): 800-813 (2011).

Sharif, T., M. Alhosin, C. Auger, C. Minker, J.H. Kim, N. Etienne-Selloum, P. Bories, H. Gronemeyer, A. Lobstein, C. Bronner, G. Fuhrmann, and V.B.Schini-Kerth, Aronia melanocarpa juice induces a redox-sensitive p73-related caspase 3-dependent apoptosis in human leukemia cells, PLoS One 7(3): e32526 (2012).

E. Q. Ye et al., "Greater Whole Grain Intake Is Associated with Lower Risk of Type 2 Diabetes, Cardiovascular Disease, and Weight Gain," Journal of Nutrition 142 (7) (2012): 1304-1313, doi: 10.3945/jn.111.155325.

Hu, H., X.P. Zhang, Y.L. Wang, C.W. Chua, S.U. Luk, Y.C. Wong, M.T. Ling, X.F. Wang, and K.X. Xu, Identification of a novel function of Id-1 in mediating the anti-cancer responses of SAMC, a water-soluble garlic derivative, in human bladder cancer cells, Mol Med Rep 4(1): 9-16 (2011).

Dierlamm, I., M. Baens, I. Wiodarska, M. Stefanova-Ouzounova, J.M. Hernandez, D.K. Hossfeld, C. De Wolf-Peters, A. Hagemeijer, H. Van den Berghe, and P. Marynen, The apoptosis inhibitor gene AP 12 and a novel 18g gene, MLT, are recurrently rearranged in the t(11;18) (q21;21) associated with MALT lymphomas, Blood 93(11): 3601-3609 (1999).

A. D. Liese et al., Whole Grain Intake and Insulin Sensitivity: The Insulin Resistance Atherosclerosis Study" American Journal of Clinical Nutrition 78 (5) (2003): 965-971.

Lamm, D. L, and D.R. Riggs, The potential application of Allium sativum (garlic) for the treatment of bladder cancer, Urol Clin North Am 27 (1): 157-162 (2000).

Ly V, Bottelier M, Hoekstra PJ, Arias Vasquez A, Buitelaar JK, Rommelse NN. Elimination diets' efficacy and mechanisms in attention deficit hyperactivity disorder and autism spectrum disorder. Eur Child Adolesc Psychiatry. 2017 Feb 11.

Park SW, Kim JY, Kim YS, Lee SJ, Lee SD, Chung MK. A milk protein, casein, as a proliferation promoting factor in prostate cancer cells. World J Mens Health. 2014;32(2):76-82.

Cecconi, D., A. Zamò, A. Parisi, E. Bianchi, C. Parolini, A.M. Timperio, L. Zolla, and M. Chilosi, Induction of apoptosis in Jeko-1 mantle cell lymphoma cell line by resveratrol: A proteomic analysis, J Proteome Res 7(7): 2670-2680 (2008).

Cohen, E.W. and C.M. Rudin, Molecular biology of esophageal cancer, Pos-ner, M.C., E.E. Vokes, and R.R. Weichselbaum (Eds.), in Cancer of the Upper Gastrointestinal Tract, London: BC Decker (2002).

Cakir, Z., G. Saydam, F. Sahin, and Y. Baran, The roles of bioactive sphingolipids in resveratrol-induced apoptosis in HI60: Acute myeloid leukemia cells, J Cancer Res Clin Oncol 137(2): 279-286 (2011).

Stockwell T, Zhao J, Naimi T, Chikritzhs T. Stockwell et al. response: Moderate use of an "intoxicating carcinogen" has no net mortality benefit—is this true and why does it matter?. J Stud Alcohol Drugs. 2016 Mar; 77(2):205-207.

Wang, Q., Y. Wang, Z. Ji, X. Chen, Y. Pan, G. Gao, H. Gu, Y. Yang, B.C. Choi, and Y.Yan, Risk factors for multiple myeloma: A hospital-based case-control study in northwest China. Cancer Epidemiol 36(5): 439-444 (2012).

Yang M, Kenfield SA, Van Blarigan EL, et al. Dairy intake after prostate cancer diagnosis in relation to disease-specific and total mortality. Int J Cancer. 2015;137(10):2462-2469.

Stein, H., I. Marafioti, H.D. Foss, H. Laumen, M. Hummel, I. Anagnosto-poulos, I. Wirth, G. Demel, and B. Falini, Down-regulation of BOB.1/OBE.1 and Oct2 in classical Hodgkin disease but not in lymphocyte predominant Hodgkin disease correlates with immunoglobulin transcription, Blood 97(2): 496-501 (2001).

Tzonou, A., L. Lipworth, A. Garidou, L.B. Signorello, P. Lagiou, C. Hsieh, and D. Trichopoulos, Diet and risk of esophageal cancer by histologic type in a low-risk population, Int J Cancer 68(3): 300-304 (1996).

NIH Medical Encyclopedia - antigen https://medlineplus.gov/ency/article/002224.htm

Cao, H., K. Zhu, L. Qiu, S. Li, H. Niu, M. Hao, S. Yang, Z. Zhao, Y. Lai, J.L. Anderson, J. Fan, H.J. Im, D. Chen, G.D. Roodman, and G. Xiao, Critical role of AKT in myeloma-induced osteoclast formation and osteolysis, / Biol Chem 288(42): 30399-30410 (2013).

Park, M.H. and S. Min Do, Quercetin-induced downregulation of phospho-lipase D1 inhibits proliferation and invasion in U87 glioma cells, Biochem Biophys Res Commun 412(4): 710-715 (2011).

Mandal, S. and G.D. Stoner, Inhibition of N-nitrosobenzylmethylamine-induced esophageal tumorigenesis in rats by ellagic acid, Carcinogenesis 11(1): 55-61 (1990).

Tatman, D. and H. Mo, Volatile isoprenoid constituents of fruits, vegetables and herbs cumulatively suppress the proliferation of murine B16 melanoma and human HL-60 leukemia cells, Cancer Lett 175(2): 129-139 (2002).

Hou, D.X., T. Ose, S. Lin, K. Harazoro, I. Imamura, M. Rubo, I. Uto, N. Terahara, M. Yoshimoto, and M. Fujii, Anthocyanidins induce apoptosis in human promyelocytic leukemia cells: Structure-activity relationship and mechanisms involved, Int J Oncol 23(3): 705-712 (2003).

Alidina, A., T. Siddiqui, I. Burney, W. Jafri, F. Hussain, M. Ahmed, Esophageal cancer — a review, J Pak Med Assoc 54(3): 136-141 (2004).

Mishra, S. and M. Vinayak, Ellagic acid checks lymphoma promotion via regulation of PKC signaling pathway, Mol Biol Rep 40(2): 1417-1428 (2013).

Takeuchi, H., S. Ozawa, N. Ando, C.H. Shih, K. Koyanagi, M. Ueda, and M. Kitajima, Altered p16/MTSI/CDKN2 and cyclin D1/PRAD-1 gene expression is associated with the prognosis of squamous cell carcinoma of the esophagus, Clin Cancer Res 3(12 Pt. 1): 2229-2236 (1997).

Zheng, B., P. Fiumara, Y.V. Li, G. Georgakis, V. Snell, M. Younes, J.N. Vauthey, A. Carbone, and A. Younes, MEK/ERK pathway is aberrantly active in Hodgkin disease: A signaling pathway shared by CD30, CD40, and RANK that regulates cell proliferation and survival, Blood 102(3): 1019-1027 (2003).

Stoner, G.D., T. Chen, L.A. Kresty, R.M. Aziz, T. Reinemann, and R. Nines, Protection against esophageal cancer in rodents with lyophilized berries: Potential mechanisms, Nutr Cancer 54(1): 33-46 (2006).

Adelaide,]., G. Monges, C. Derderian, J.F. Seitz, and D. Birnbaum, Oesophageal cancer and amplification of the human cyclin D gene CCND1/PRADI, Br J Cancer 71(1): 64-68 (1995).

Spagnuolo, C., M. Russo, S. Bilotto, I. Tedesco, B. Laratta, and G.L. Russo, Dietary polyphenols in cancer prevention: The example of the flavonoid quercetin in leukemia, Ann NY Acad Sci 1259: 95-103 (2012).

Nielsen TS, Höjer A, Gustavsson AM, Hansen-Møller J, Purup S. Proliferative effect of whey from cows' milk varying in phyto-oestrogens in human breast and prostate cancer cells. J Dairy Res. 2012;79(2):143-149.

Barch, D.H. and C.C. Fox, Dietary ellagic acid reduce the esophageal microsomal metabolism of methylbenzylnitrosamine, Cancer Lett 44(1): 39-44 (1989).

De Bruijn, M.F. and N.A. Speck, Core-binding factors in hematopoiesis and immune function, Oncogene 23(24): 4238-4248 (2004).

Breastfeeding provides passive and likely long-lasting active immunity https://www.ncbi.nlm.nih.gov/pubmed/9892025

Salesse, S. and C.M. Verfaillie, BCR/ABL: From molecular mechanisms of leukemia induction to treatment of chronic myelogenous leukemia, Oncogene 21(56): 8547-8559 (2002).

There are more references available on the p53diet website at p53diet.com.

REFERENCES

INDEX

A

F

G

M

O

Q

W

X

NOTES:

NOTES:

www.ingramcontent.com/pod-product-compliance
Lightning Source LLC
Chambersburg PA
CBHW051707020426
42333CB00014B/880
9781733043700